桑原史成写真集

水俣事件

The MINAMATA Disaster

Documentary Photographer **Kuwabara Shisei**

藤原書店

水俣事件

The MINAMATA Disaster

もくじ

1. 最高裁判決へ……5
2. 二つの慰霊……13
3. 「宝子」……28
4. 「生ける人形」……37
5. 隣村の網元二世代を襲った奇病……44
6. 奇病発見のきっかけとなった船大工一家……51
7. 中村荒蔵網……60
8. 役者をもしのぐ茂道の女網元……65
9. チッソ水俣工場……70
10. 胎児性患者たちの成人とその後……75
11. 水俣病専用病棟や自宅の患者たち……81
12. 新潟水俣病事件……101
13. 労働争議の町と化した水俣……107

- 14 熊本水俣病一次訴訟　水俣病の底辺　慢性微量汚染の取り組み……藤野糺 … 110
- 15 苦海地獄　磁力ということ……高峰武 … 114
- 16 行商人の魚は山間部でよく売れた　見舞金契約と細川証言……坂東克彦 … 133
- 17 隠れ患者の島　「特措法」の暑い夏……西貴晴 … 136
- 18 支援者たち　ネコ四〇〇号実験記録の発見……宇井紀子 … 138
- 19 水銀国際会議　「水俣病にはなってしまったが生きていて良かった」冥土連・設立宣言……旗野秀人 … 145
- 20 ある胎児性患者の一族 … 148

〈私の水俣病事件〉

- 「記者たちの水俣」を制作して……村上雅通 … 12
- 光と影の魔術師……原一男 … 36
- 教育と水俣病……広瀬武 … 50
- 舞台を支える裏方として……久保田好生 … 74

あとがき……桑原史成 … 162

［附］

- Kuwabara Shisei's photo-documentary *The Minamata Disaster* … 163
- 偉大なノーテンキということについて……西村幹夫 … 165
- 水俣事件と桑原史成の略年表（一九〇六〜二〇一三年）… 169
- 不知火海の地図／Minamata and the Shiranui Sea Area … 173

- An Abridged Chronology of the Human-made Minamata Disease Disaster … 176
- Photograph Explanation … 180
- *The Minamata Disaster* Abridged translation of the expository essay on photographer Kuwabara Shisei …Nishimura Mikio … 182

「水俣事件」は半世紀を超えて

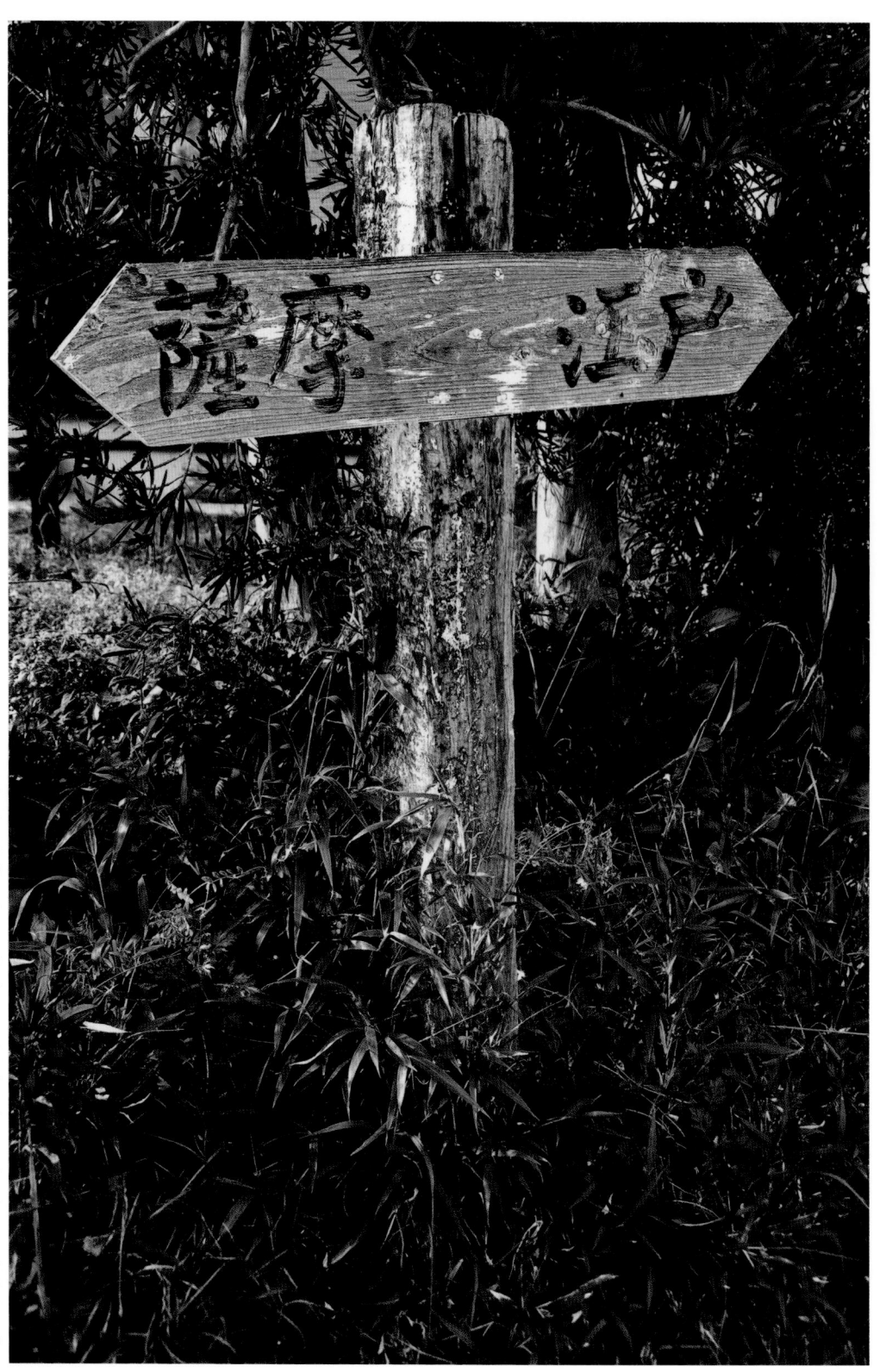

旧薩摩街道の標識。道沿いの海辺に奇病恐怖が広がってから、すでに六〇年を経た

1 最高裁判決へ

二〇一三年四月一六日、最高裁は二つの行政訴訟で熊本県の水俣病認定棄却処分を不当と認めた。故・溝口チエ（水俣市、二審勝訴）で県の上告を棄却し、故・F（水俣市出身、二審敗訴）で控訴審判決を破棄、差し戻した。

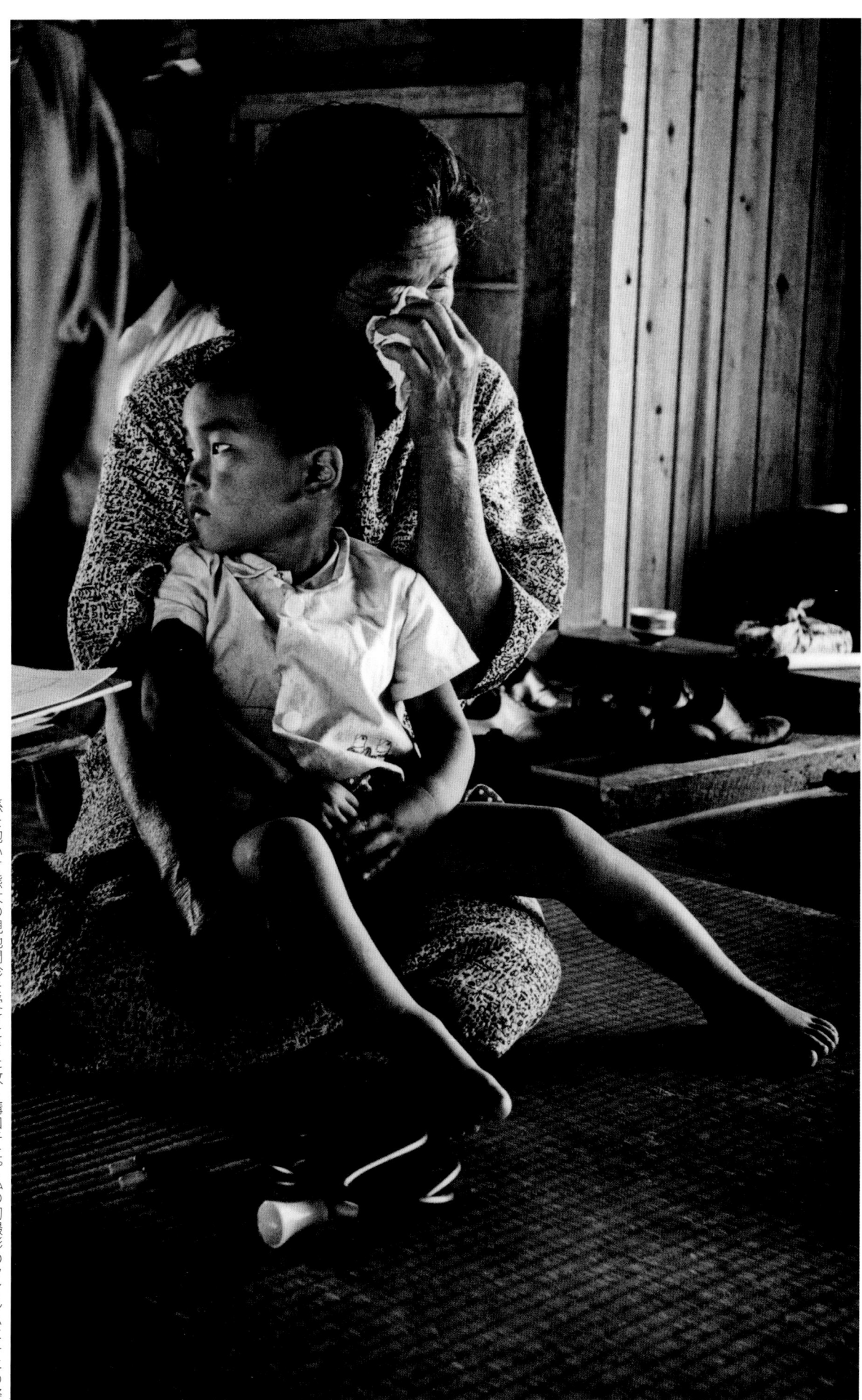

孫を抱いて熊大の現地問診を受けにきた故・溝口チエ。私の初撮影のフィルムにチエの姿があると知ったのは撮影の五〇年後だった　水俣市袋　一九六〇年七月

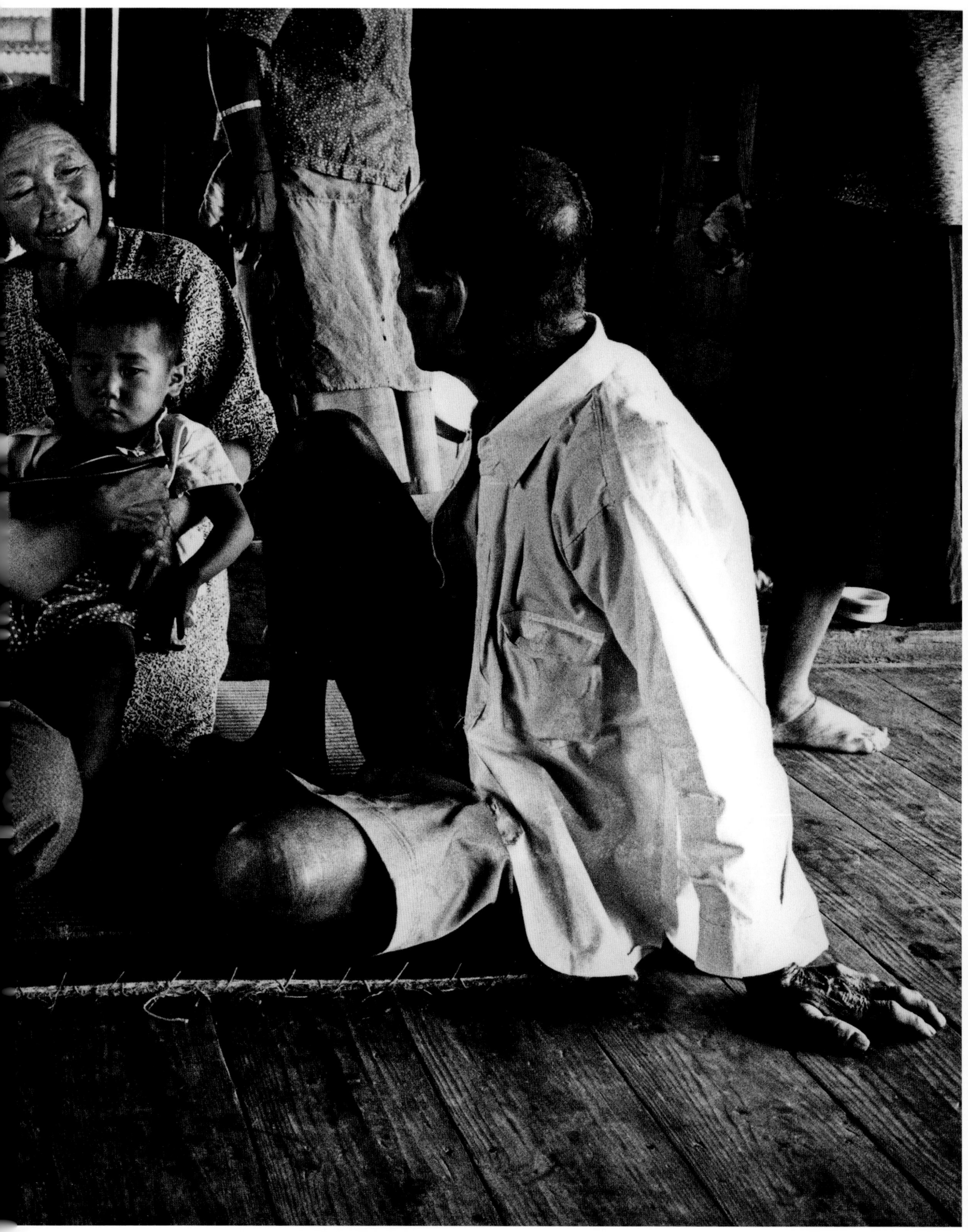

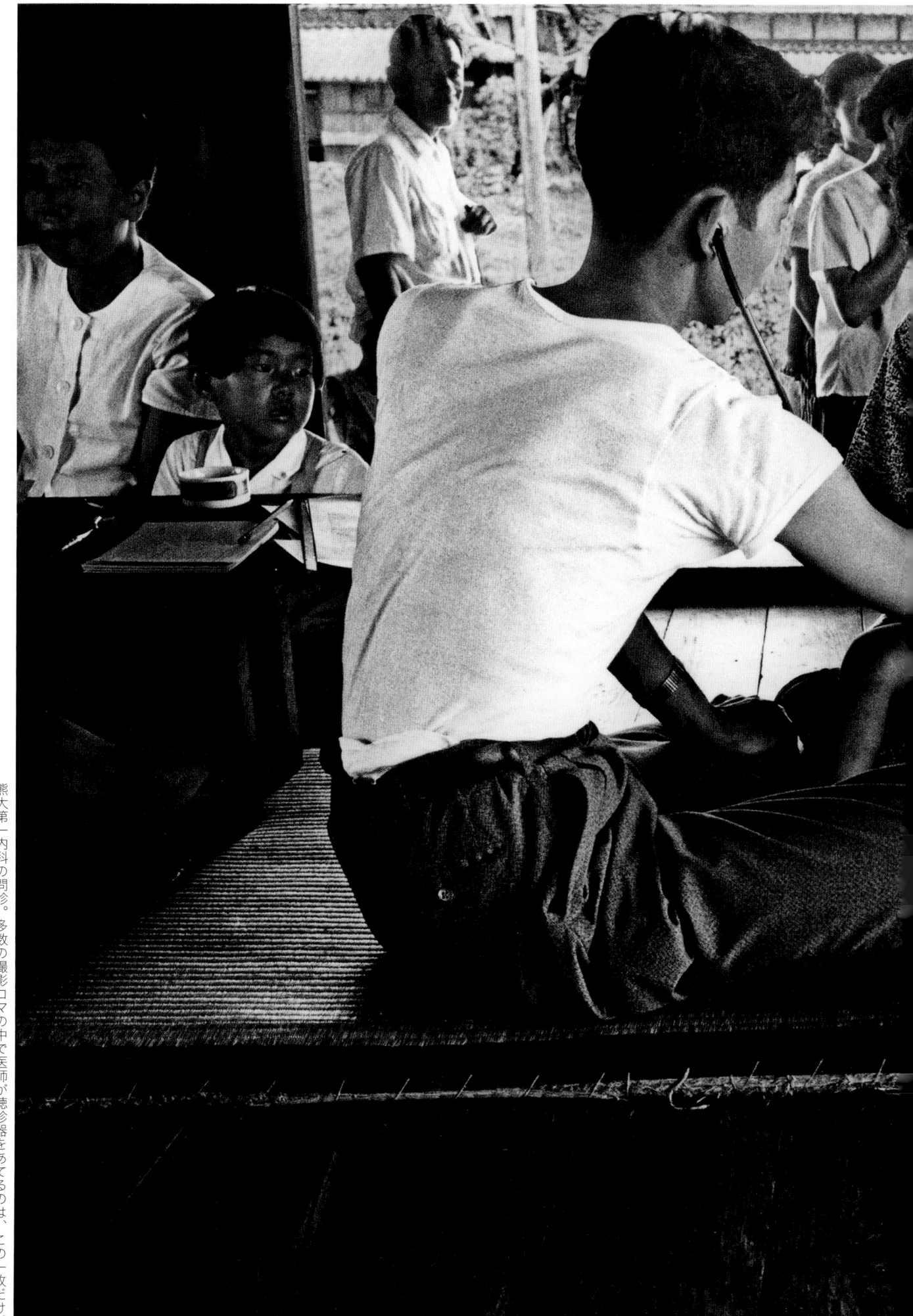

熊大第一内科の問診。多数の撮影コマの中で医師が聴診器をあてるのは、この一枚だけ。「孫のからだを診て」とチエが特にせがんだのだろう 一九六〇年七月

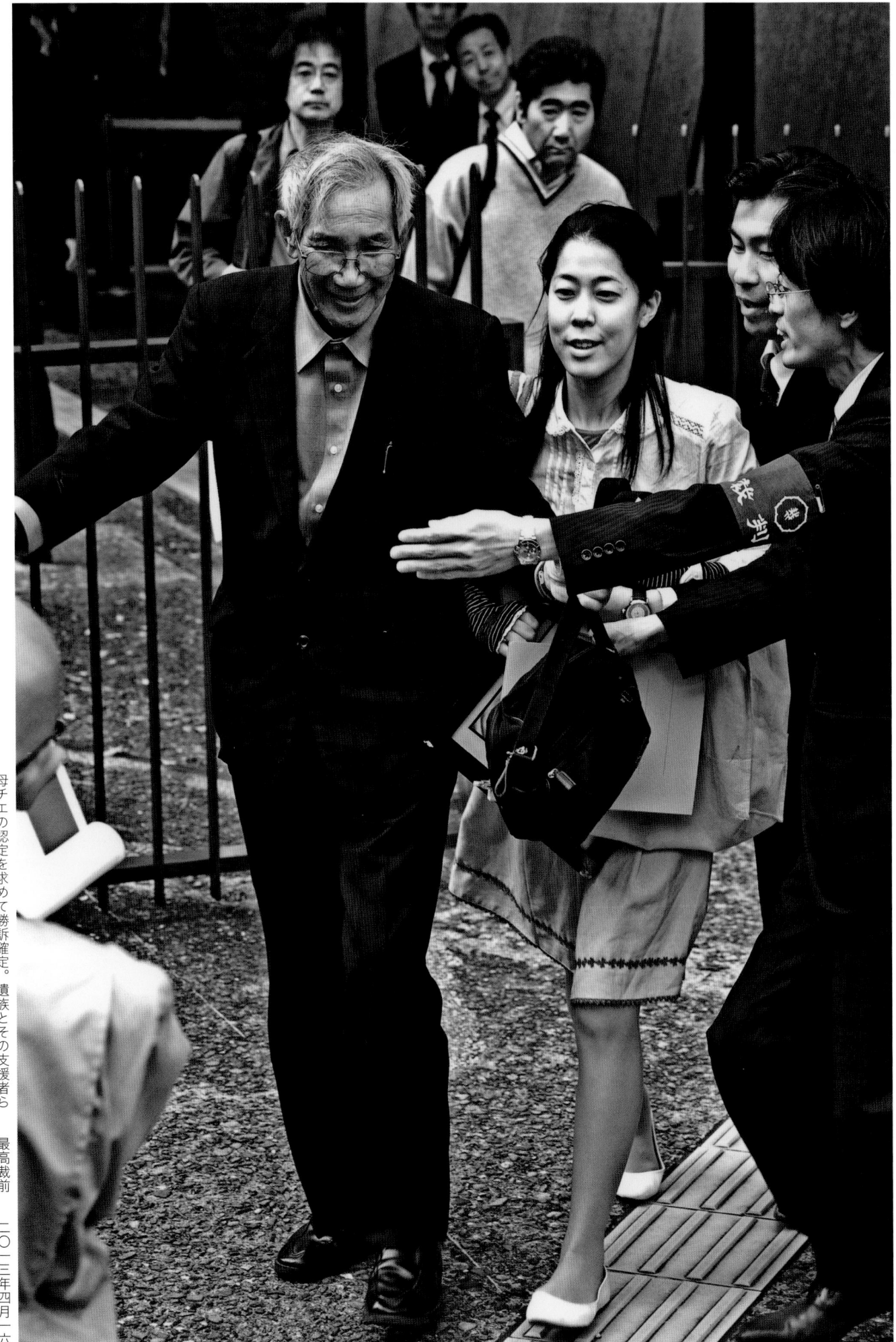

母チエの認定を求めて勝訴確定。遺族とその支援者ら　最高裁前　二〇一三年四月一六日

←（次頁）原告患者敗訴の二審判決を破棄、差し戻しの判決を得た故・F（匿名）の遺族にも報道取材がつめかける　最高裁前　二〇一三年四月一六日

私が撮影した生前のチエの写真を手に、ある遺族の一家　水俣市袋の自宅　二〇一三年五月

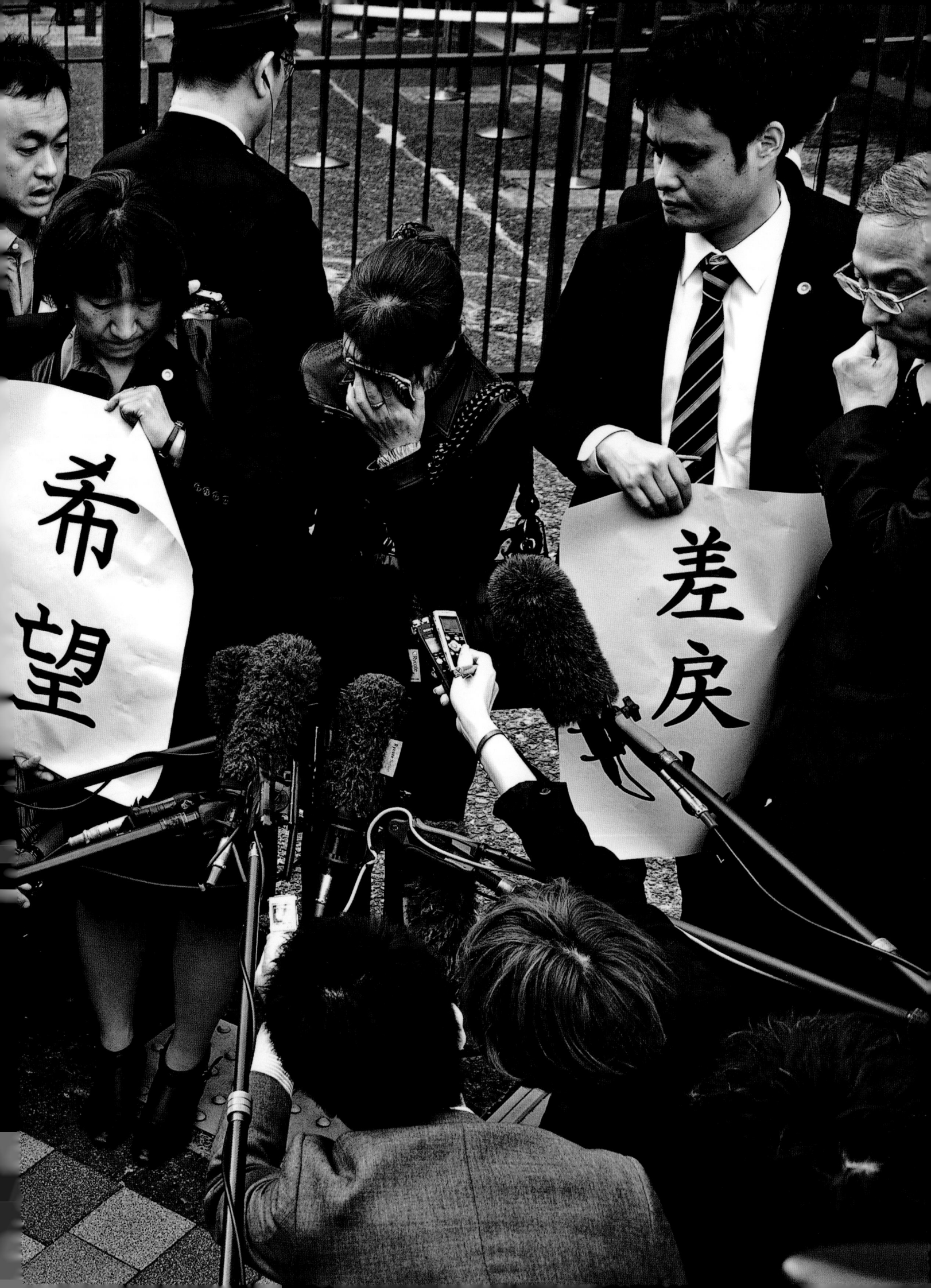

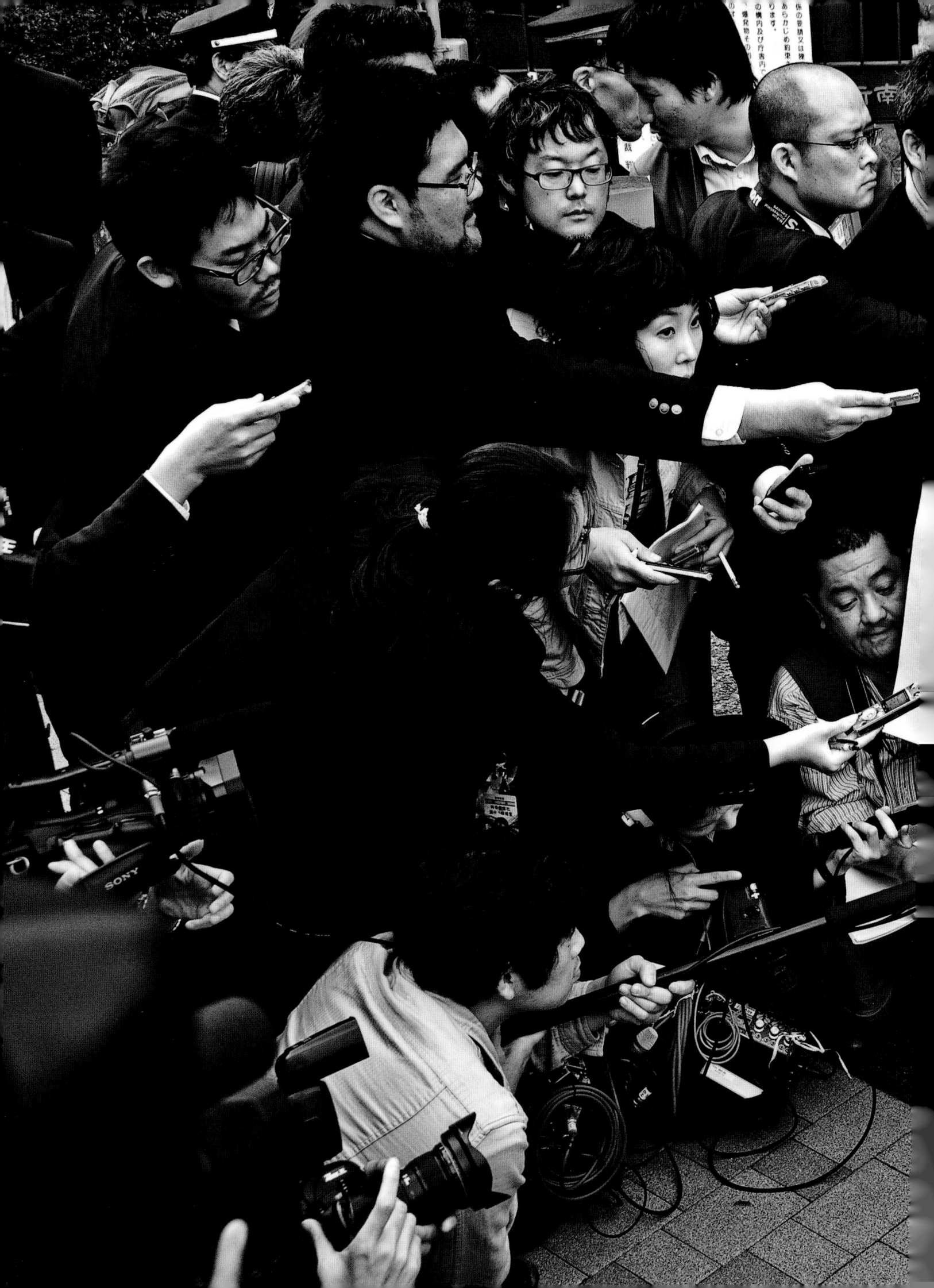

私の水俣病事件

「記者たちの水俣」を制作して

村上雅通

チッソに支えられた我が家

「水俣の人は生理的に、水俣病を語りたくないんですよ」。私が制作したテレビドキュメンタリー「記者たちの水俣病」の東京での記者発表で、桑原史成さんは、こう言って私の気持ちを代弁してくれた。四〇歳代になるまで水俣病をテーマに掲げなかった理由を聞かれ、答えに窮していた私への助け舟でもあった。

「記者たちの水俣病」は、水俣病報道を検証した番組だ。"伝染病"の誤報、見舞金契約以降の空白、第三水俣病の過熱など、水俣病を巡る報道がメディアに突き付ける課題は多い。そんな中、核心に迫る取材をした数少ないジャーナリストの一人として桑原さんを取り上げた。

記者会見の冒頭部分に出た質問が、私の水俣病事件に対するスタンスだった。水俣出身の私が、何故、長年故郷に目を向けようとしなかったか、という疑問だ。明確な答えが出せない私を見かねたのか、桑原さんが発したのが「生理的」という言葉だったのだ。私が水俣病事件の取材をためらっていた理由の全てを抱合した言葉だったからだ。

私は、一九五三（昭和二八）年水俣市で生まれた。実家は水俣駅から歩いて三〇秒、駅前に聳え立つチッソ水俣工場は、物心ついたころから故郷を象徴する誇りだった。父親はチッソの下請け鉄工所に勤め、母親が経営する洋装店の客の九割はチッソの従業員やその家族だった。我が家の経済は、まさに、チッソに支えられていたと言っても過言ではない。

子供の頃、水俣川の河口でアサリ貝を採って食べていた位だから、少なくとも我が家に、水俣病が郊外の漁村で多発し、患者のほとんどが経済的に貧しいという話は、親から聞こえてきた。

それに水俣で進められていた"もやいなおし運動"を取材したのだが、元気だと思っていた故郷には、水俣病事件の後遺症から逃れられない一般市民たちの苦悩があふれていたのだ。

この現実が、水俣病事件に取り組むきっかけとなった。テーマに据えたのは、一般市民と水俣病だ。テーマに据えたのは、一般市民と水俣病だ。私が目を背けていた間、患者ではない市民たちは、どう水俣病に向き合ったのかを解きほぐす内容だった。両親や親族からの情報を元に取材対象者を探した。しかし、水俣病の認定申請をした父親を叱責し、自殺に追い込んでしまったチッソ下請け工場の従業員、親族から認定患者が出たため退職を余儀なくされたチッソ社員、補償金を巡りいがみ合う兄弟。私が無視してきた故郷の現実が、次々と浮上した。

「市民たちの水俣病」が完成した一九九七年だった。以降、水俣病をテーマにしたテレビ番組一三作に関わったが、チッソが株式上場を廃止した一九七八（昭和五三）年。五年後には司法記者として水俣病裁判を担当する立場になったが、患者支援につながるような報道は、無意識のうちに避けるようになっていた。

こうした環境で、私の水俣病に対するスタンスは醸成されていった。しかし、自らの思いを吐露することはしなかった。公の場ではもちろん、家族の間でさえ水俣病、患者の悪口を封印してしまった。どう擁護しても、チッソの責任は揺るぎないものだったからだ。熊本放送に入社したのは、チッソが株式上場を廃止した一九七八（昭和五三）年。五年後には司法記者として水俣病裁判を担当する立場になったが、患者支援につながるような報道は、無意識のうちに避けるようになっていた。

一般市民の苦悩を番組に

そんな私が取材者として故郷に目を向けるようになったのは、一九九五年に村山内閣が実施した政治決着がきっかけだった。ようやく故郷に目を向けるようになったからだ。私は地域再生に取り組む元気な水俣を伝えるバラエティー番組を企画し、取材者として初めて故郷に出向いた。温泉、グルメ、

鮮明に覚えている。その一方で悪化するチッソの経営。「中風のおじさんまでもが水俣の物価を釣り上げている」「水俣病御殿」が建てられていった。「患者地区には"水俣病御殿"が建てられていった。患者を誹謗する言葉は母の洋装店の客は減り続けた。その一方で病気の多発俣の景気は落ち込んでいった。父の鉄工所への発注や、水は厳しい状況に追い込まれ、比例するかのように、水うになってからだ。補償金の支払いで、チッソの経営は、認定患者にチッソから補償金が支払われるよのは、認定患者にチッソから補償金が支払われるよ

者会見で桑原さんが指摘した「生理的」一面は、わずかではあるが、今も私の中に存在する。

二年前に熊本放送を退職し長崎の大学で教鞭をとっている。水俣病問題と私の取材者としてのスタンスは、全ての授業に取り入れた。ほとんどの学生が、水俣病を歴史上の出来事としてしか考えていなかったが、卒論で取り上げる学生も現れた。熊本放送の後輩と組んで、番組作りも続けている。あまりにも長すぎた人生の空白を埋める作業は、生涯終わることはなさそうだ。

（むらかみ・まさみち／長崎県立大学教授）

② 二つの慰霊

毎年五月一日水俣市で同時刻に始まる。水俣病互助会が乙女塚で営む慰霊祭は、犠牲となったすべての生類の合祀、三三回目となった。一方、ずっと後の年に始まった水俣市ほか実行委主催の犠牲者慰霊式には、国と県のトップや議員らが水俣湾埋立地にズラリ列席する。

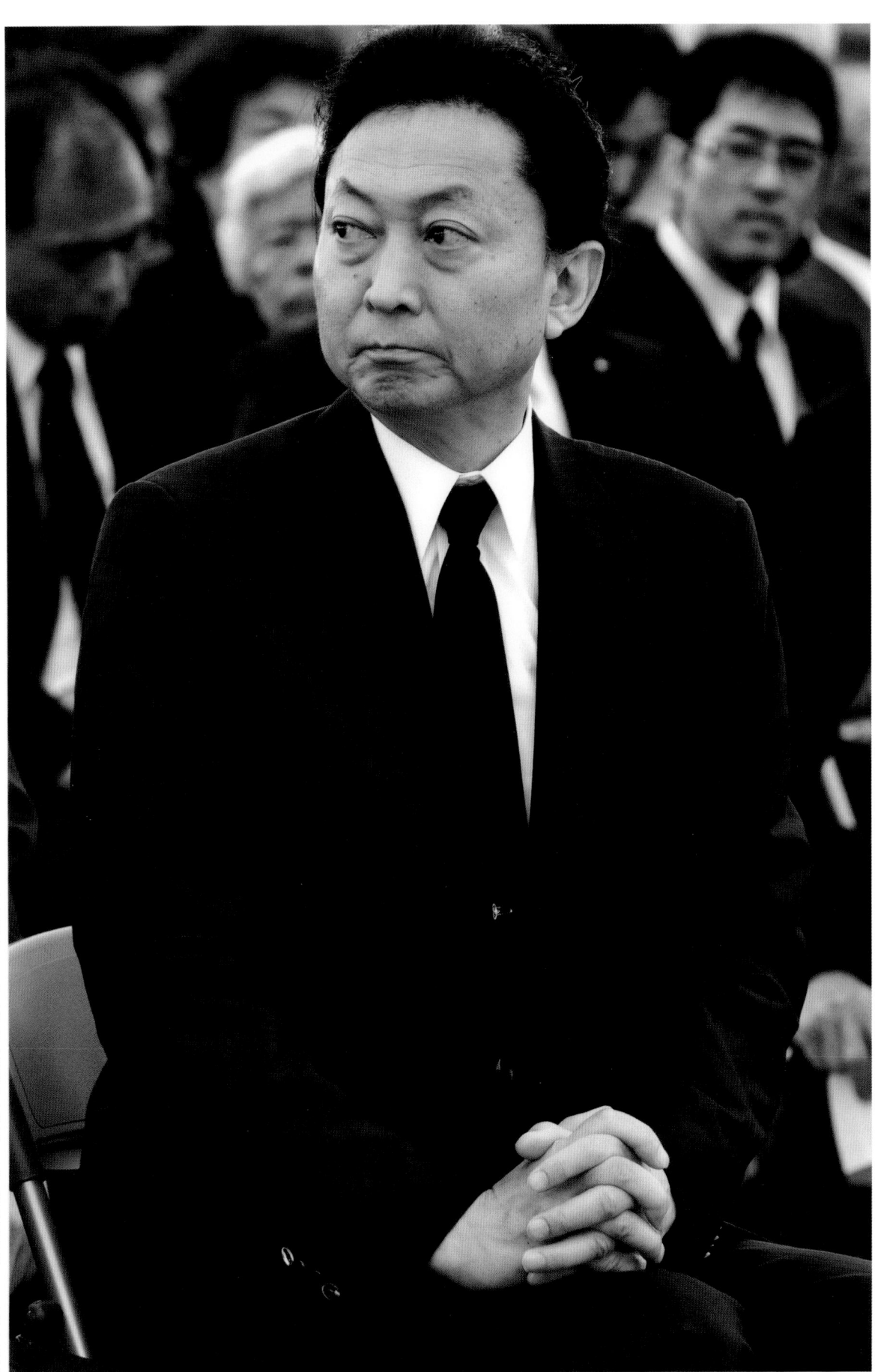

首相が初めて行政側の慰霊式に参加した。鳩山由紀夫　二〇一〇年

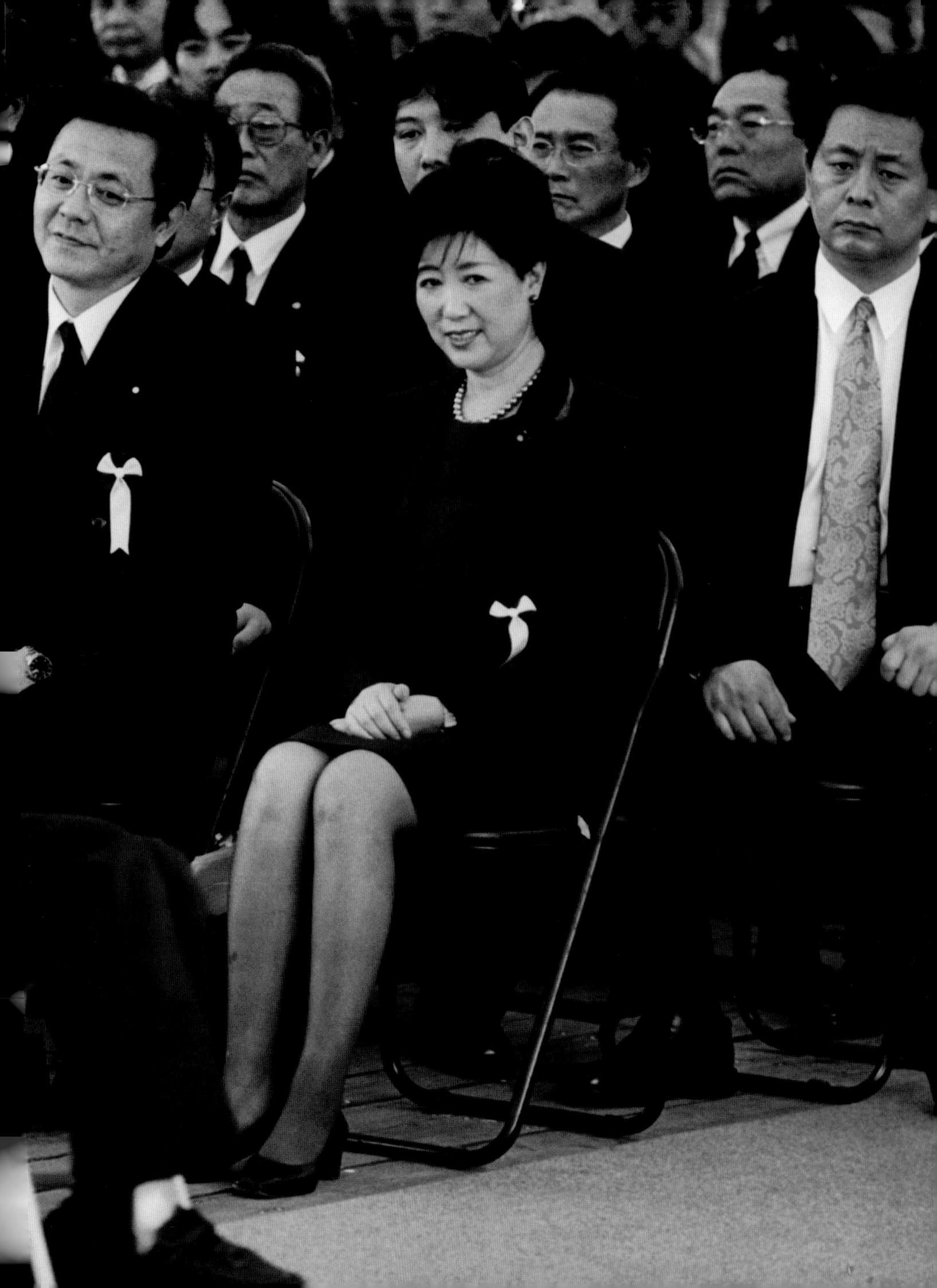

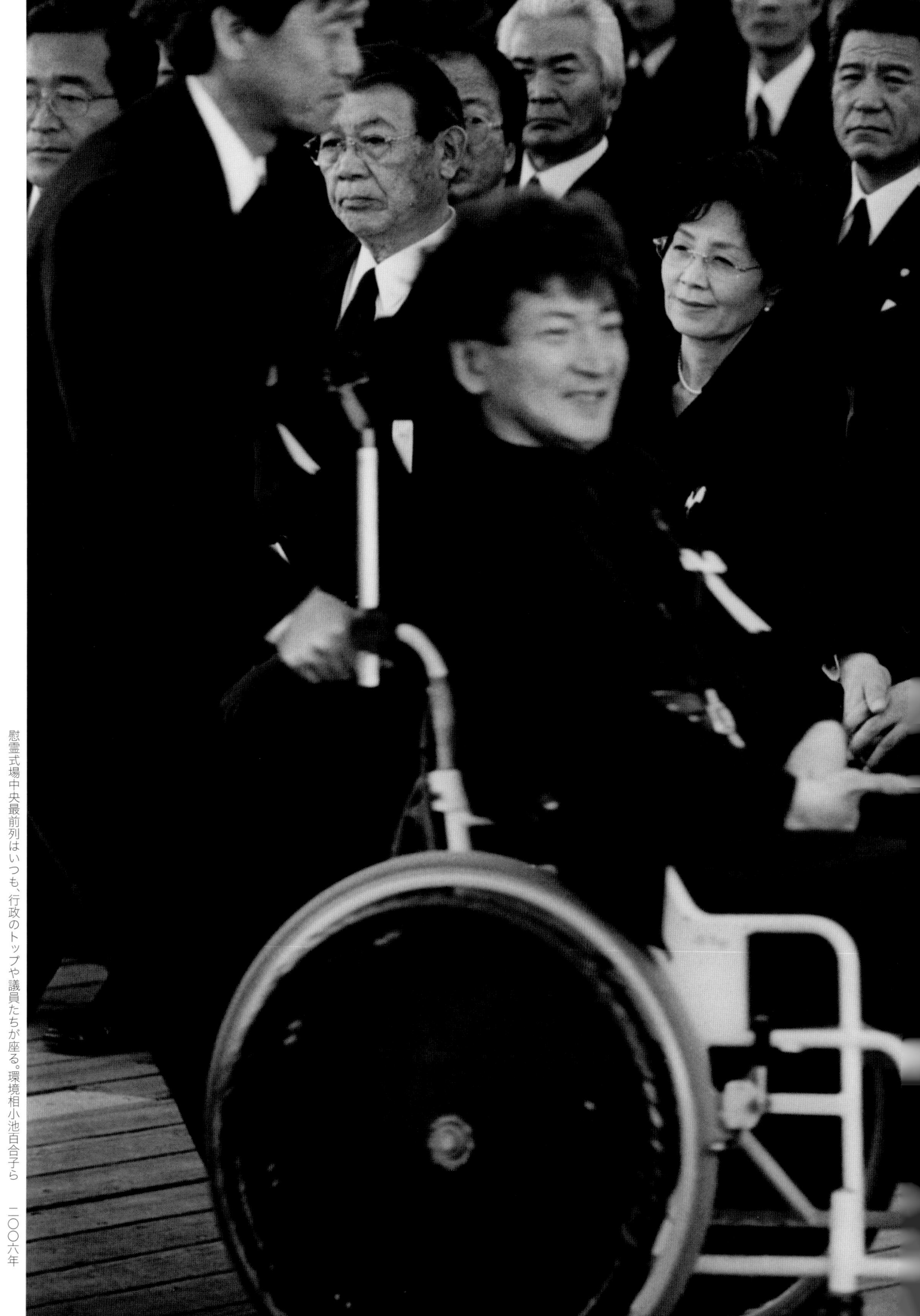

慰霊式場中央最前列はいつも、行政のトップや議員たちが座る。環境相小池百合子ら　二〇〇六年

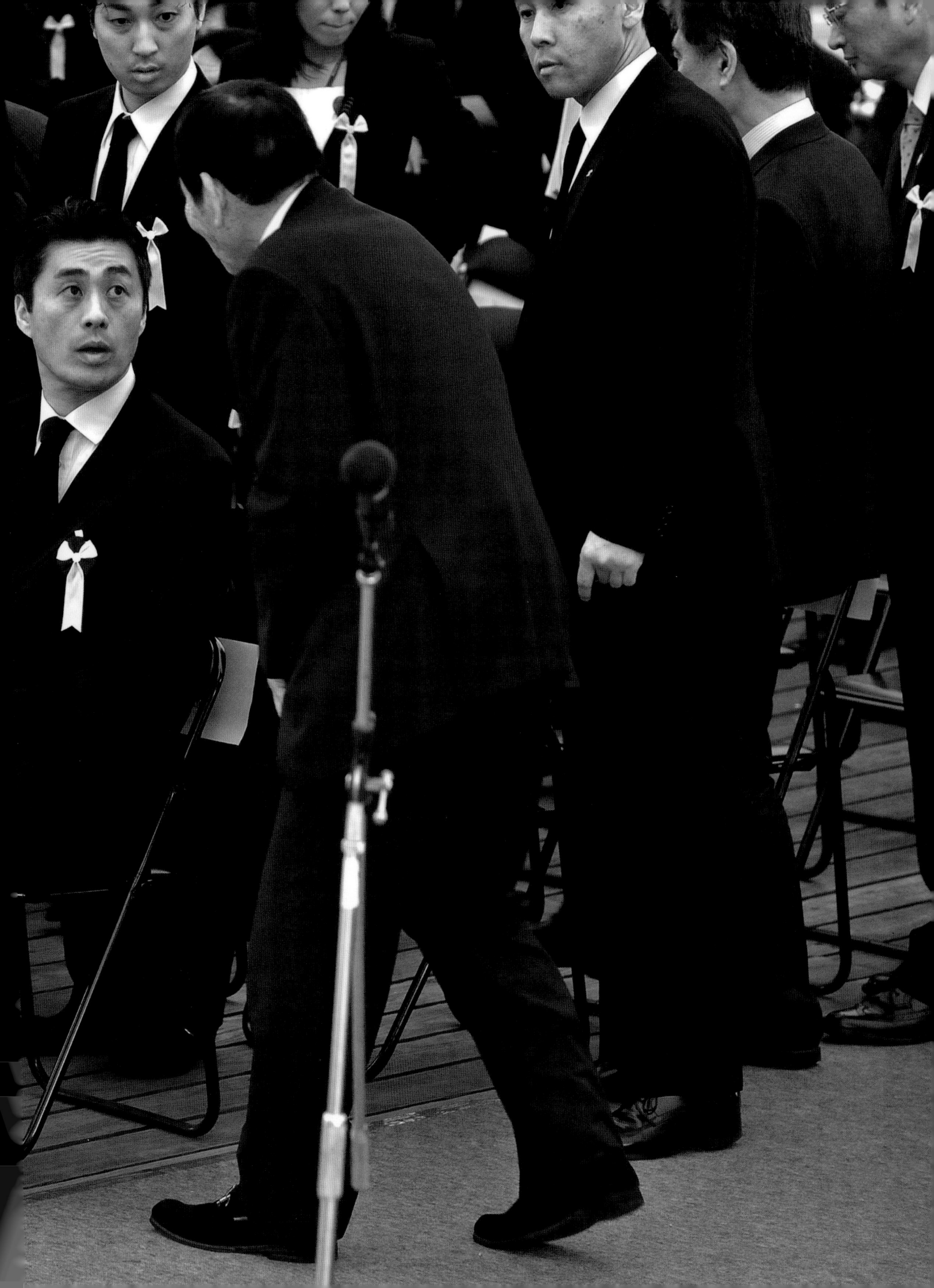

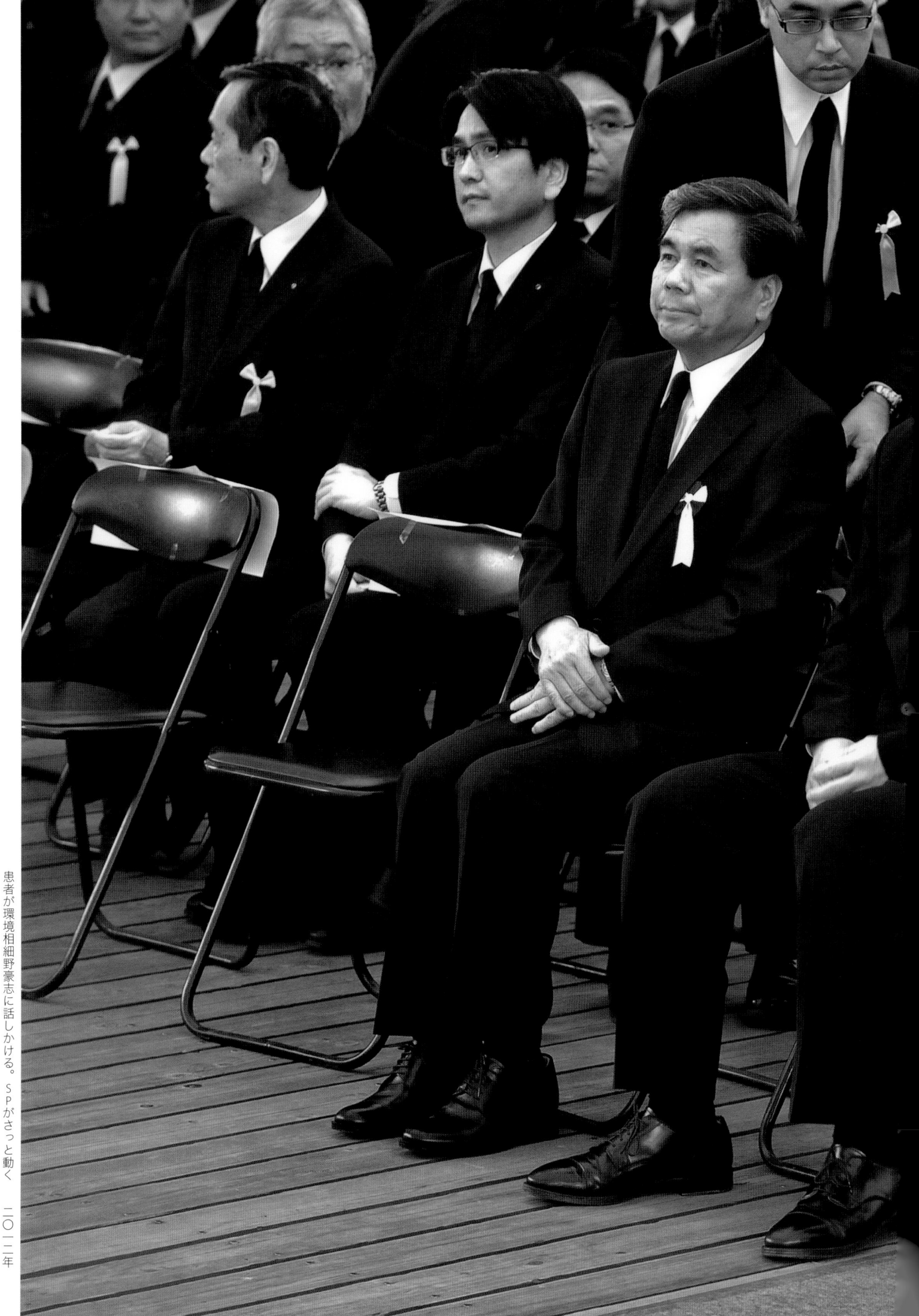

患者が環境相細野豪志に話しかける。SPがさっと動く　二〇一二年

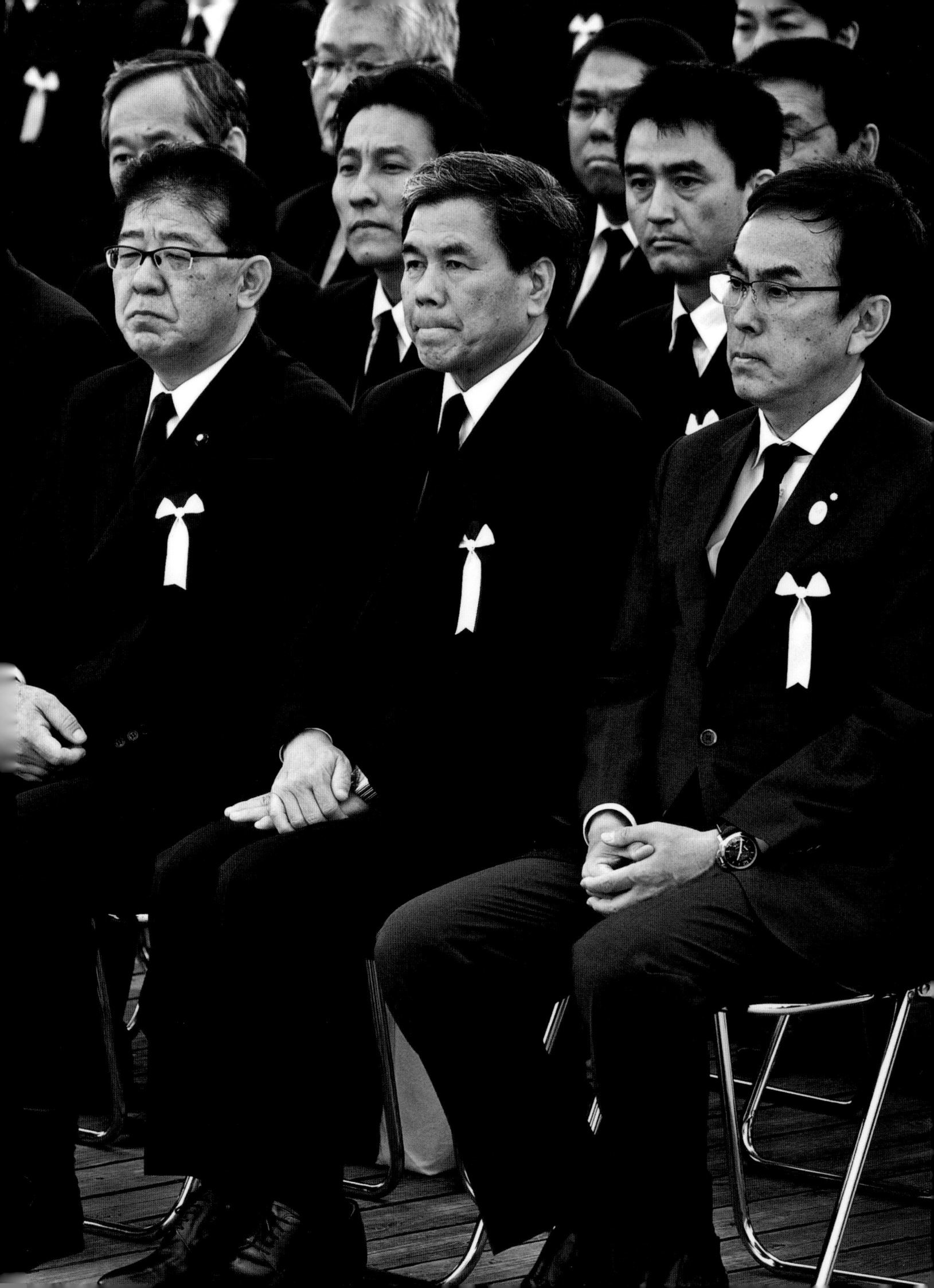

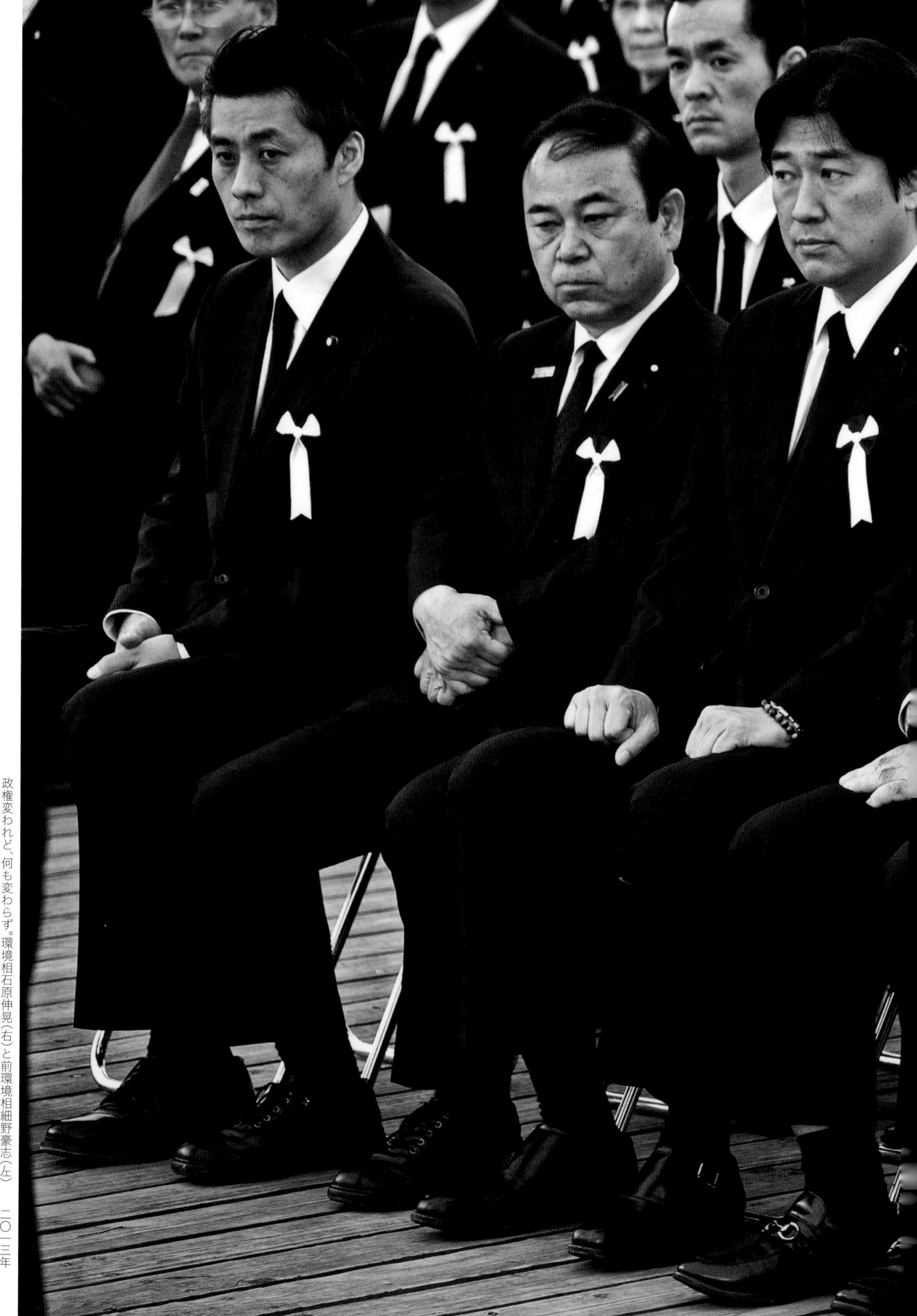

政権変われど、何も変わらず。環境相石原伸晃(右)と前環境相細野豪志(左) 二〇一三年

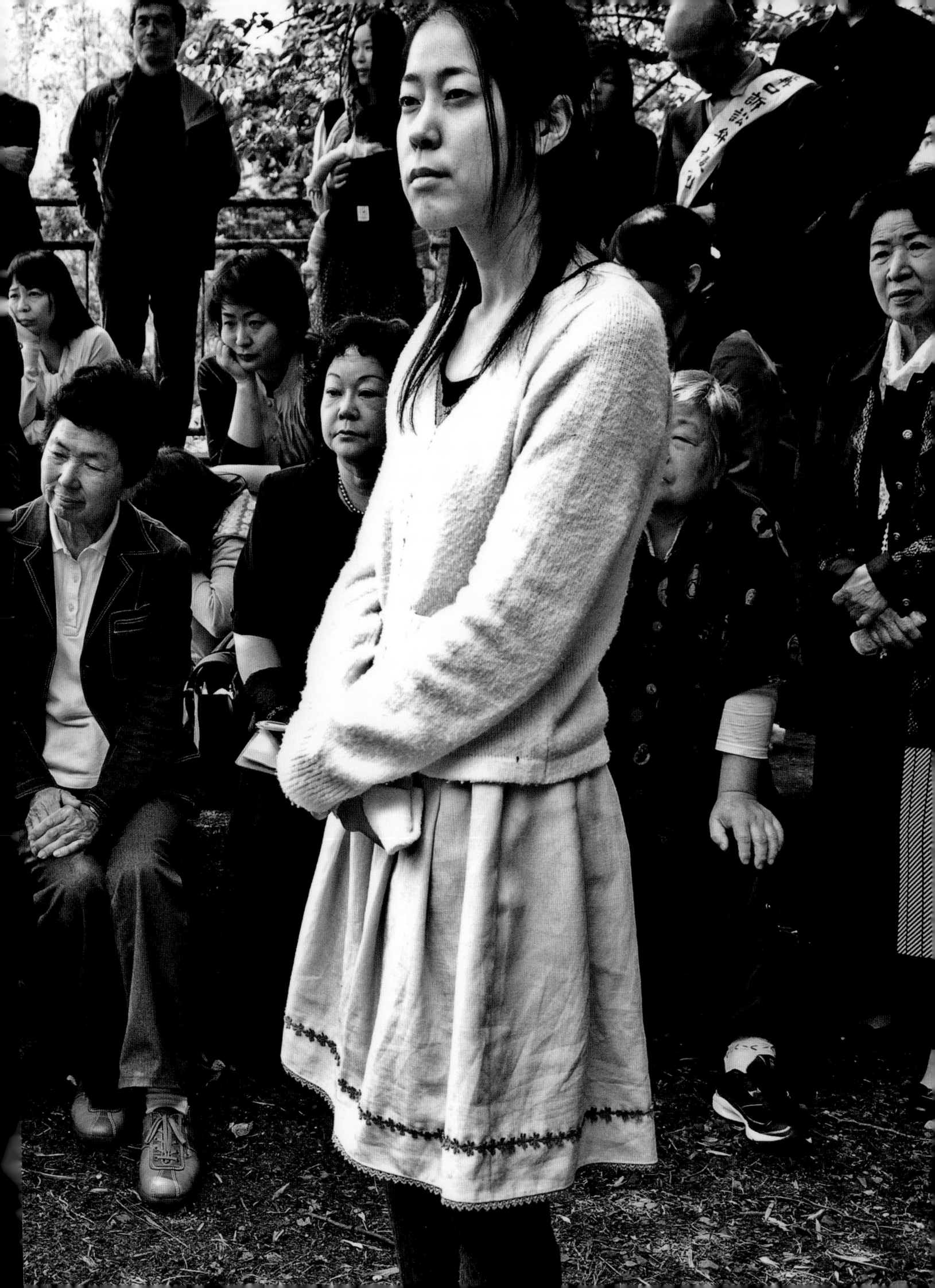

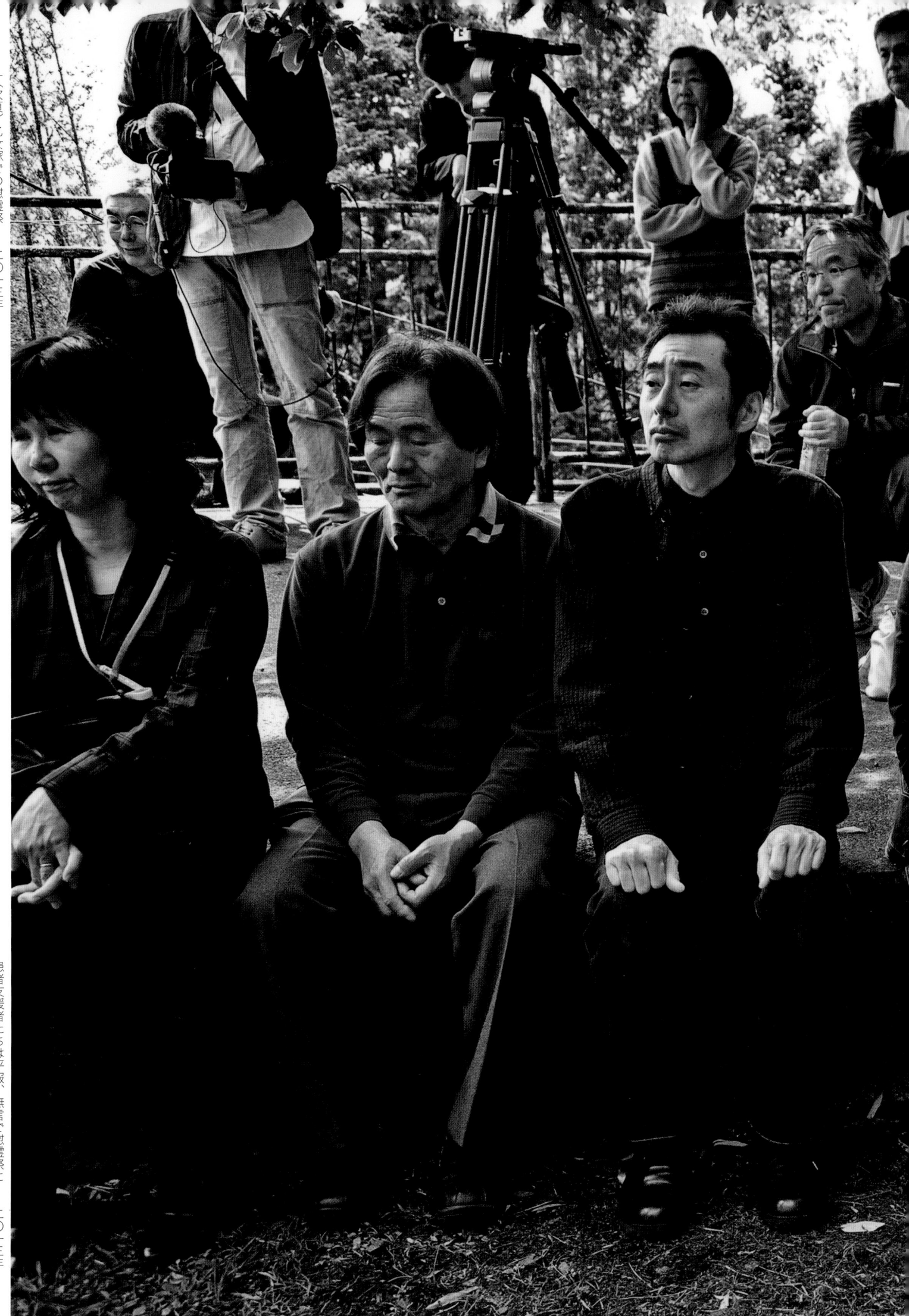

←〈次頁〉乙女塚での慰霊祭　二〇一三年

患者支援者たちは平服、無言で慰霊祭に　二〇一三年

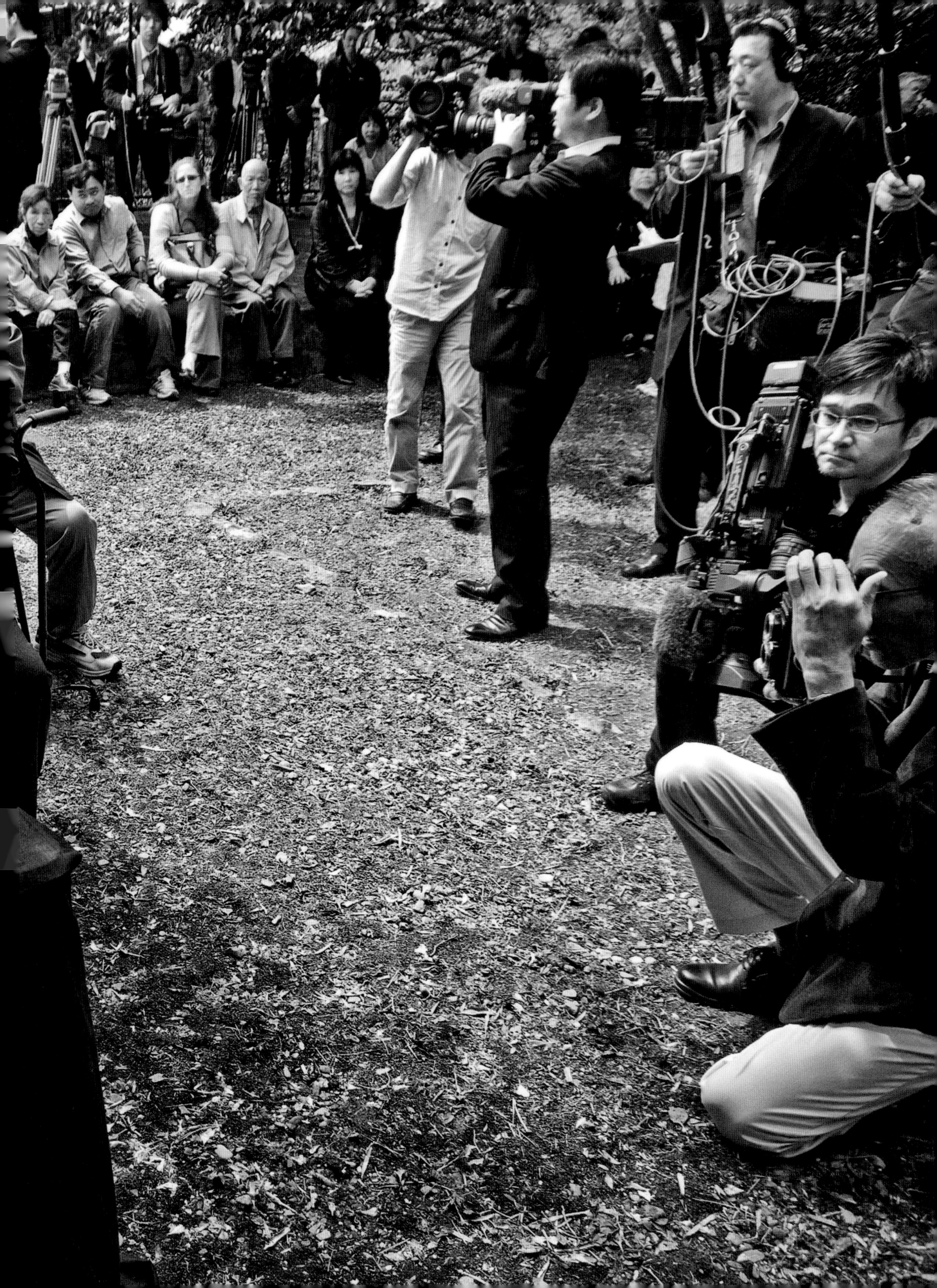

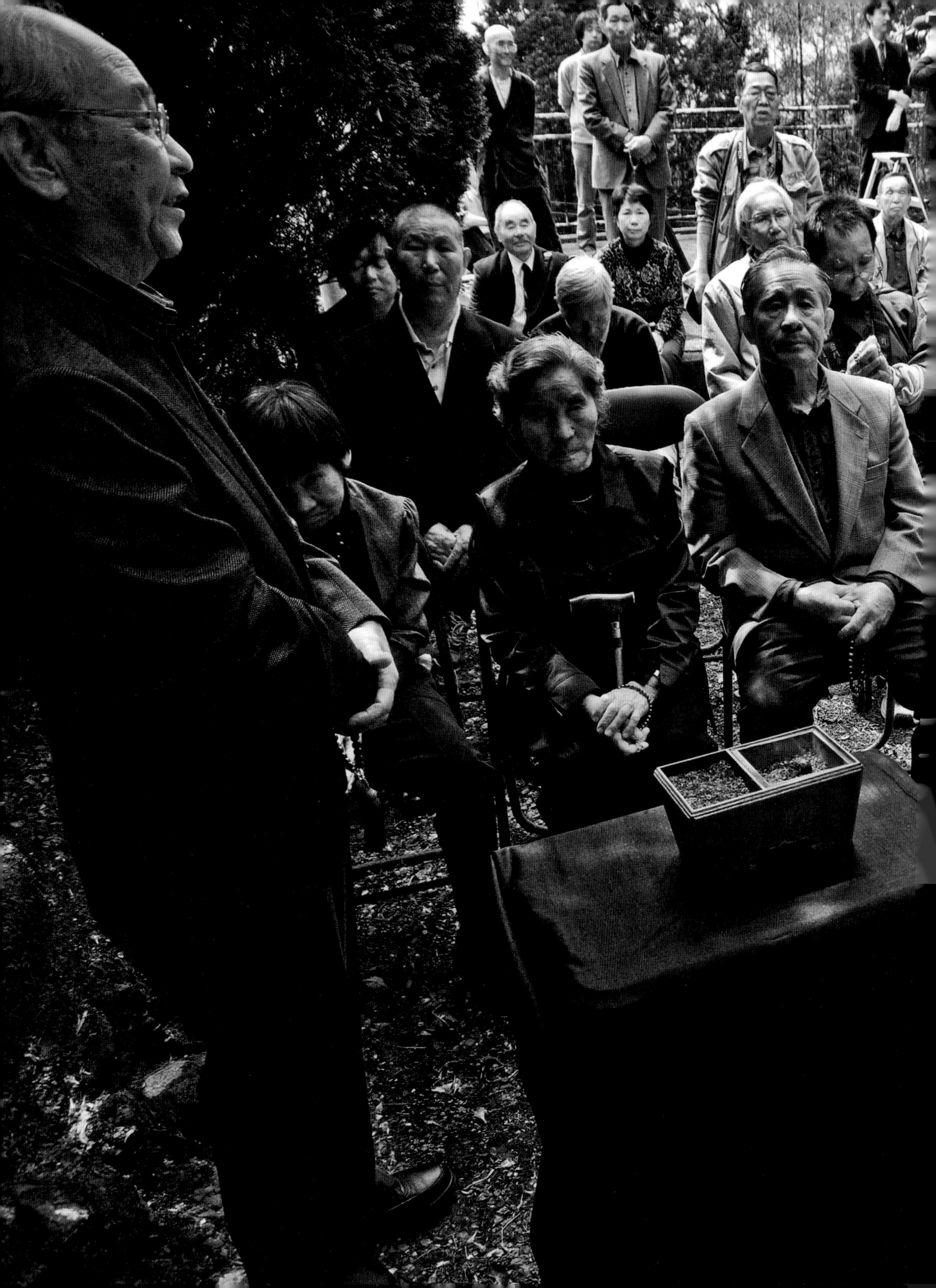

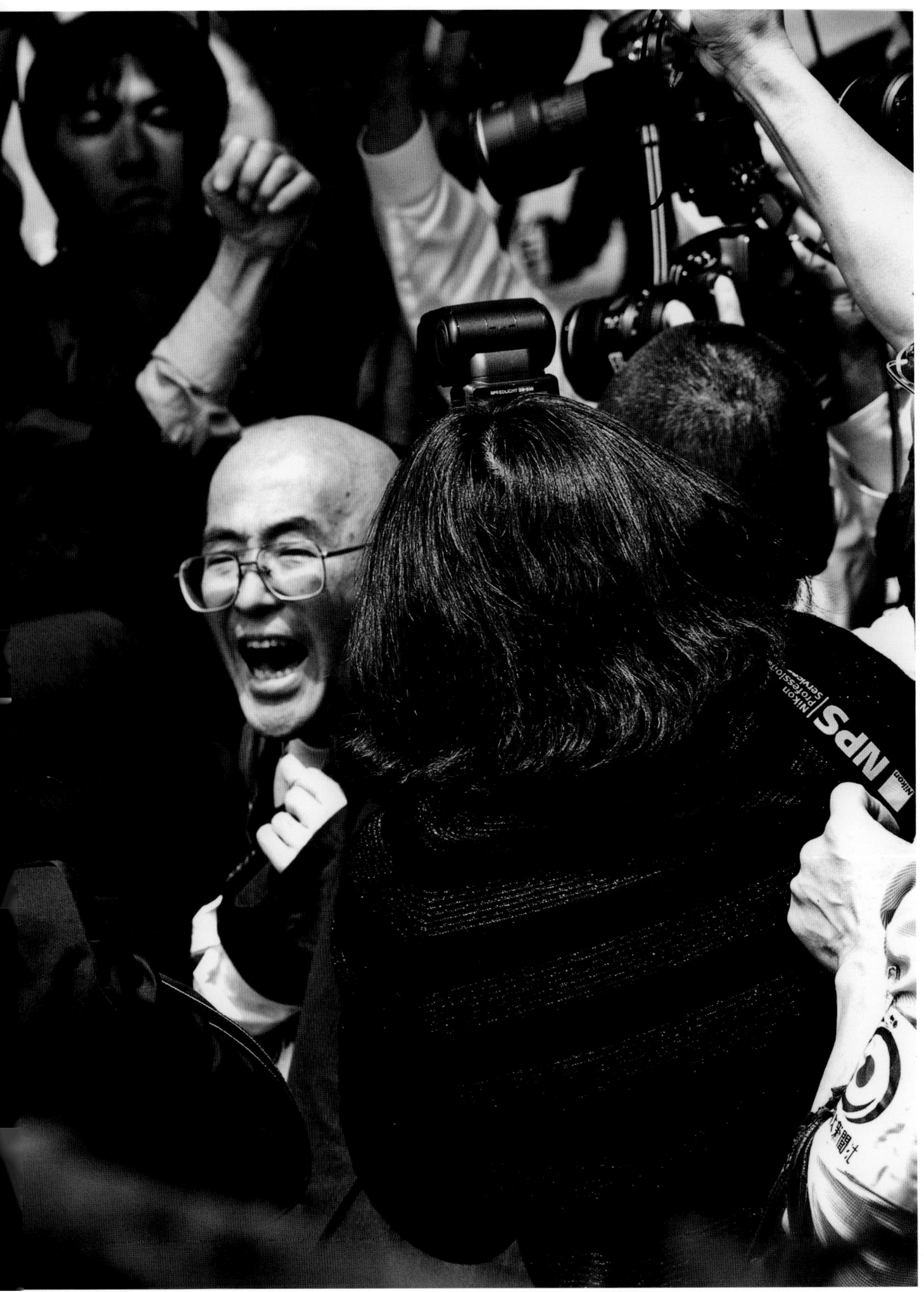

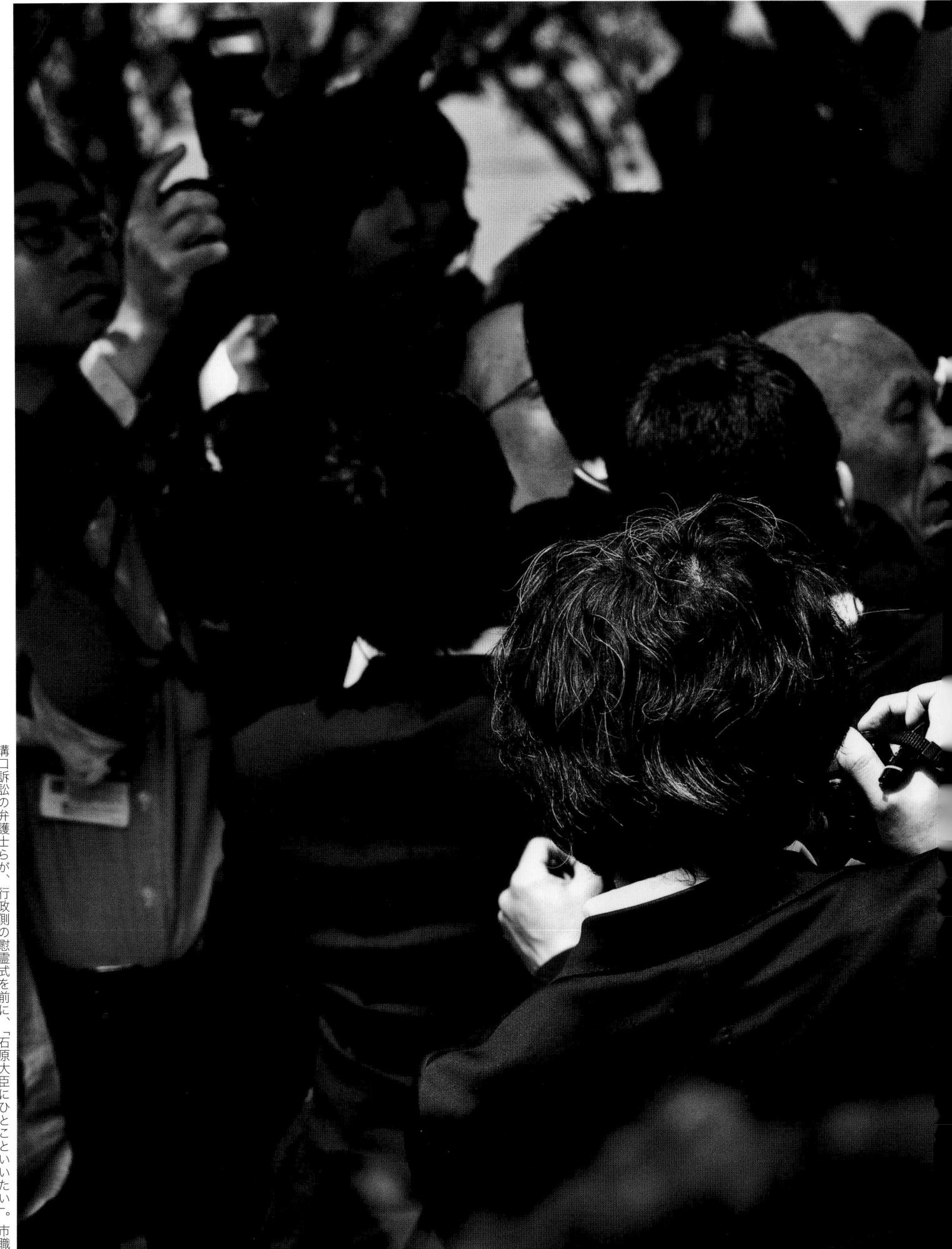

溝口訴訟の弁護士らが、行政側の慰霊式を前に、「石原大臣にひとこといいたい」。市職員が阻止した　二〇一三年

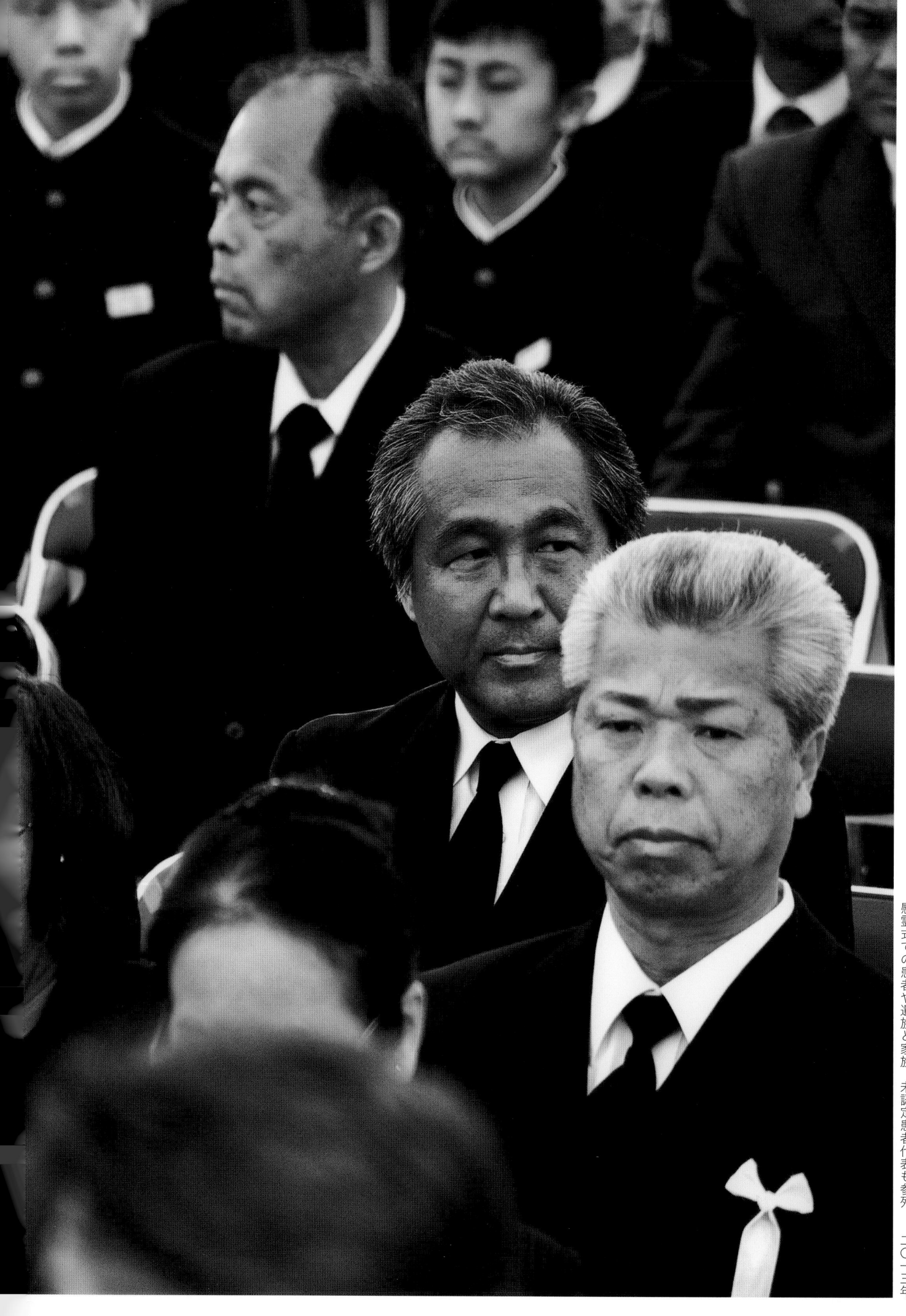

慰霊式での患者や遺族と家族、未認定患者代表も参列　二〇一三年

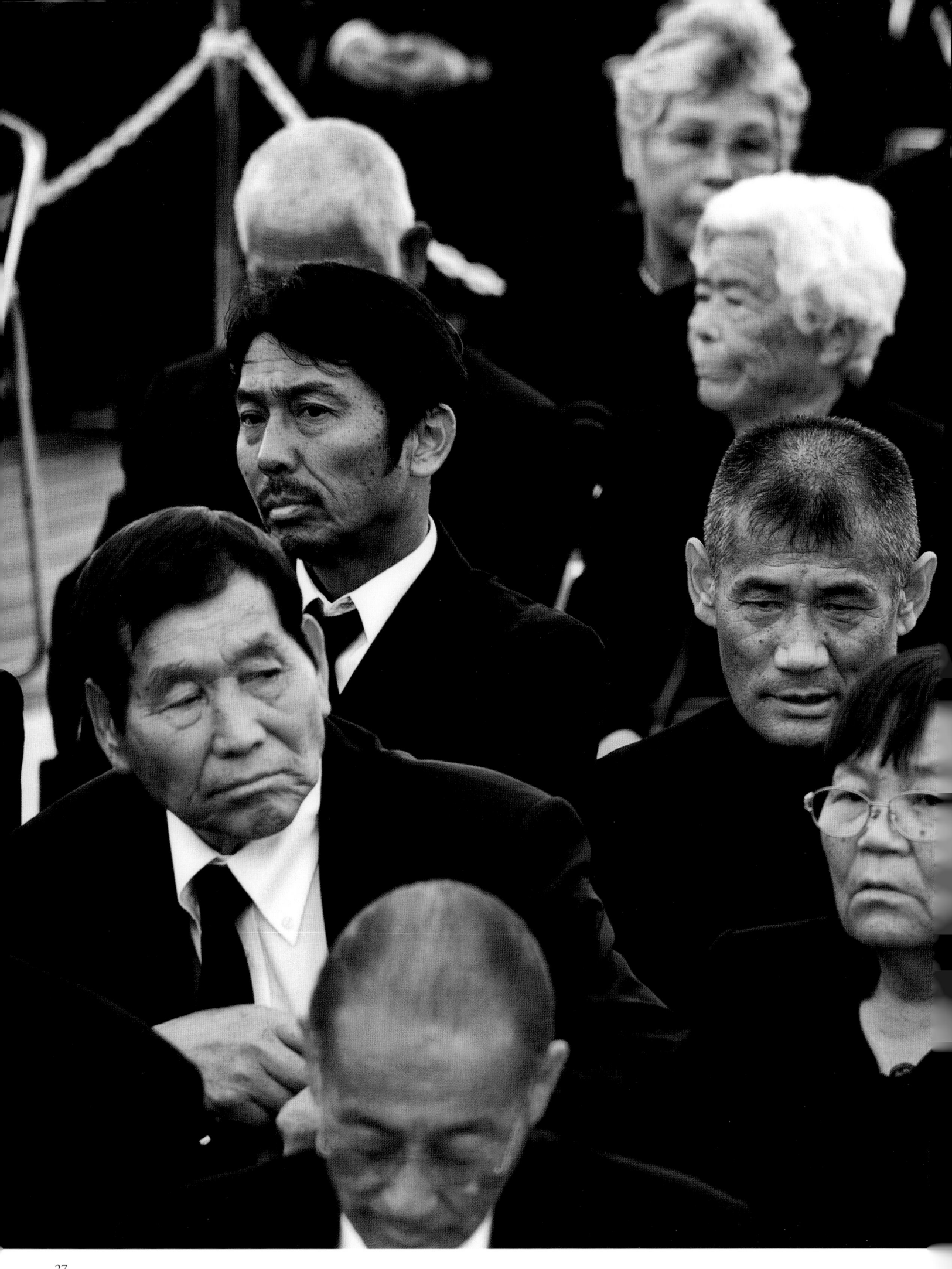

③「宝子(たからご)」

初産で胎児性患者の子をもった母は述べた。「こん子は、私の宝子です。私のからだから水銀ば吸い取ってくれたおかげで、あとの六人の妹弟たちは元気だし、私の症状も軽くすんどるとです」。宝子の上村(かみむら)智子は、両親から終始自宅で介護され、21歳6カ月で他界した。

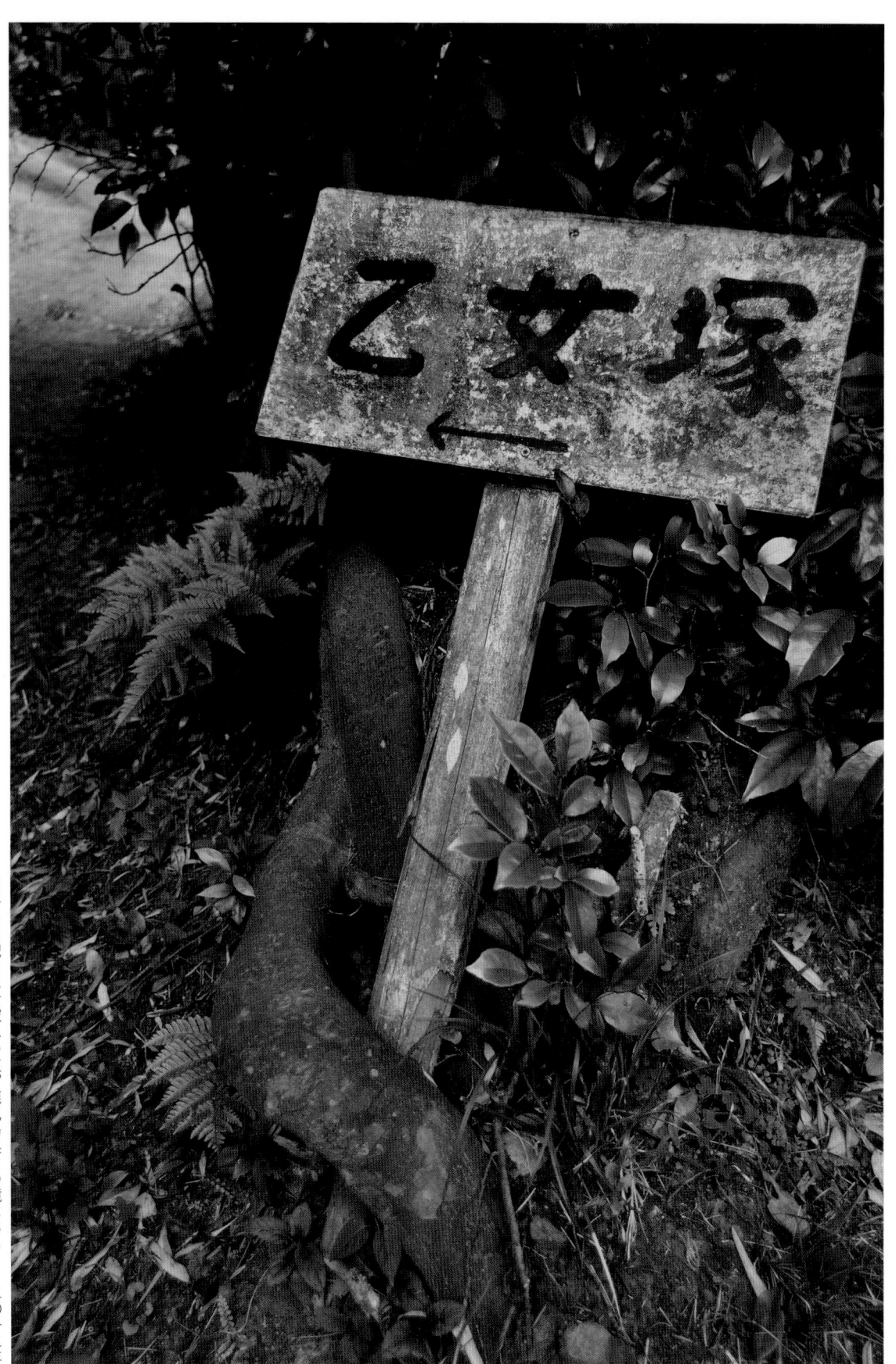

智子らを祀る乙女塚への道。鹿児島県との境にある　二〇一二年

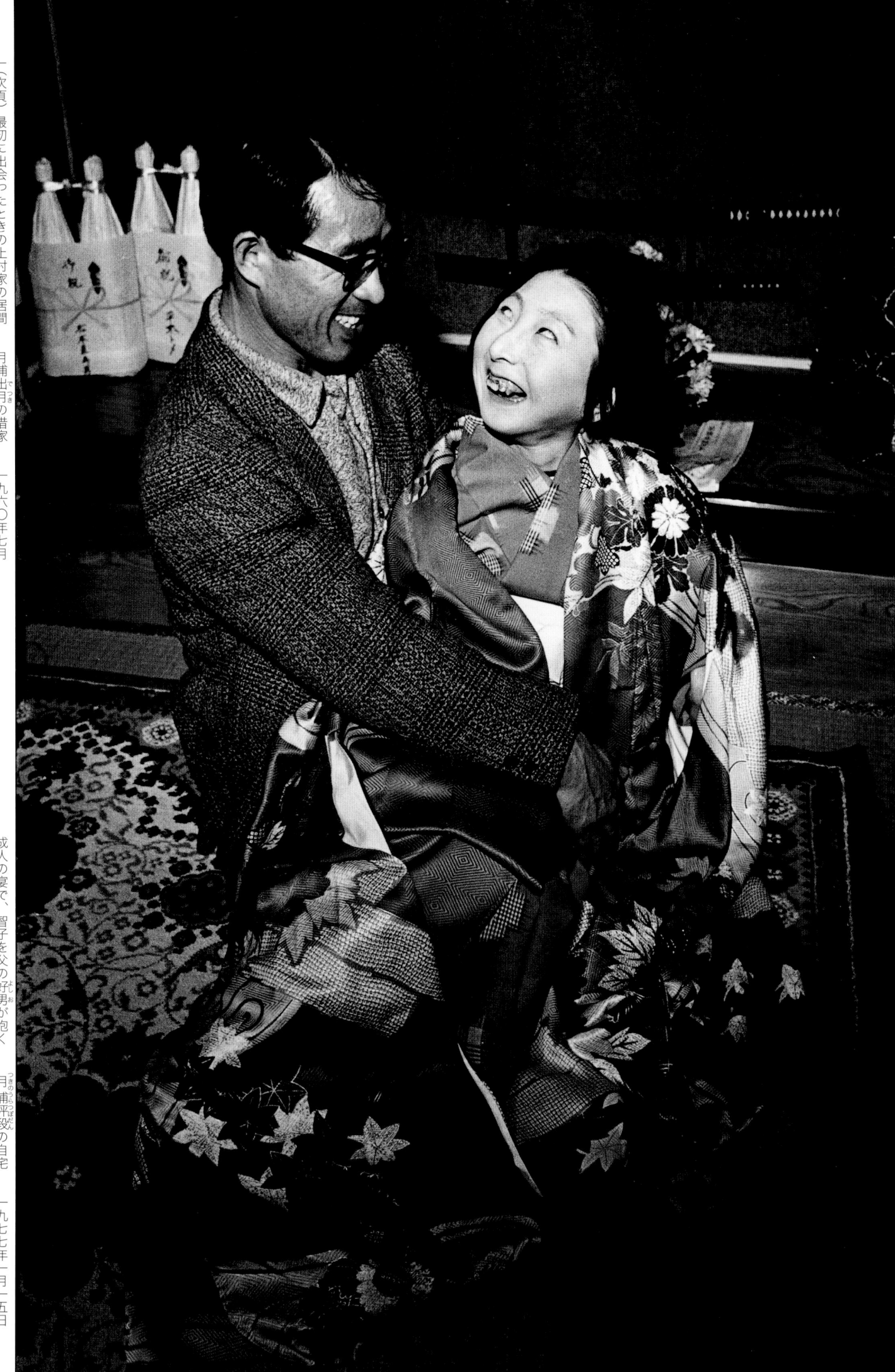

←〈次頁〉最初に出会ったときの上村家の居間　月浦出月の借家　一九六〇年七月

成人の宴で、智子を父の好男が抱く　月浦坪段の自宅　一九七七年一月一五日

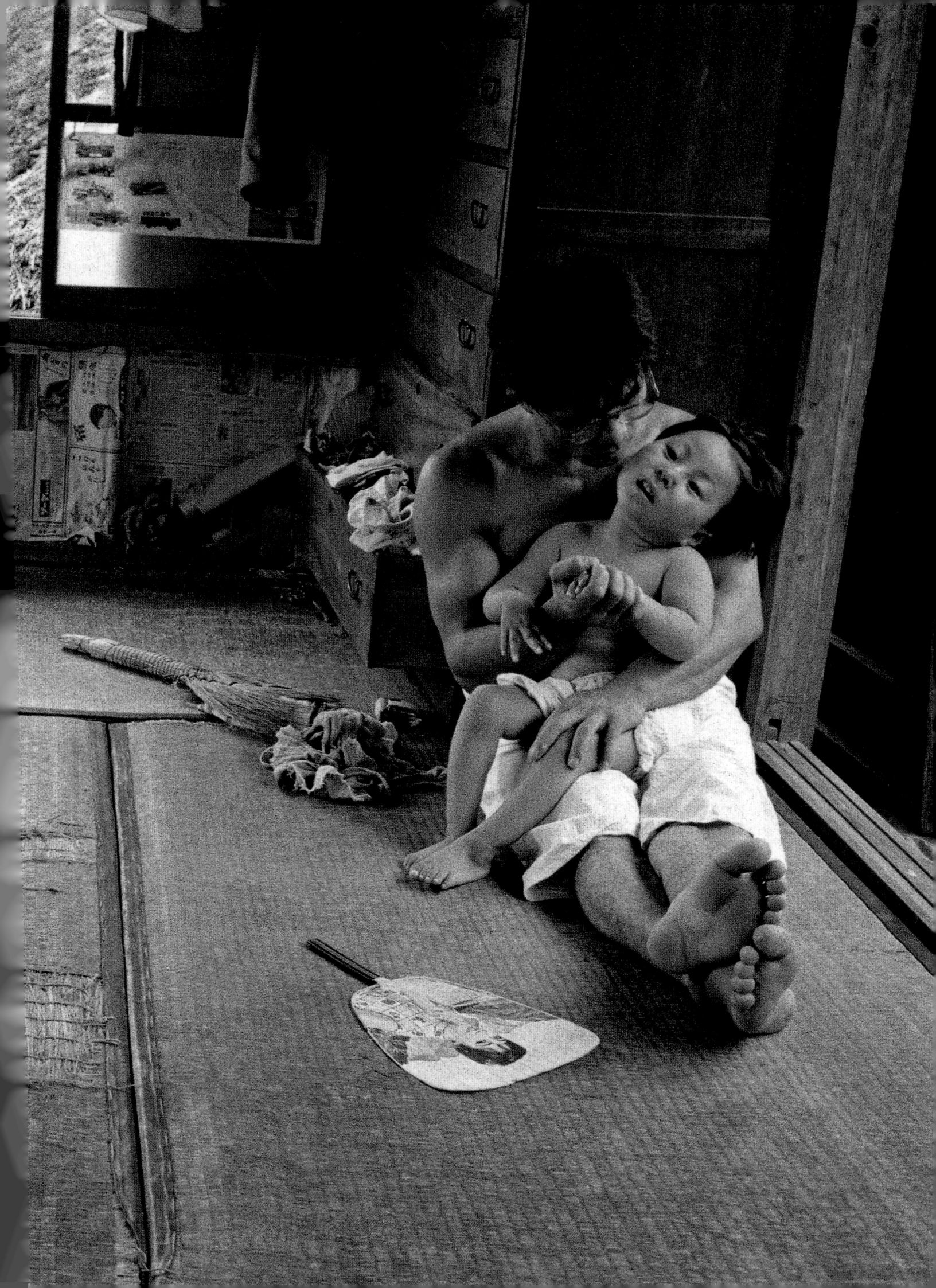

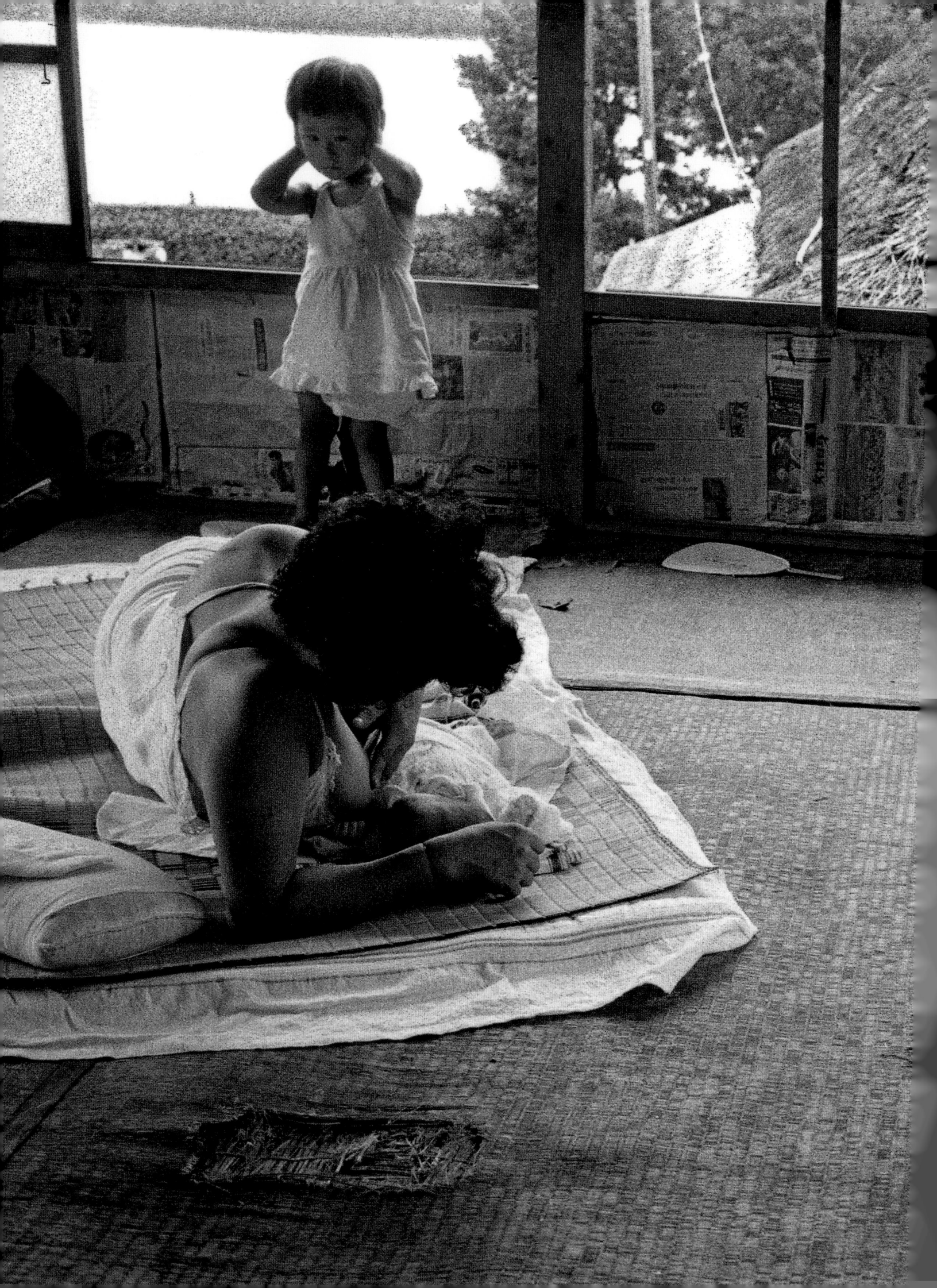

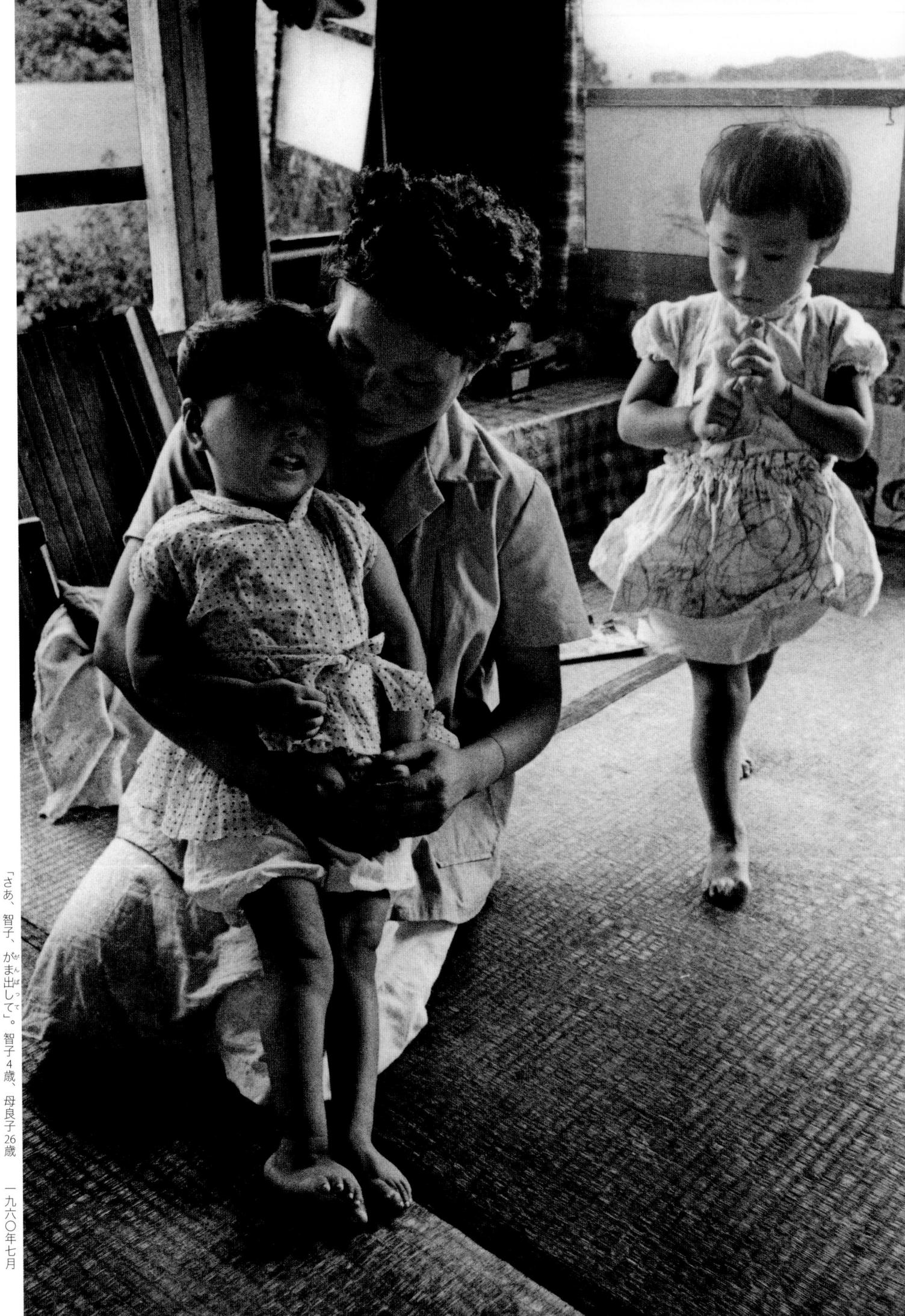

「さあ、智子、がまん出して」。智子4歳、母良子26歳 一九六〇年七月

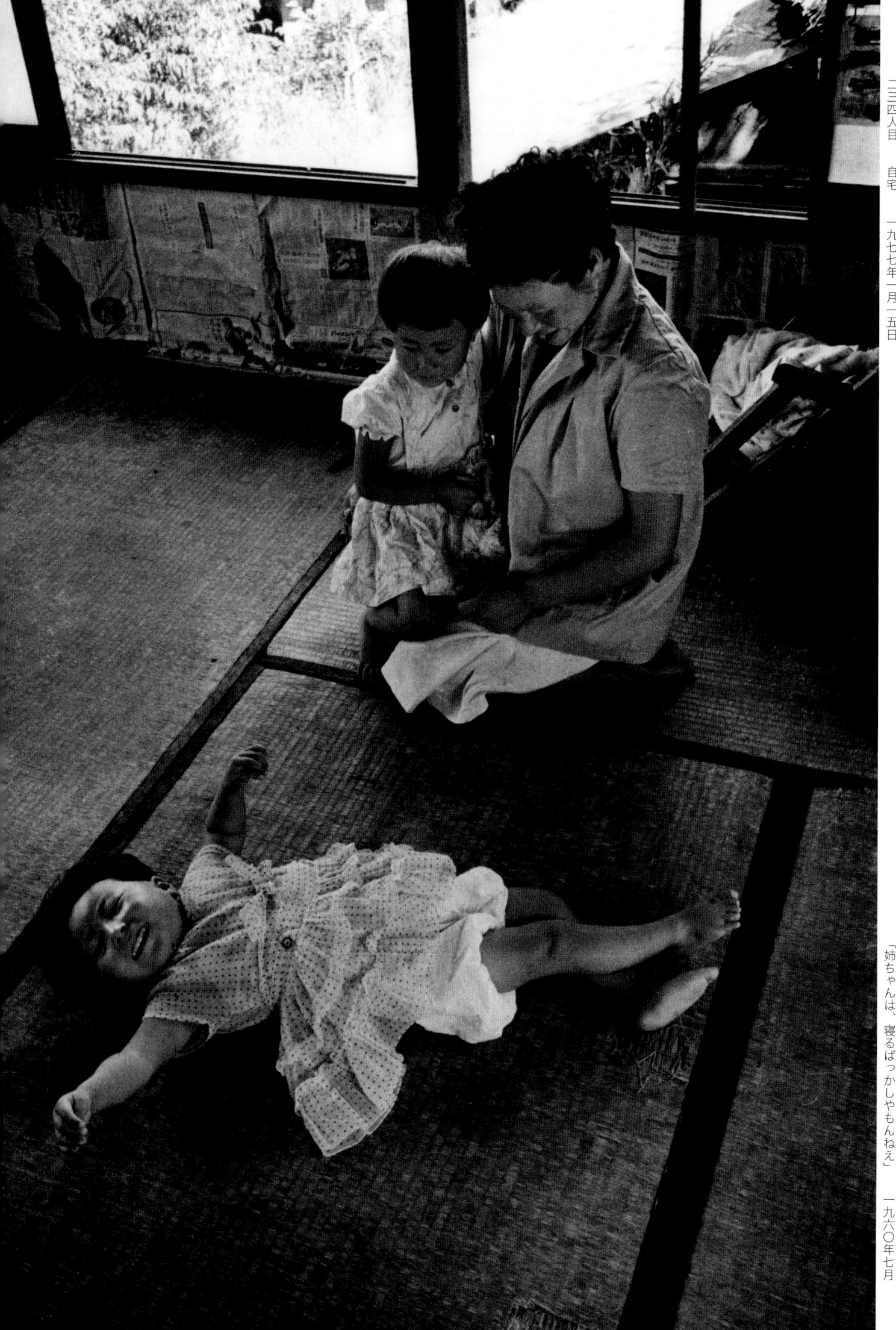

←（次頁）成人の宴に集う親類や縁者。智子はこの後、三三四日で死亡した。認定死者二三四人目　自宅　一九七七年一月一五日

「姉ちゃんは、寝るばっかしやもんねえ」　一九六〇年七月

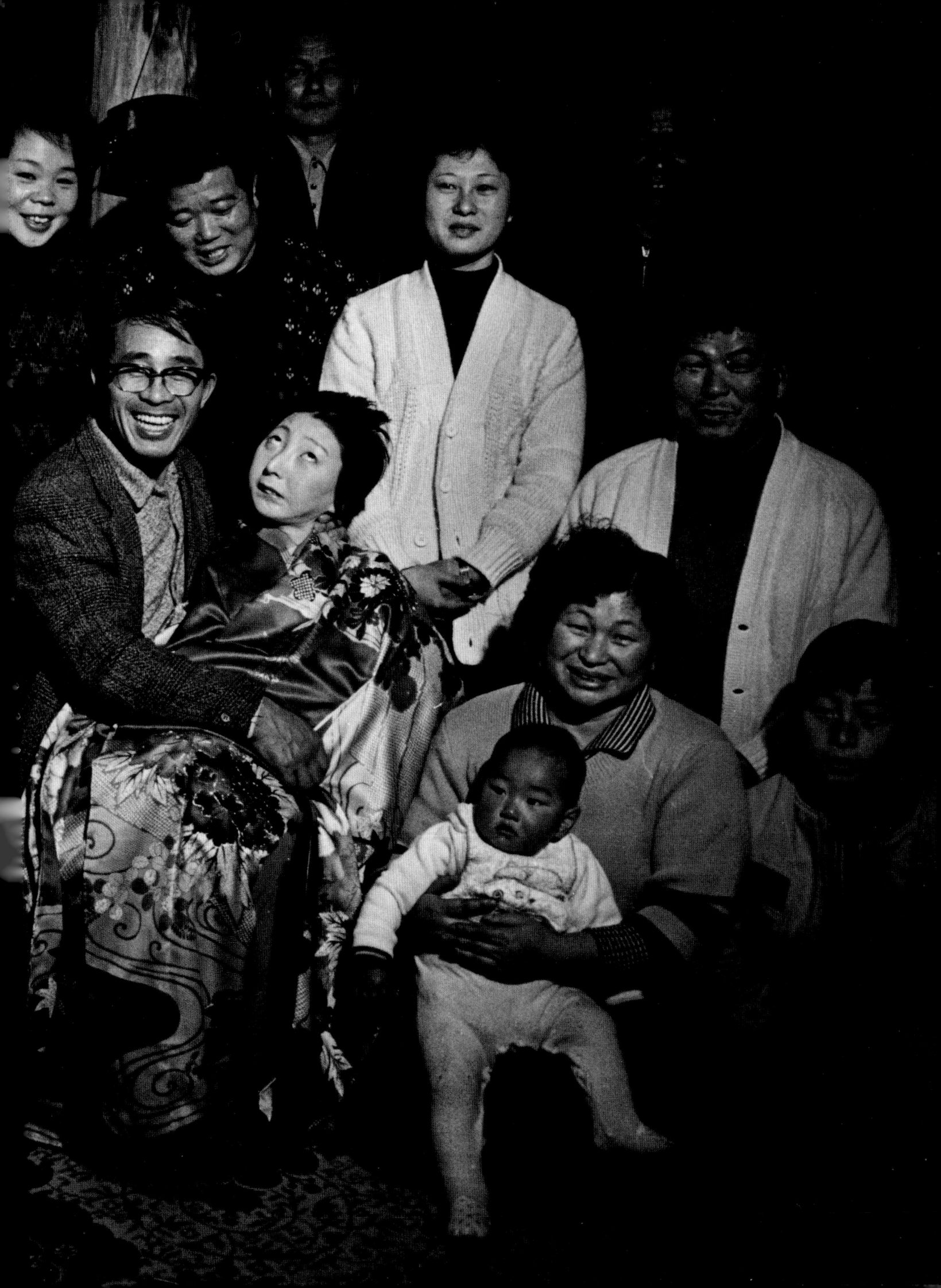

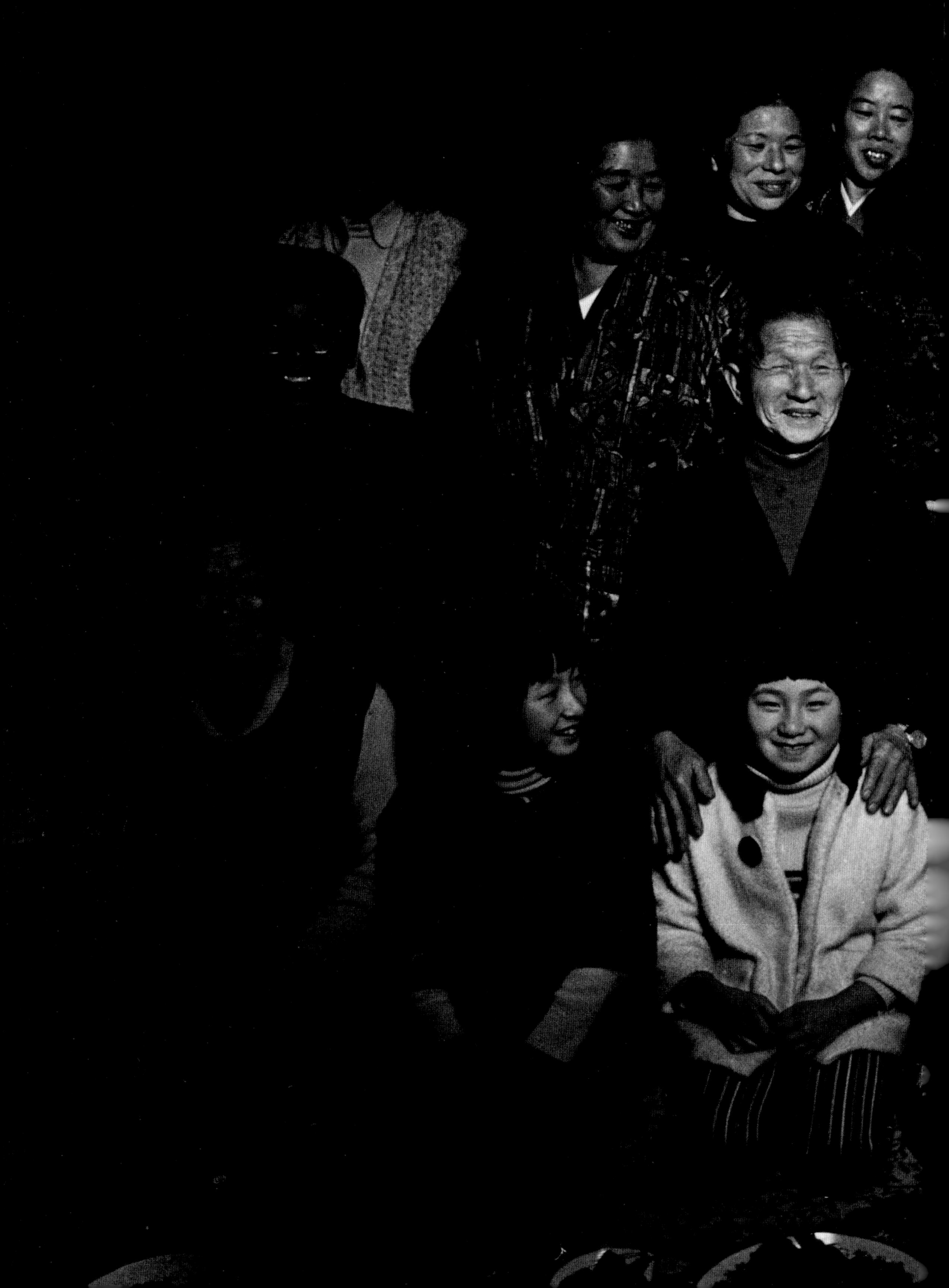

私の水俣病事件
光と影の魔術師

原　一男

水俣病事件を撮りはじめて

水俣の現地へ、私が初めて出向いたのは、一〇年前のことだろうか。「水俣病」に関わってみませんか？と、ある人（名前を伏せる特別な理由があるわけではないが）から誘われたからだ。現地を案内されながら、水俣病の問題は全面的に解決されたわけではないんだ、と実感。そのことに驚いた。どうやら、新たな局面を迎えているようなのだ。胎児性水俣病の子どもだった患者たちの老齢化、さらに第二世代の患者が増えているという。

水俣病患者たちの運動と三里塚闘争は、六〇年代から七〇年代にかけて大きな盛り上がりを見せ、それらを記録した小川プロダクションの「三里塚シリーズ」と土本典昭監督の「水俣病シリーズ」は、日本のドキュメンタリー史上の金字塔であって、当時、私を含めて多くの若者たちの血を騒がせたものだ。あれから四〇年もの時間は経過していた。

「水俣病シリーズ」を長く、心血を注いで作ってきた土本監督は、新たな局面を迎えつつある事態に対してどうするんだろうか？と気になった。私の中で、水俣病は〝土本さんの縄張り〟であり、私なんぞがシャシャリでるべきではない、という妙な意識があった。だが、土本監督もまた高齢になり、対応は難しいという。ならば、自分がやってもいいかな、と思ったのだ。こんなやつがやってきて私は、新たなる水俣病事件の展開の映像化に関わることになった。

桑原史成は憧れの存在

四〇年前、私が二十歳の頃。報道写真家、フォトジャーナリストになり世界を駆けることを夢見て、東京綜合写真専門学校に入学。

この頃、憧れていたのが、桑原史成だった。「桑原さんは、この学校の先輩なんだぜ。」とクラスメイトと自慢し合ったものだった。同じ学校に学んだといっても、こちらの実力に何の関係もないのは百も承知。ただ訳もなく誇らしかったのだ。桑原さんのような写真家になりたいと目標にしていたことは確かだった。その頃、桑原さんは「水俣病」の仕事が評価されて日本写真家批評家協会新人賞を受賞、次の傑作になる「韓国」のシリーズに取り組んでいた。

桑原史成の写真の魅力に触れておきたい。桑原作品の魅力の最も大きなポイントは、凄くドラマチックであることだ。一枚の写真の中に、よくもこんなに濃密な世界を凝縮できるもんだといつも感心させられる。写された人の感情を、ギュッとそのエキスを画面に絞り出していてエネルギーが観る側にビシビシ伝わってくる。そのドラマチックな世界を構築するために、まず第一に、光の処理、いかし方が、舌を巻くほどうまい。映画作りの現場のように、スタジオの中で、ライティングで光と影の世界を創っていくわけではない。

名作「水俣病シリーズ」においても、患者たちの日々の暮らしの中での光を、映像にどう活かすかを桑原さんは常に考えていたのではないだろうか。これはもう動物的な感覚としか言いようがないと思うが、桑原さんはとりわけ斜光の生かし方は抜群にうまい！　一瞬の判断で構図とサイズを決めてしまうセンスは、天才の技だと思う。写真は光と影の芸術である、と言わるが、桑原さんは、まさに〝光と影の魔術師〟である。二番目に、レンズワークのうまさ。私はその中でも、望遠を使った画が大好きだ。望遠レンズ独特の遠近感をギュッと圧縮したような描写が持つ世界の、近さをヒシヒシと感じさせてくれる。そこに写された人たちの運命の過酷さをヒシヒシと感じさせてくれる。もちろん、ワイド系のレンズワークも見事だ。映画の場合は、一つのシーンをいくつかのカットに分解して撮り、編集でつなぐことによって、よりドラマチックな場面＝シーンとして成立するわけだが、桑原さんの一枚の写真は、そのまま映画の一シーンに匹敵するくらい、いや、それ以上にドラマチックなのである。私がムービーカメラを回すときに脳裡に浮かべるのは桑原さんの写真である。私が「水俣病問題」と関わることになってからなおのこと、桑原さんの写真集のページを繰ることが多くなった。

私は、二〇〇四年一〇月一四日「チッソ水俣病関西訴訟最高裁勝利判決」の日から川上敏行さんをメインにカメラを回し始めた。それからさらに足掛け九年という時間が過ぎた。そして二〇一三年四月一六日、「水俣病認定義務付け溝口訴訟＋Fさん訴訟」判決の日、舞台は同じ最高裁。この日、新聞社のスチールカメラマン、TV各局のカメラマンが大勢、押し合いへし合い、ひしめき合ってる中に飄々とファインダーを覗きシャッターを押している桑原さんの姿を見た。知名度や実績から言えば巨匠とも呼ばれてもおかしくない桑原さんだが、驕りなど微塵も感じさせない、軽快な動きを見て私は胸が熱くなる思いだった。写真学校に入学したときから四七年が経っていた。

（はら・かずお／映画監督・大阪芸術大学教授）

1989年11月創立 1990年4月創刊

月刊 機

2013.9 No.258

発行所 株式会社 藤原書店
〒162-0041
東京都新宿区早稲田鶴巻町五二三
電話 〇三・五二七二・〇三〇一（代）
FAX 〇三・五二七二・〇四五〇
◎本冊子表示の価格は消費税込の価格です。

編集兼発行人 藤原良雄
頒価 100円

一九九五年二月二七日第三種郵便物認可 二〇一三年九月一五日発行（毎月一回一五日発行）

「セレクション 竹内敏晴の『からだと思想』」発刊！

「からだ」から「生きる」ことを考え抜いた、稀有の哲学者の精選集！

一九七五年刊『ことばが劈かれるとき』で、聴覚障害者としての生いたちから、ことばが劈かれた瞬間の経験を鮮烈に描いた演出家、竹内敏晴(1925-2009)。『からだ』を通じて、「他者」とは、そして「主体」とは何かを掘り下げ続けた、竹内敏晴の軌跡とは何であったのか。本セレクションでは、約四十年にわたる竹内敏晴の著作を精選する。「からだ」という根幹を喪失しつつある戦後日本社会の問題を人と人との関係の根源を粘り強く問い続けることから照らし出してきた竹内敏晴の仕事のエッセンスを読者に贈る。

編集部

● 九月号 目次 ●

「からだ」から「生きる」ことを考え抜いた、稀有の哲学者
「セレクション 竹内敏晴の『からだと思想』」発刊！ 1

『岡田英弘著作集』待望の第2巻刊行！
世界史はモンゴル帝国から始まった 岡田英弘 6

写真家・桑原史成が撮り続けた水俣病事件の半世紀！
水俣事件 The MINAMATA Disaster 10

『易経』とは何か 黒岩重人 14

内務省とは何だったのか？ 黒澤 良 16

〈リレー連載〉今、なぜ後藤新平か96 ア主義者——後藤新平と大倉喜八郎 〈村上勝彦〉18

いま「アジア」を観る128「日中で価値観の共有を」増田寛也 21

〈連載〉ル・モンド 紙から世界を読む126「GPIIとは？」〈加藤晴久〉20 女性雑誌を読む65「女の世界」（一九）〈尾形明子〉22 ちょっとひと休み6「回線故障」〈山崎陽子〉23

8・10月刊案内/書店様へ/イベント報告/読者の声・書評日誌/刊行案内/告知・出版随想

本セレクションを推す

谷川俊太郎（詩人）

──野太い声とがっちりしてしなやかな肢体

アタマとココロとカラダの三位一体から、コエが生まれ、それがコトバとして他者に投げかけられるという、人間が群れとして生きていく基本を、竹内さんは繰り返しおのが肉体を原点として他者に働きかけ、またそれを文字化して飽きなかった。あの野太い声と、がっちりしてしかもしなやかな肢体の記憶は、竹内さんが遺した書き物とともに、この時代にますます新しい。

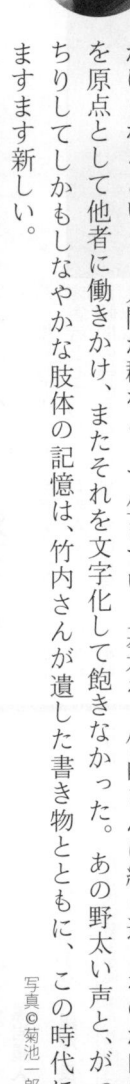

写真©菊池一郎

木田 元（哲学者）

──「からだ」によって裏打ちされた「ことば」

結局のところ竹内さんとは、二〇〇二年の晩秋に対談をして本にしてもらったとき、一度お会いしただけに終わってしまったが、初対面だというのに懐かしいという思いをさせられるお人柄に深く心を惹かれた。「からだ」によって裏打ちされていないような「ことば」には人を動かす力はないといったところで、強く共感し合ったことが今も忘れられない。

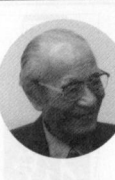

4 「生ける人形」

水俣病専用病棟で、私は一人の美少女に釘付けとなった。松永久美子、当時9歳8カ月。まさに"天女"かと思った。元気に生まれたが、5歳7カ月で突然寝たきりに。失外套症候群、大半を無動無言の一八年。23歳9カ月で死亡、一〇〇人目の認定死者だった。

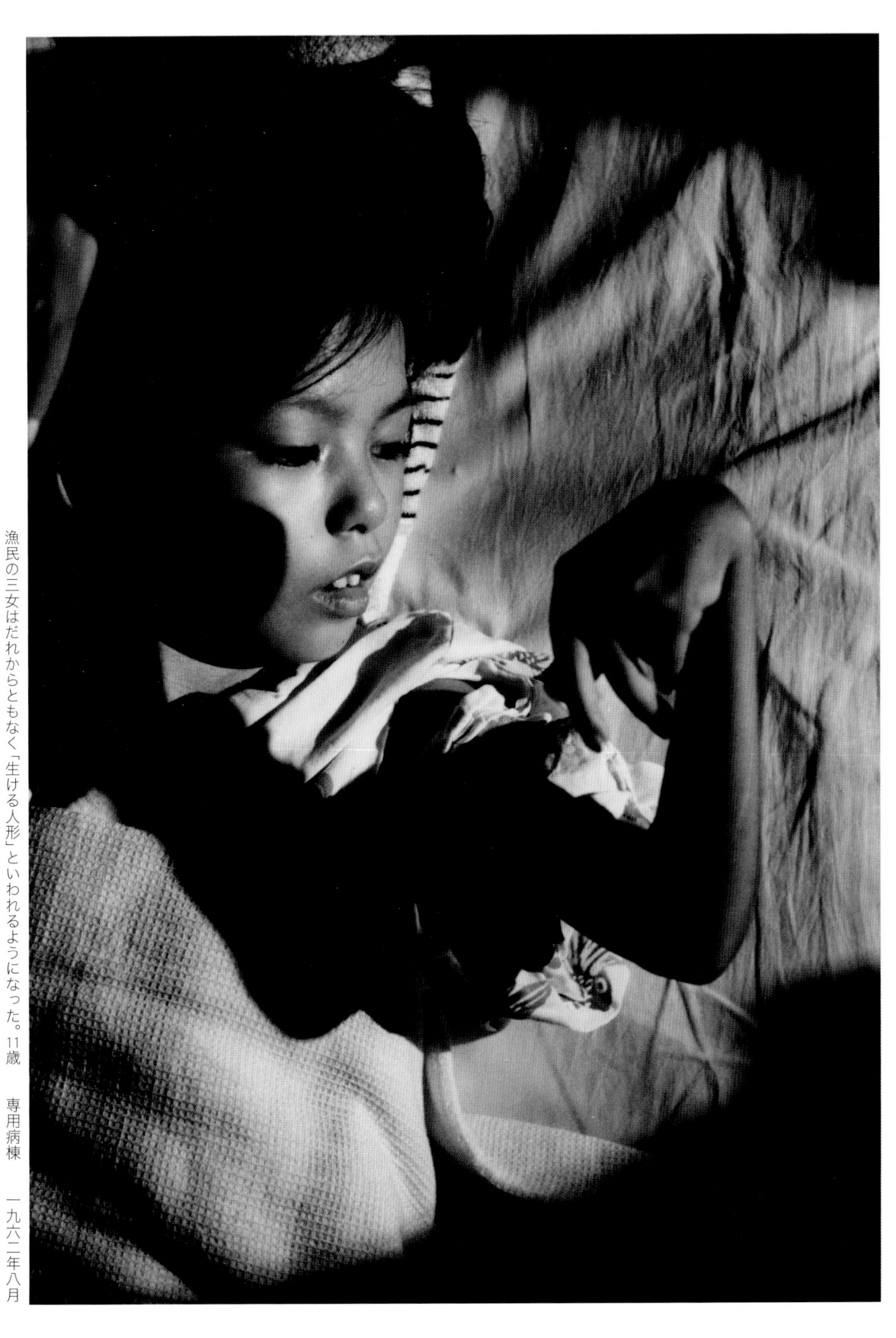

漁民の三女はだれからともなく「生ける人形」といわれるようになった。11歳　専用病棟　一九六二年八月

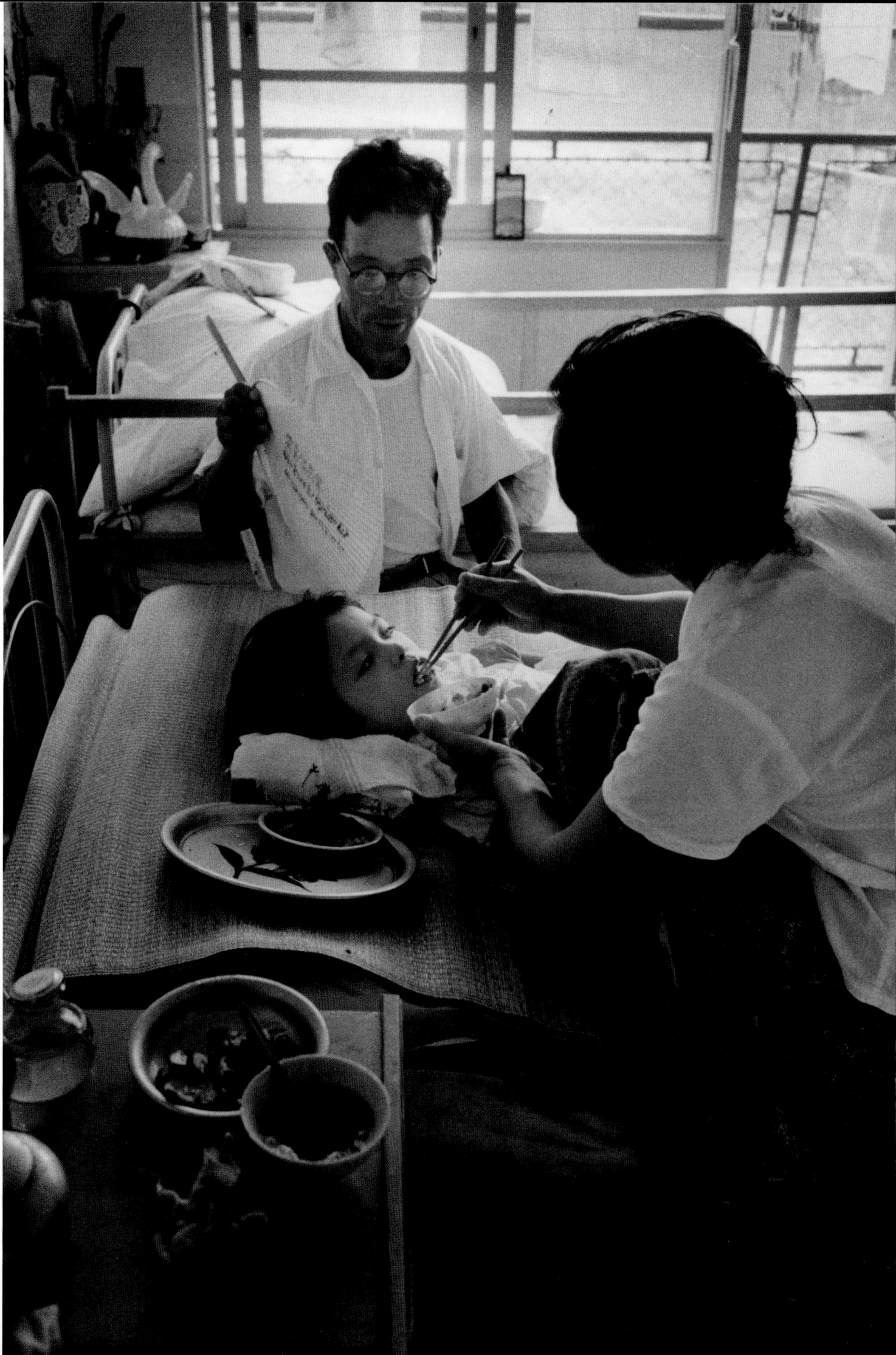

しばし娘に寄り添う父善一44歳と母マサ44歳　専用病棟　一九六〇年八月

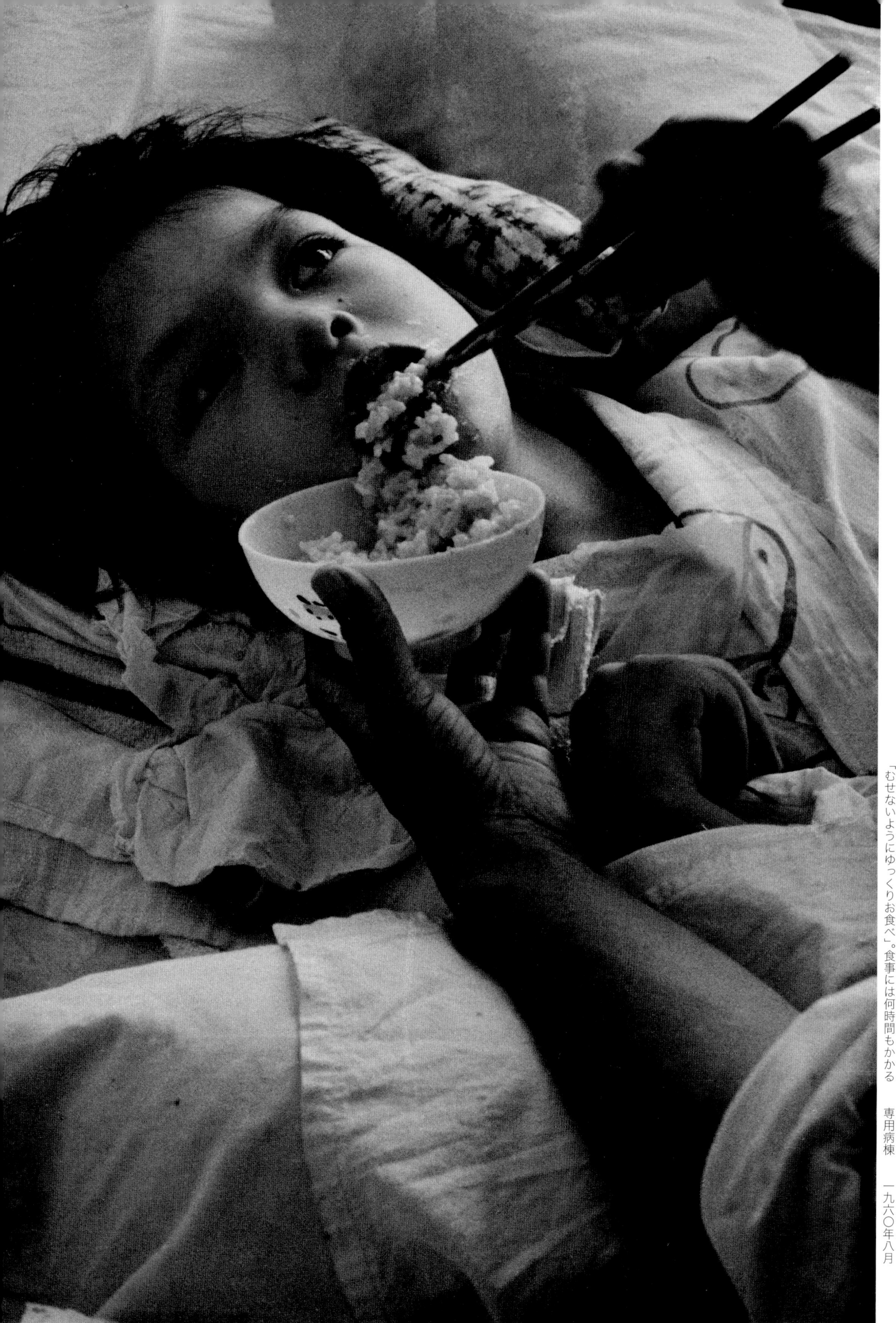

「むせないようにゆっくりお食べ」。食事には何時間もかかる　専用病棟　一九六〇年八月

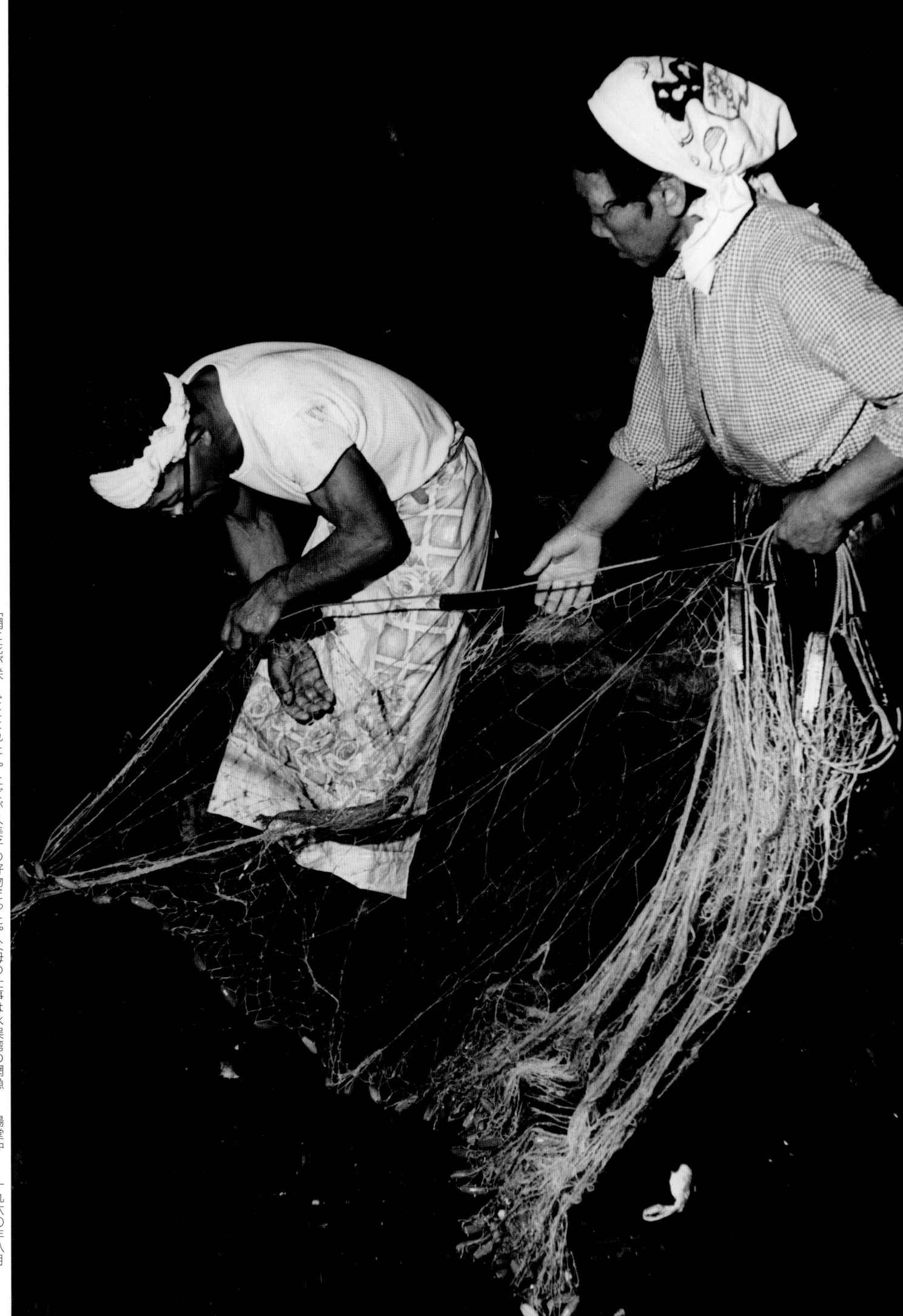

「網に花が咲くごととれた」。エビが久美子の好物だった。父母の仕事は水俣湾の網漁　湯堂沖　一九六〇年八月

← (次頁)「久美ちゃん、今日はいいお顔をしていますねえ」専用病棟　一九六〇年八月

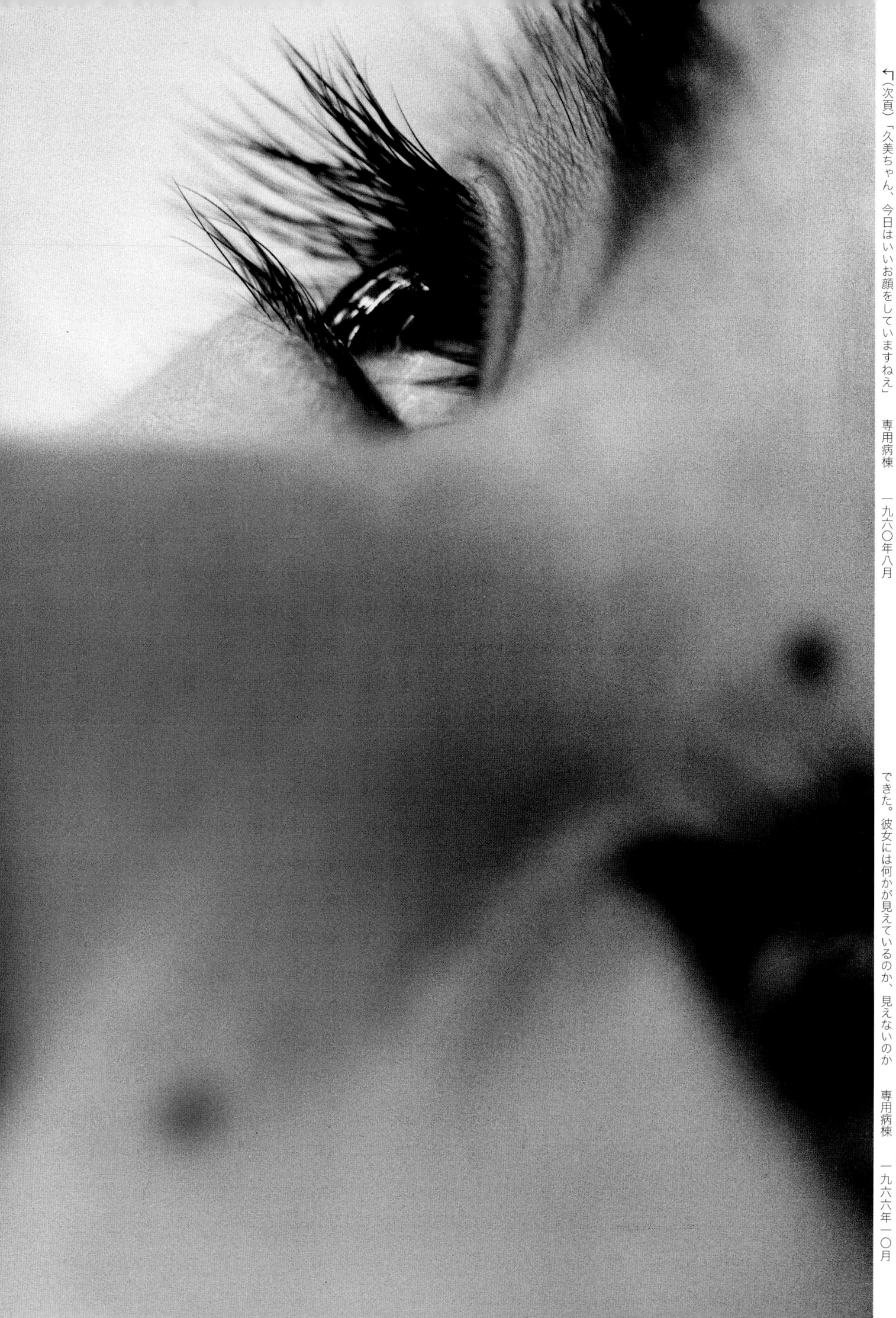

私は久美子を美しく撮りたかった。五度目の水俣取材で、15歳の「人形」の瞳を被写体にできた。彼女には何かが見えているのか、見えないのか　専用病棟　一九六六年一〇月

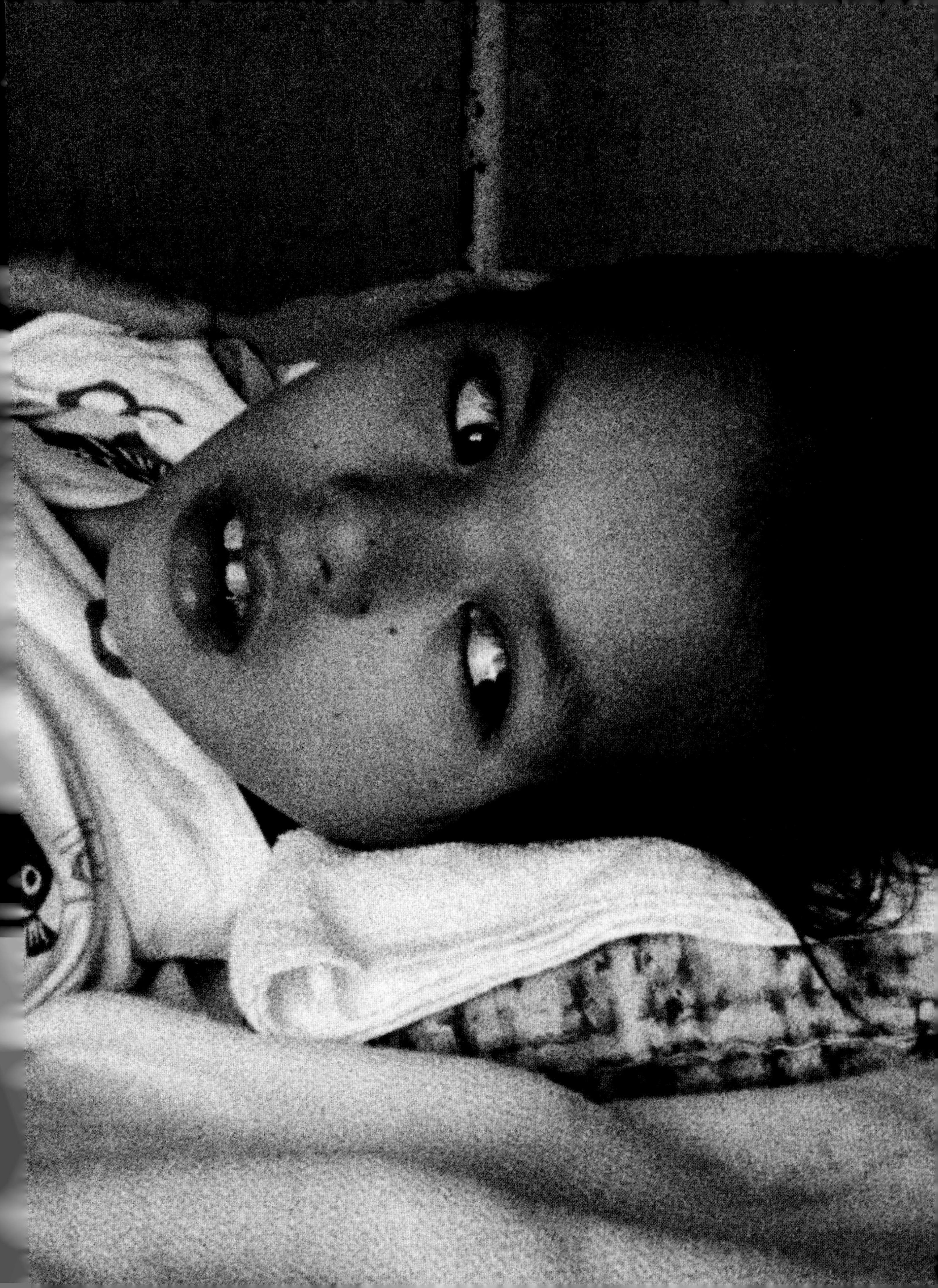

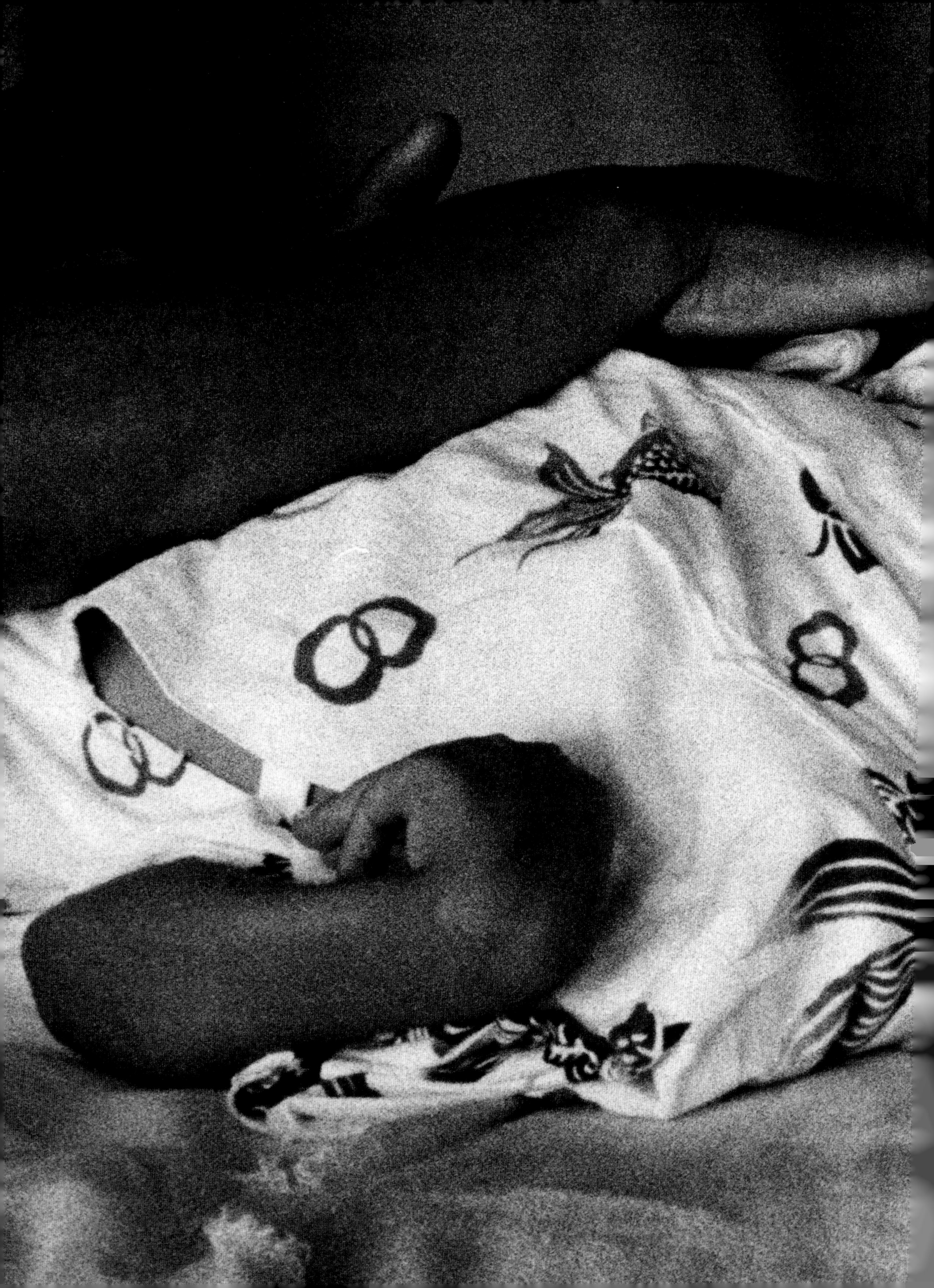

⑤ 隣村の網元二世代を襲った奇病

新日窒（後のチッソ、JNC）水俣工場は、水銀排水の放出先を一九五八年九月、水俣湾から水俣川河口へと密かに変更した。翌年、河口周辺から北隣の津奈木(つなぎ)村に劇症患者が続発した。事実上の人体実験である。津奈木の網元船場藤吉の入院では、村人挙げて見送りに出た。「出征のごとあった」と妻恵美香。藤吉の父岩蔵もすぐに後を追って入院だった。一九五九年一二月藤吉死亡、**34**歳。岩蔵は一二年間寝た切りの後、一九七一年一二月に死亡、**79**歳。ともに二度と家には帰れなかった。私が一九六〇年一〇月に恵美香からもらった手紙にこうあった。「政治の中心地である東京から一人でも多く報道員のお方が来られ、実際の事をご覧になり、又未だ生きたかばねとして病床に横たわる人が一日も早く全治するよう……出来得れば、折角の取材を無意味に終らせず、この水俣病のために大きく報道して戴くことを……」

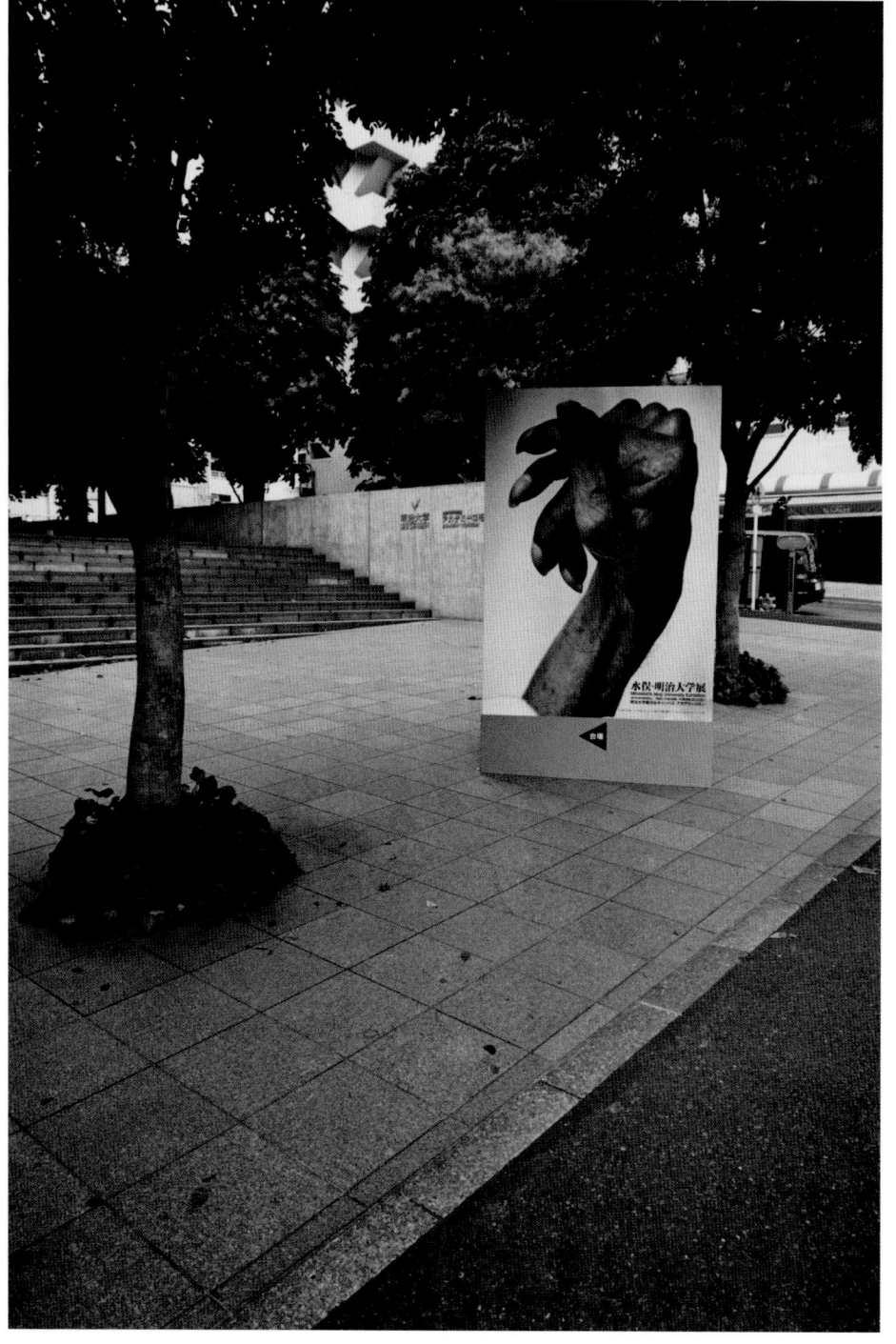

岩蔵の「手」は、ずっと後に起こった各種展示のシンボルになった　明治大学キャンパス　二〇一〇年九月

←（次頁）「手を撮っていいですか」というと、レンズの前に突き出してくれた。岩蔵はこの一年三カ月後に全身衰弱で死亡　リハビリセンター　一九七〇年九月

断末魔の藤吉が病室の壁をかき削った爪跡　水俣病専用病棟　一九六二年八月

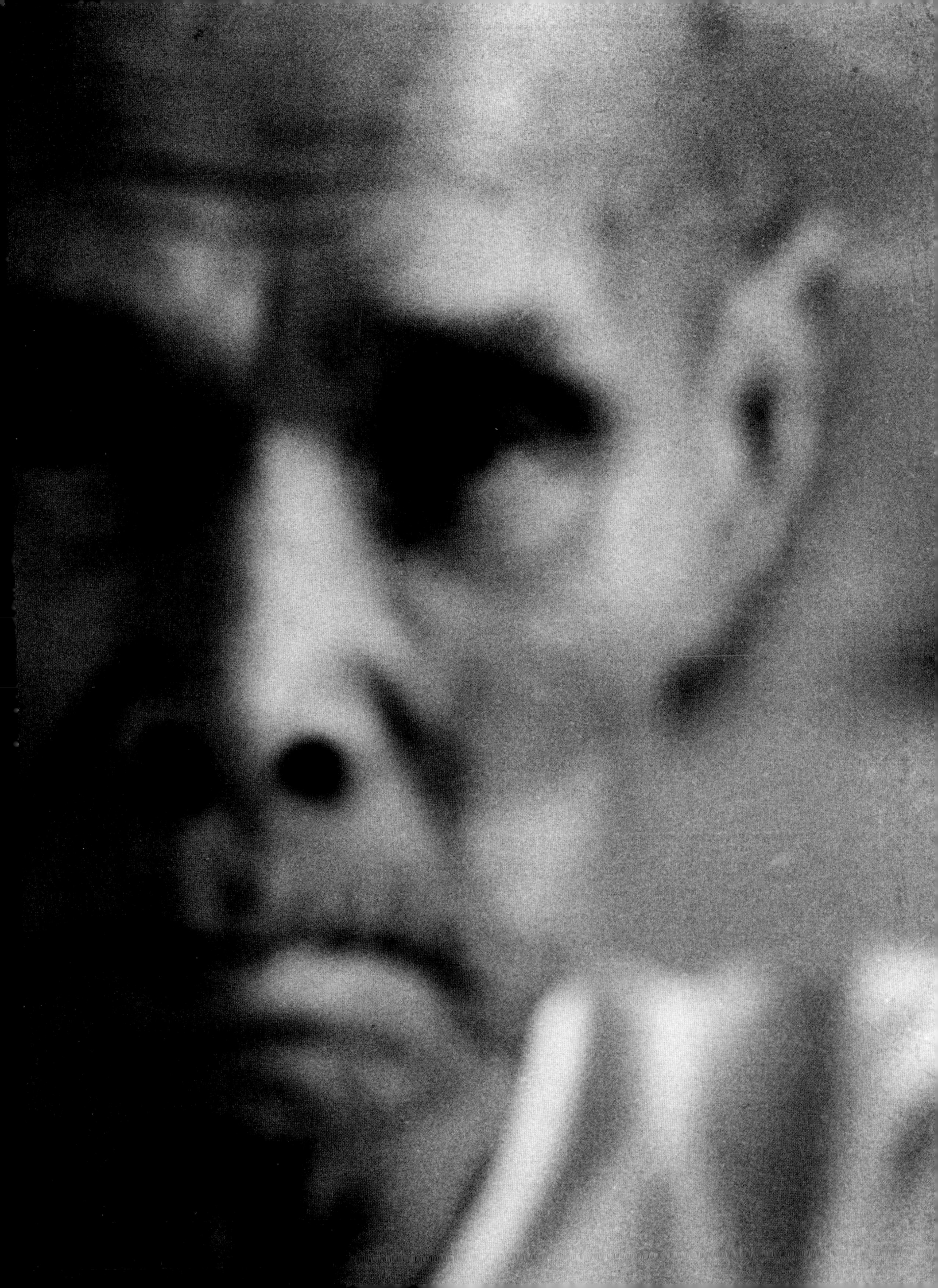

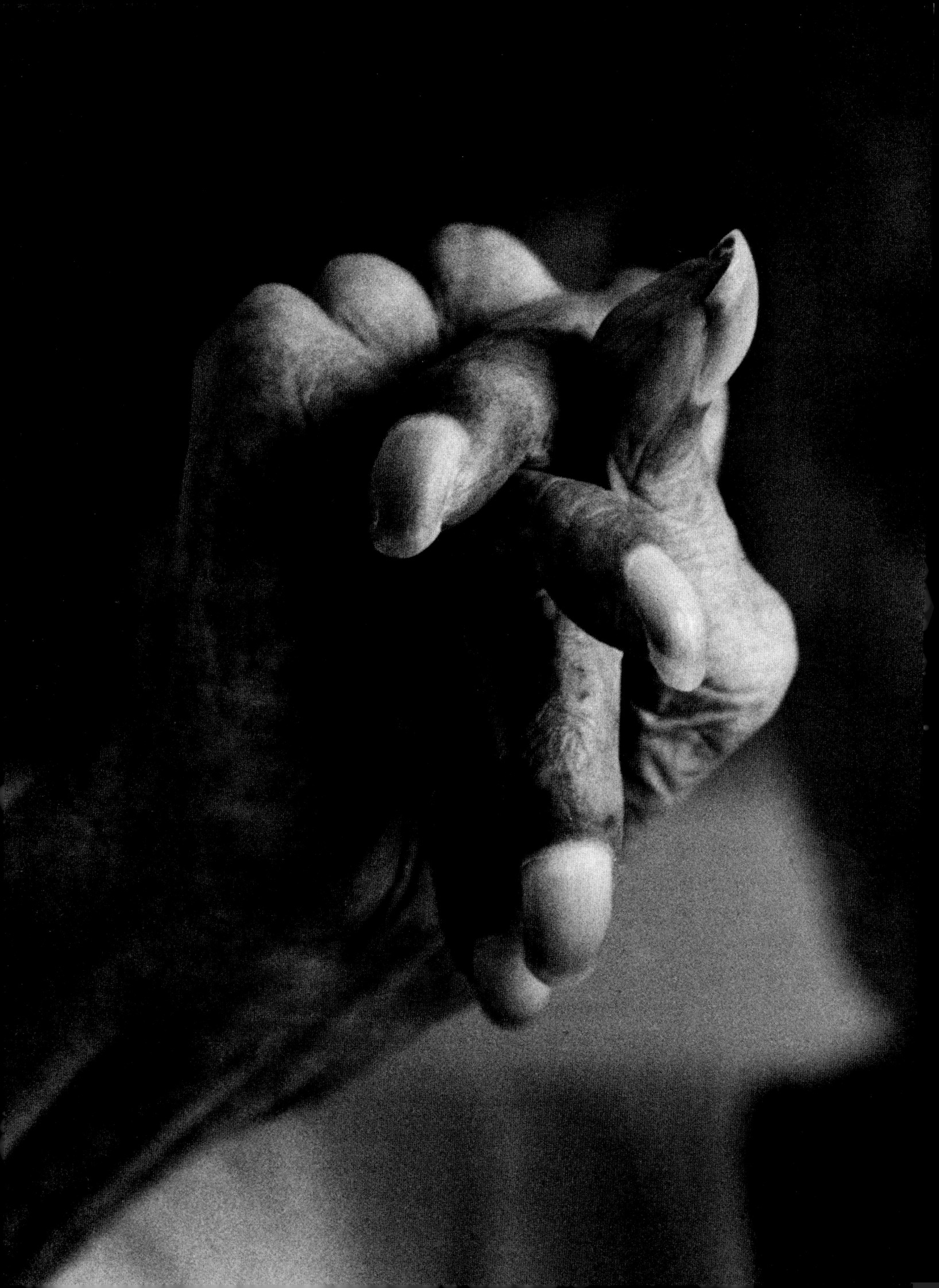

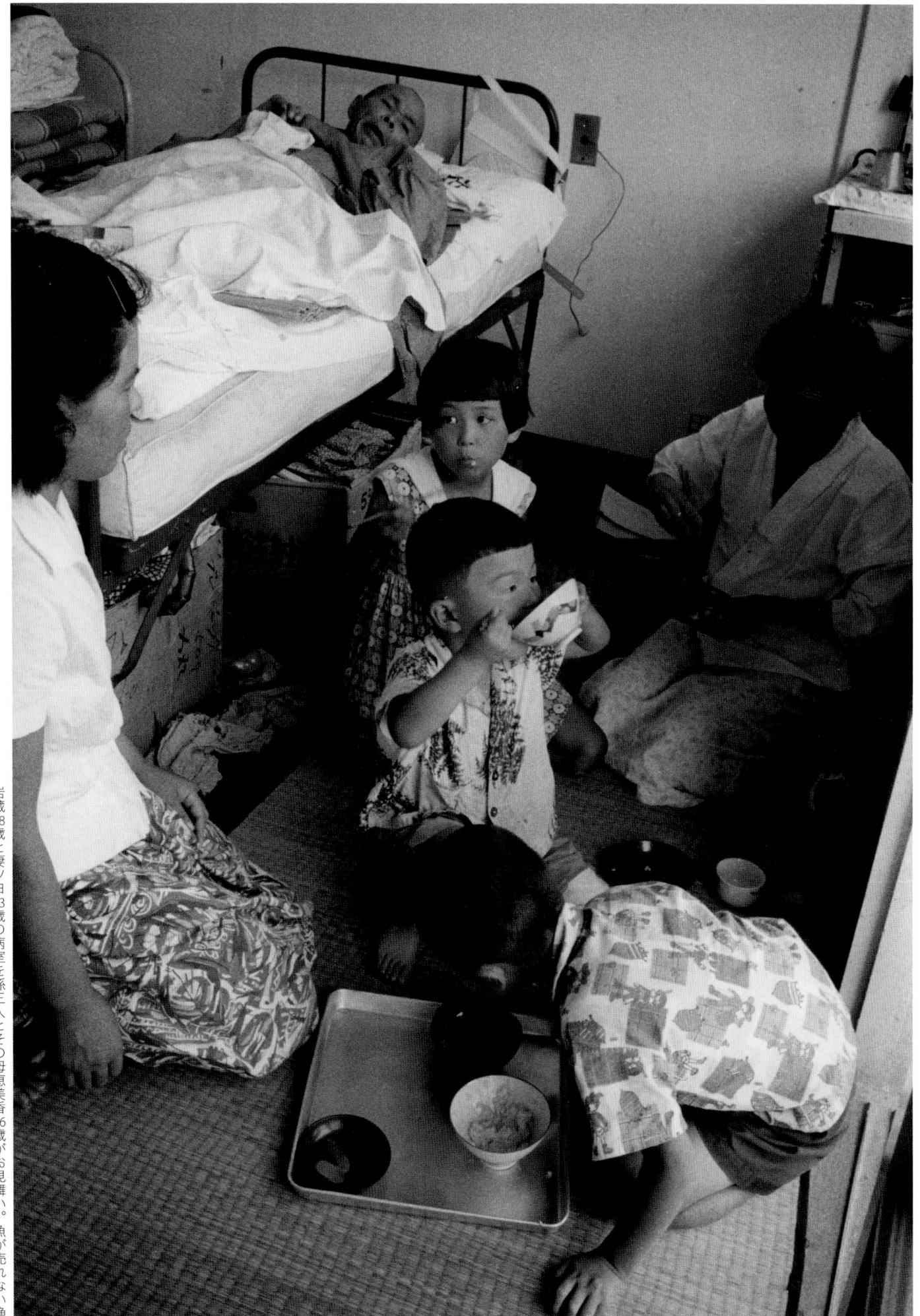

岩蔵68歳と妻ツヨ63歳の病室を孫三人とその母恵美香26歳がお見舞い。魚が売れない漁家には米の病院食はごちそうだった　専用病棟　一九六〇年八月

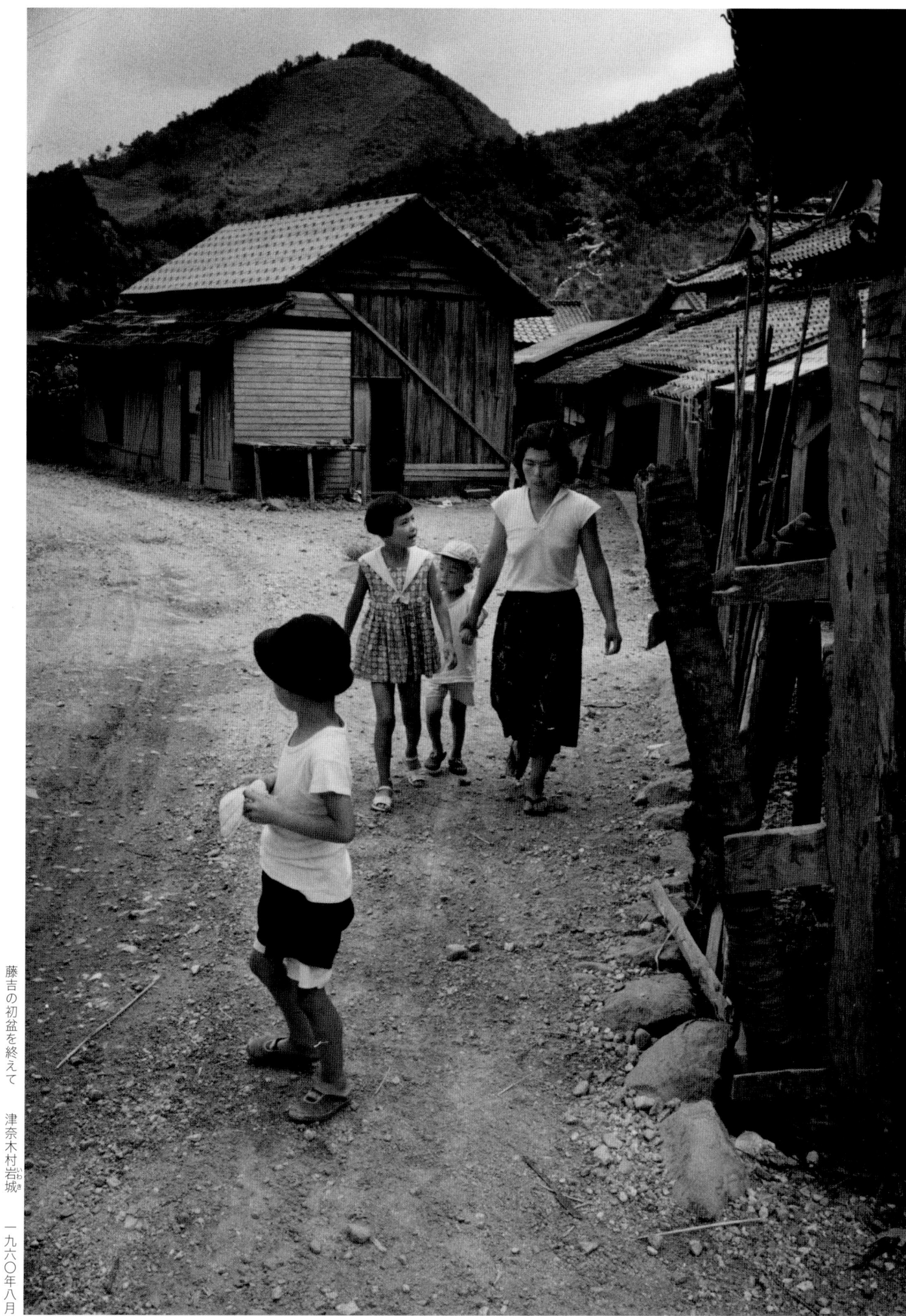

藤吉の初盆を終えて　津奈木村岩城(いわき)　一九六〇年八月

私の水俣病事件

教育と水俣病

広瀬 武

水俣病との出会い

一九六八年一月、水俣に初めて患者支援を目的とし物議を醸した。「水俣病対策市民会議」が結成され、私はそこに会員として名前を連ねた。このときから私の水俣病は始まった、と思っている。

「とうちゃんは水俣病でした」

市民会議が結成されたそのころ、新潟水俣病の患者が来水し、地元患者との交流会がもたれ、私もその会に参加したのだが、会場に中村シメさんの姿があった。中村さんから、「先生、とうちゃんは水俣病でしたもん」と告白され、私は中村さん一家が水俣病患者家庭であることを、初めて知ったのである。

娘の由美子さんを、四年生で担任していたのだが、中村さん一家は経済的に困窮していて、教材費等の納入がいつも滞っていた。私はその原因が、父親の水俣病に起因していることを知ることもなく、由美子さんに毎日どんな思いで学校生活を送っていたのか、由美子さんに思いを寄せず、「早く持って来てね」と集金を督促していたのである。今、改めて教師の罪深さを反省している。

患者を教室によぶ

山間部にある葛渡小学校で五年生を担任して、社会科「日本の工業」で水俣病を教材化した。一九七一年二月、患者の浜元二徳さんが教室に来て、自分の水俣病を語ってくれた。

この授業は朝日新聞が記事にしたので、いろいろと物議を醸した。患者を教室によぶのは生々しく行き過ぎ、裁判中であり原告を教室に入れるのは誤解を招く、といった意見が相次いで出たし、市議会ではチッソこどもたちは水俣病学習の経験は殆どなかった。多発出身の議員が授業は偏向と批判した。チッソ城下町意識の強い水俣では、水俣病をタブー視する傾向がまだ強く残っていた。

教師からも差別された

一九五六年、田中義光さん一家は三女静子、四女実子と相次いで発病した。姉妹の発病で一家は極貧に追い込まれていた。

父親の義光さんがまだ存命のころ、私はしばしば田中家を訪問して聞き書きをしていた。そのなかで「教師が差別をした」という話がある。「うちどんげ貧乏なところには、学校の先生は、いっちょんかもてくれらっさんじゃった」という言葉が、今でも私の胸につきささって離れない。

発病した娘二人の看護で母親のアサヲさんは家を留守にしていたので、長女（当時六年生）が母親代わりに、一家の切り盛りをしなければならなかった。朝から炊事や洗濯、食事の後片付けをしてから登校するので、どうしても遅刻が多くなってしまう。

学校では教師が遅刻の理由を深く問い糺すこともせず、校庭や廊下に立たせたりして罰を与えていた。こどもたちは誰ひとり一緒に遊んでくれない。それに対して教師は指導の手だてをしなかったという。まさに、教師は差別者であった。

袋校区は水俣病が最も多発している。私が赴任した七二年当時、二年から七年間勤務した。私が赴任した七二年当時、こどもたちは水俣病学習の経験は殆どなかった。多発地区であるが故に、教師も水俣病をとり上げて授業することは難しかった。

寝た子を起こす

七三年三月、水俣病一次訴訟の判決が出て、原告（患者）が勝訴した。これが契機となって袋地区でも認定申請者が増加した。

学校でも水俣病授業に取り組みやすくなっていった。熊本県教組が呼びかけた水俣病一斉授業も、県下各地で広がっていった。今では熊本県が行政として全県下の小学生に公害教育の授業をさせ、五年生を対象に水俣病資料館で語り部の話を聞かせるなどしている。私が一九七〇年代に参加した水俣芦北公害研究サークルの活動が認知された結果である。

私たち地元市民が水俣病問題に気づくよりはるかに早い時期に桑原さんが水俣病に取り組んだことを知って驚くとともに、彼の最初の写真集を私は授業で子供たちにも見せた。その本には私の義母日吉フミコの蔵書との書き込みがある。それを借りて授業したのだった。水俣からほとんど出たことがない私は、桑原さんの故郷の津和野になぜか三回ほど行ったことがある。別の用事があって津和野の桑原写真美術館には行く時間がなかった。津和野が好きになったので、今度こそ行って桑原作品に会いたいと思っている。

（ひろせ・たけし／元小学校教諭・水俣芦北地区退職教職員協議会役員）

6 奇病発見のきっかけとなった船大工一家

一九五六年四月、田中義光とアサヲは、箸も手にできなくなった5歳の三女しず子を新日窒付属病院へ担ぎ込んだ。2歳の四女実子も続いて発病。細川一院長らは、月浦坪谷へ調査に出て、小児の類似患者を発見、五月一日保健所へ届ける。後に水俣病の公式発見の日となった。

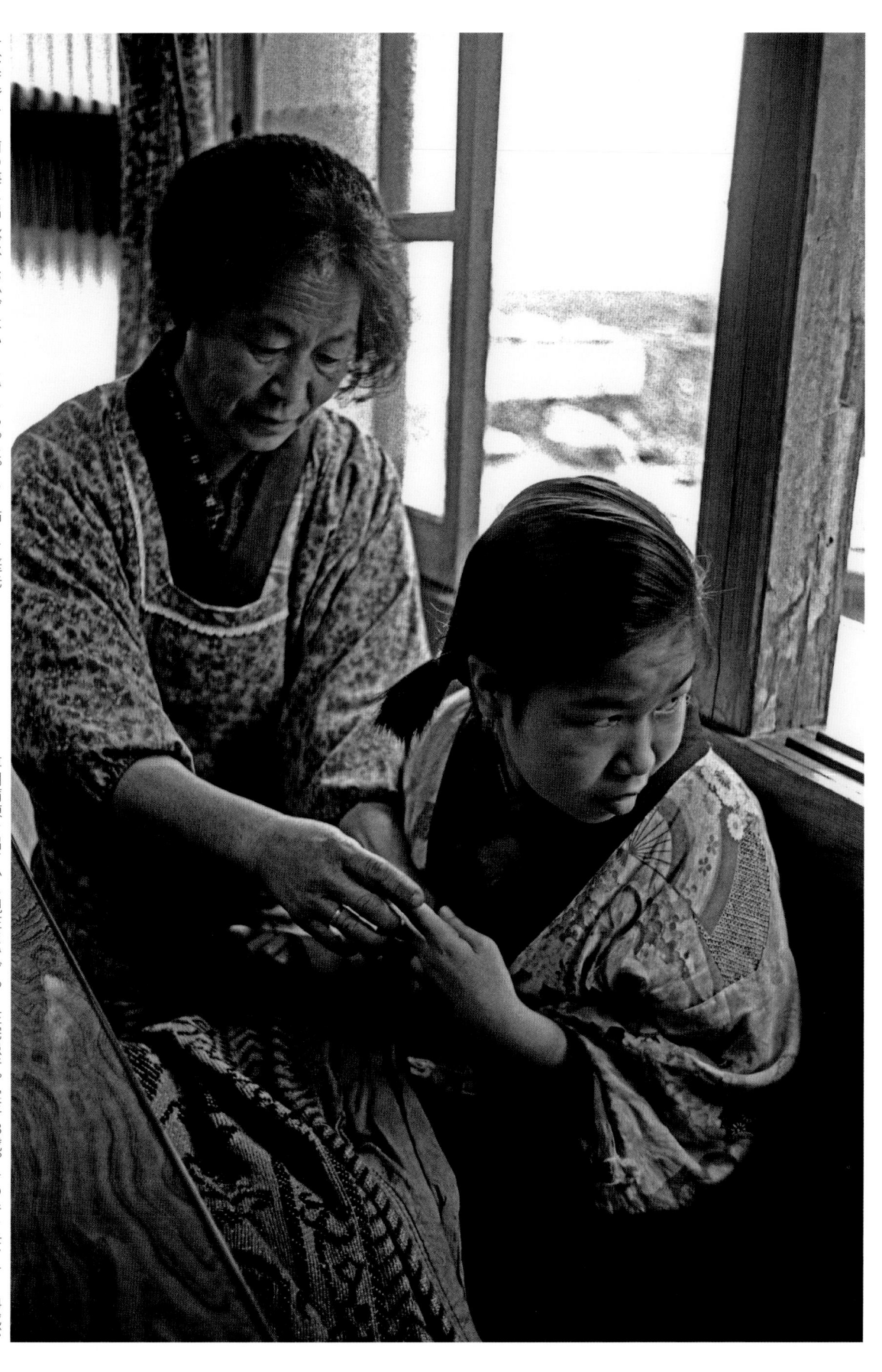

← (次頁) すぐ前の海に出れば、おかずはいくらでもあった。もう怖くて庭先漁業はできない
自宅 一九六〇年七月

専用病棟を出てから現在までずっと在宅患者。実子13歳。その手を母アサヲ44歳がもみほぐす
自宅 一九六六年一〇月

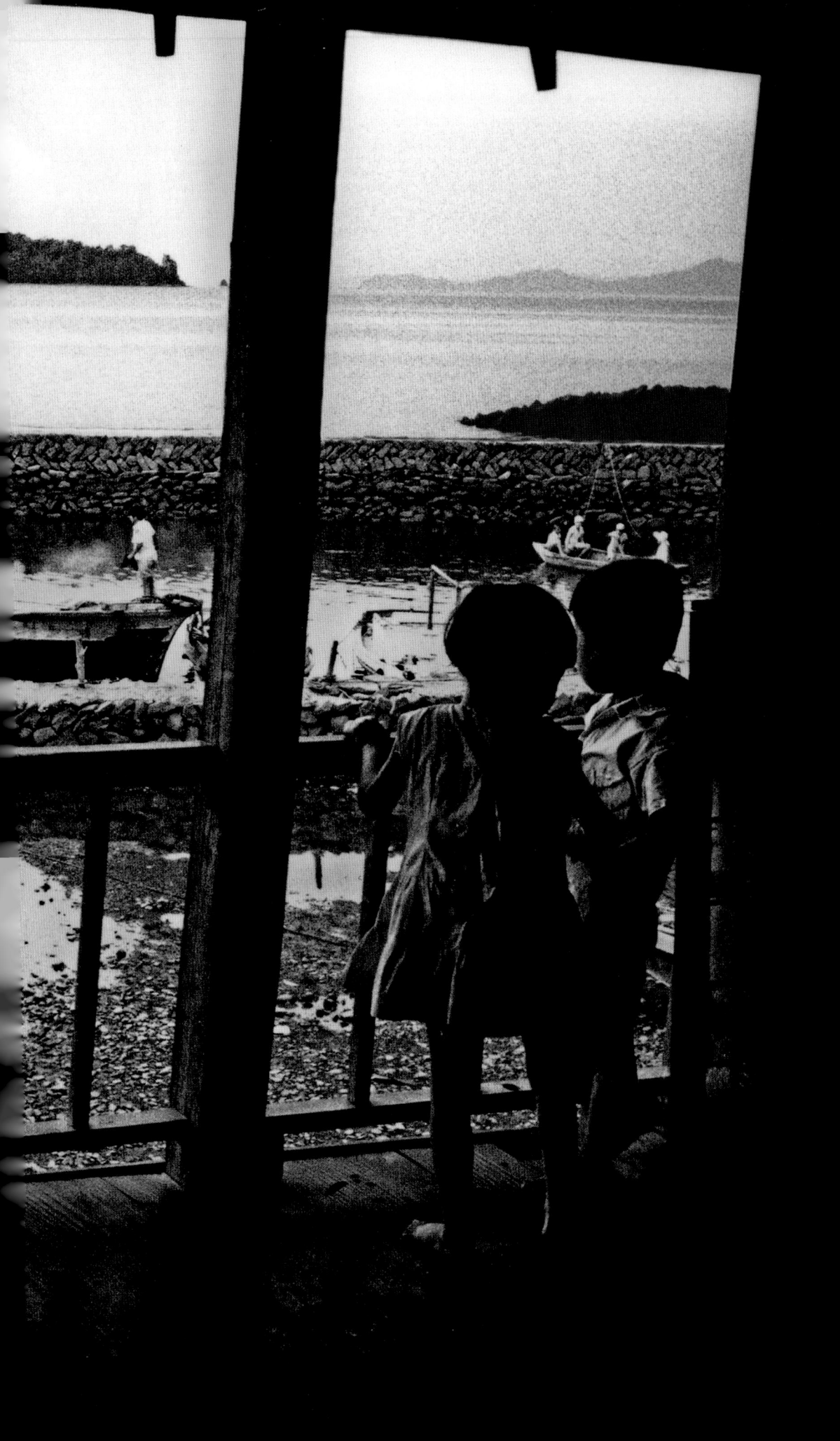

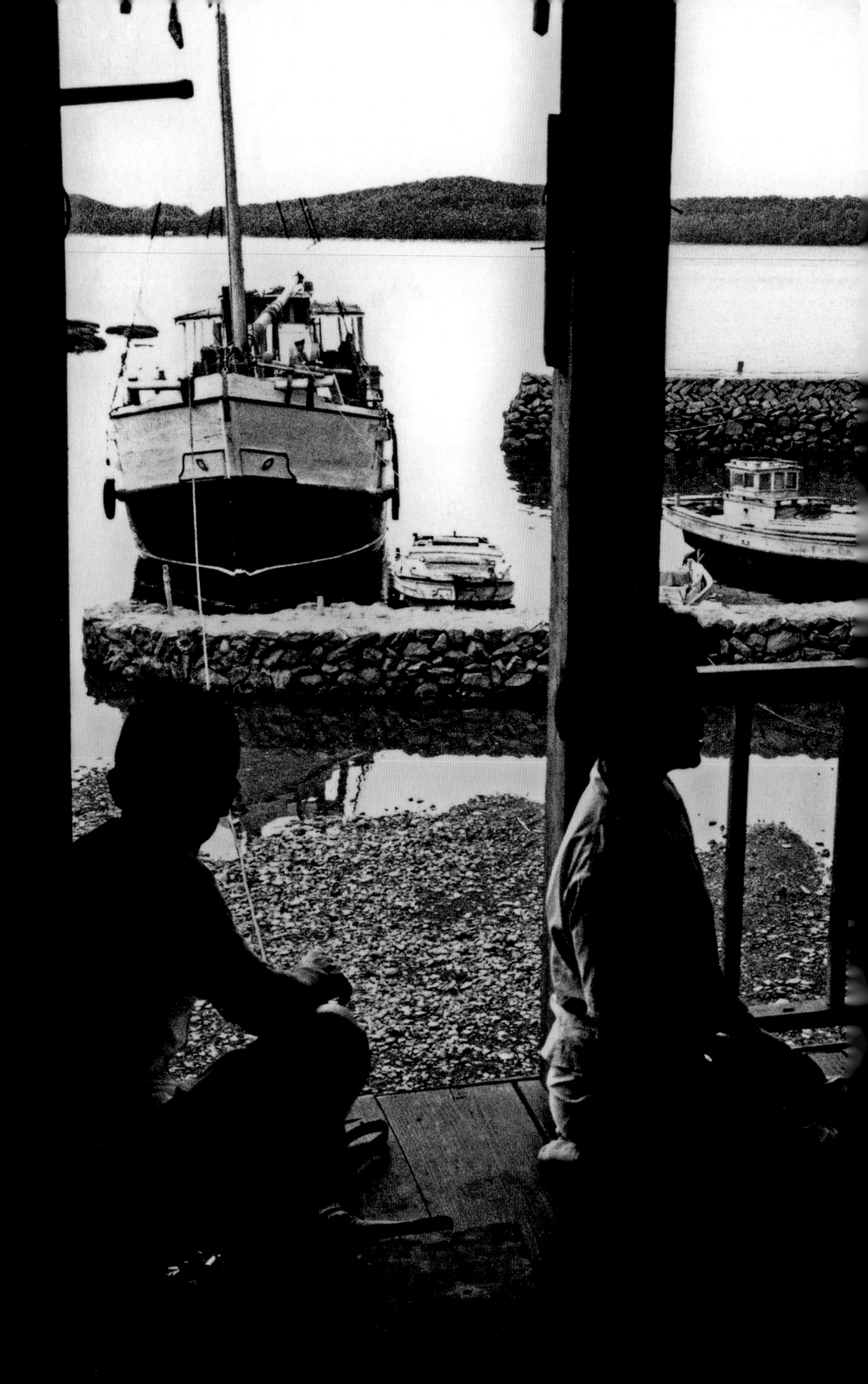

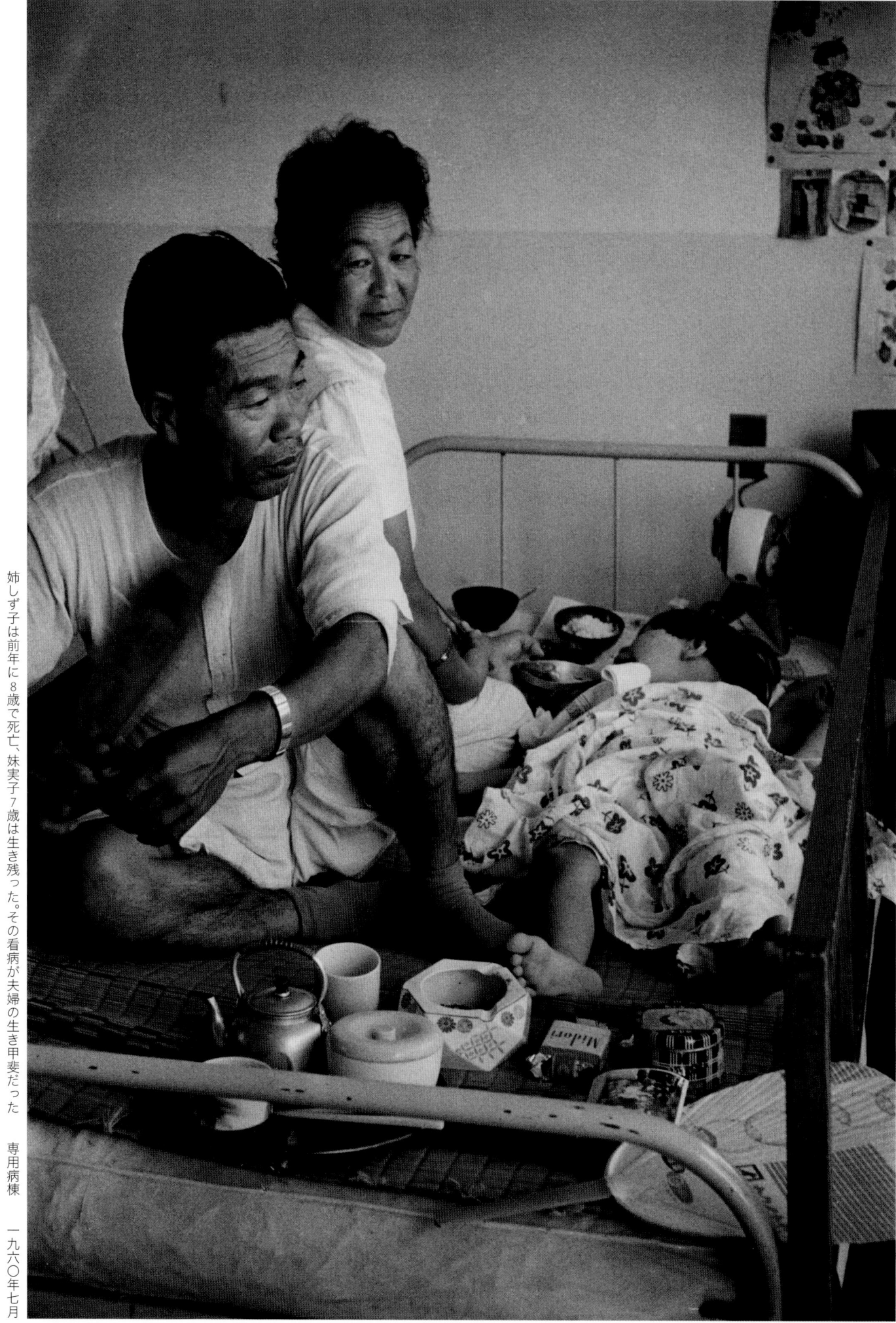

姉しず子は前年に8歳で死亡、妹実子7歳は生き残った。その看病が夫婦の生き甲斐だった　専用病棟　一九六〇年七月

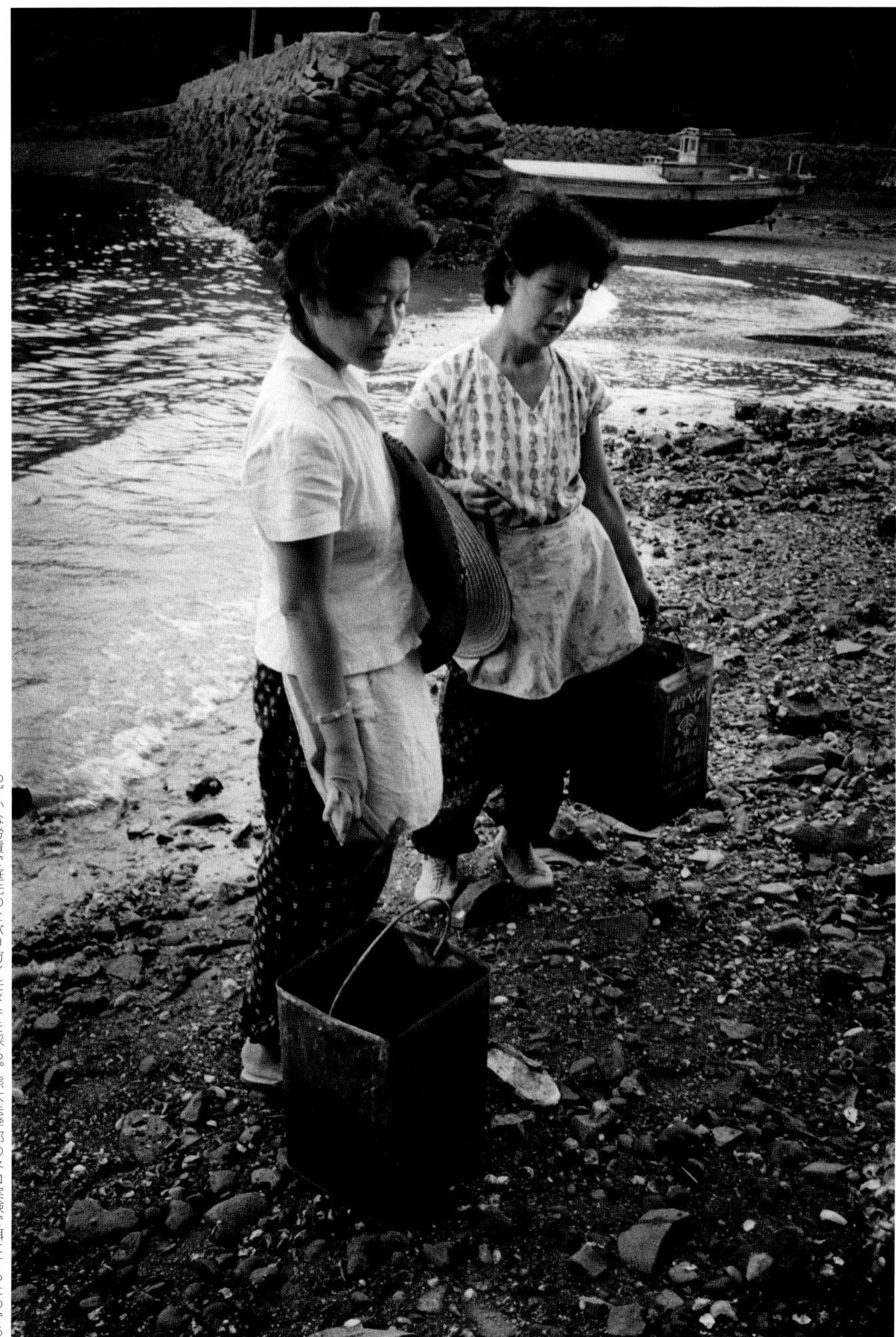

わずかな労賃で庭先のヒバリガイモドキを採る。熊大医学部のネコ実験で餌にするためである

月浦坪谷の波戸　一九六〇年七月

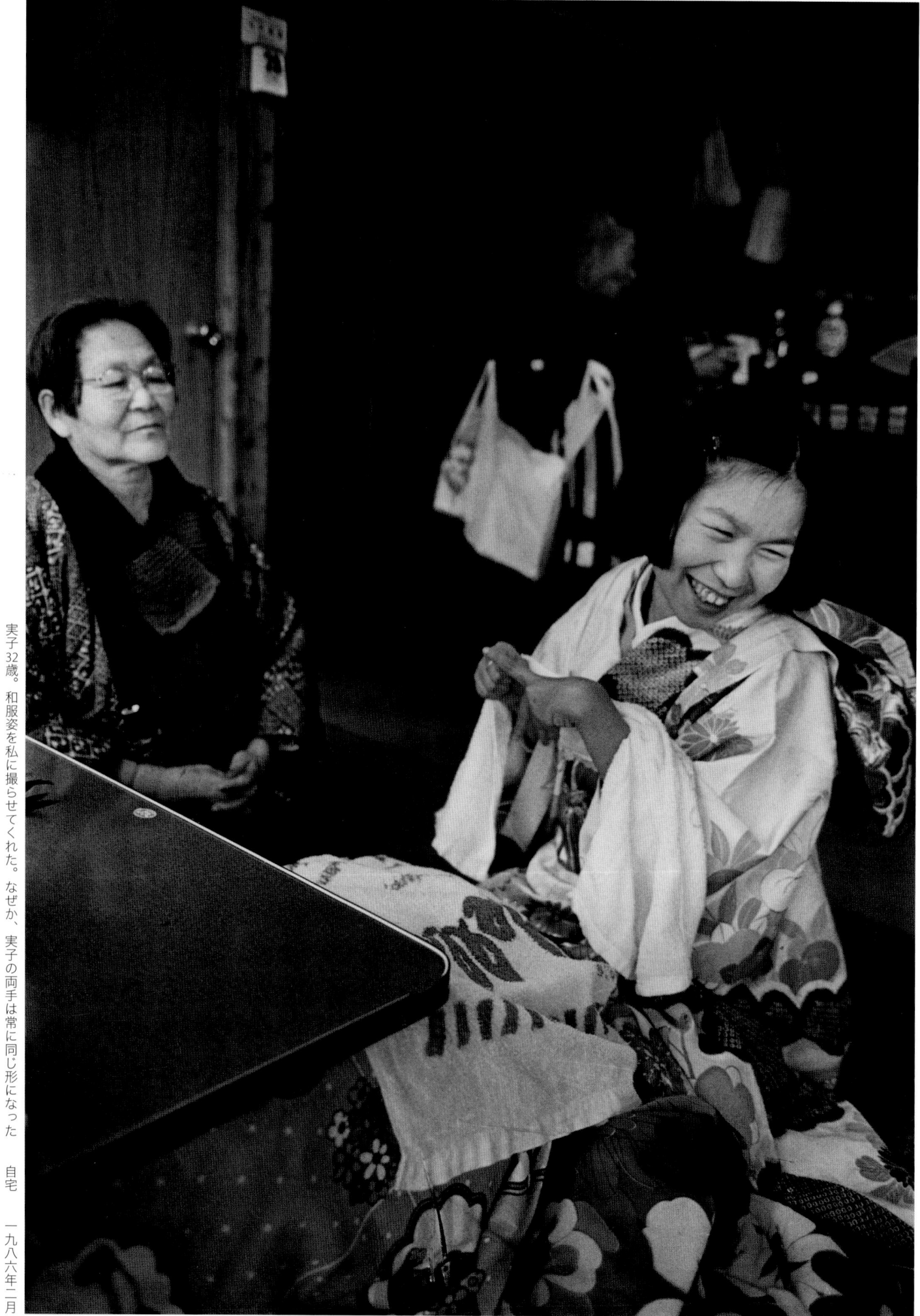

実子32歳。和服姿を私に撮らせてくれた。なぜか、実子の両手は常に同じ形になった 自宅 一九八六年二月

（次頁）実子が歩くとき姉綾子42歳が抱きついて支えた　自宅前の波戸　一九八六年二月

実子の和服姿を見た翌年に、父義光は76歳で、母アサヲは69歳で死亡　自宅　一九八六年二月

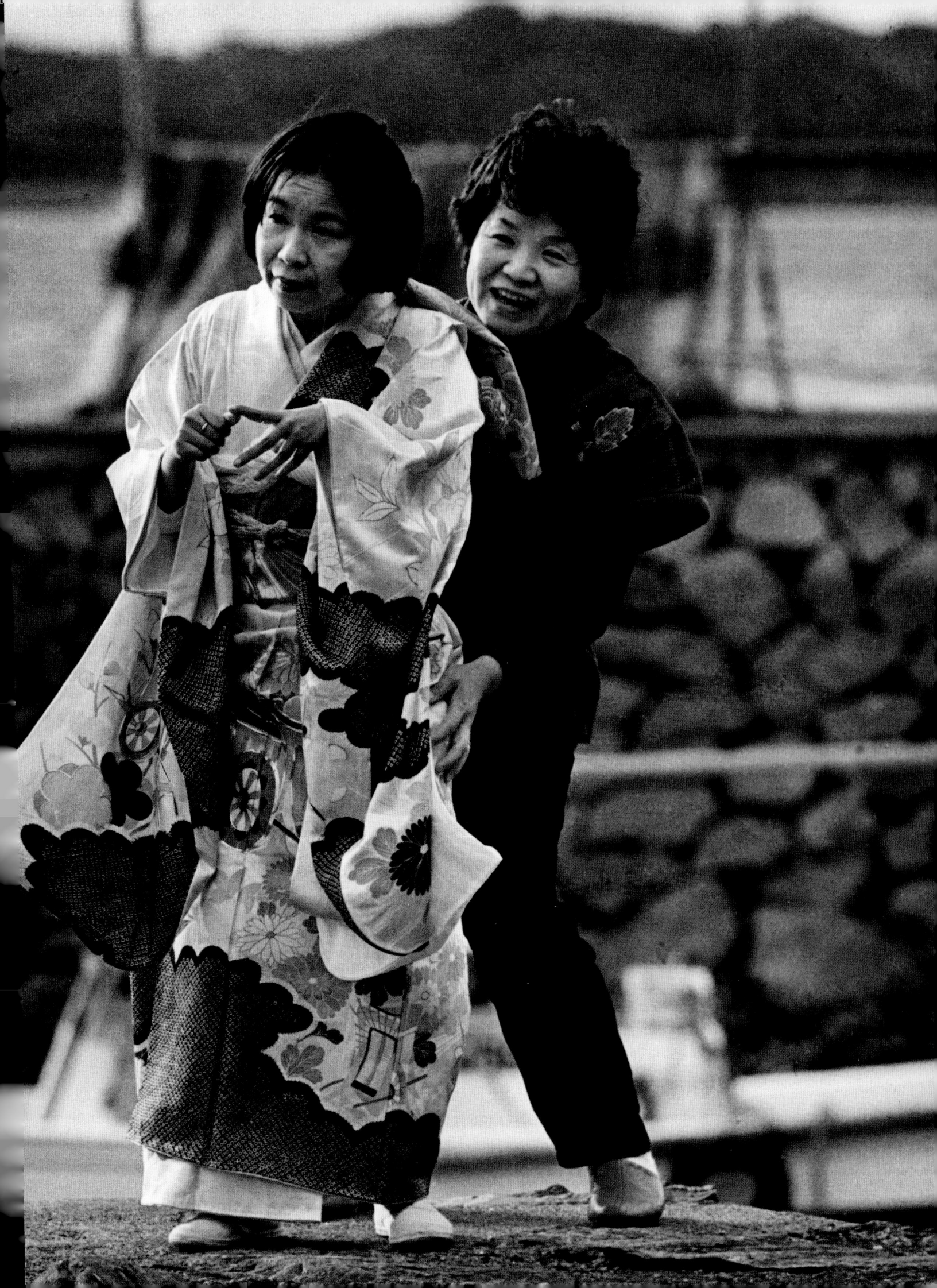

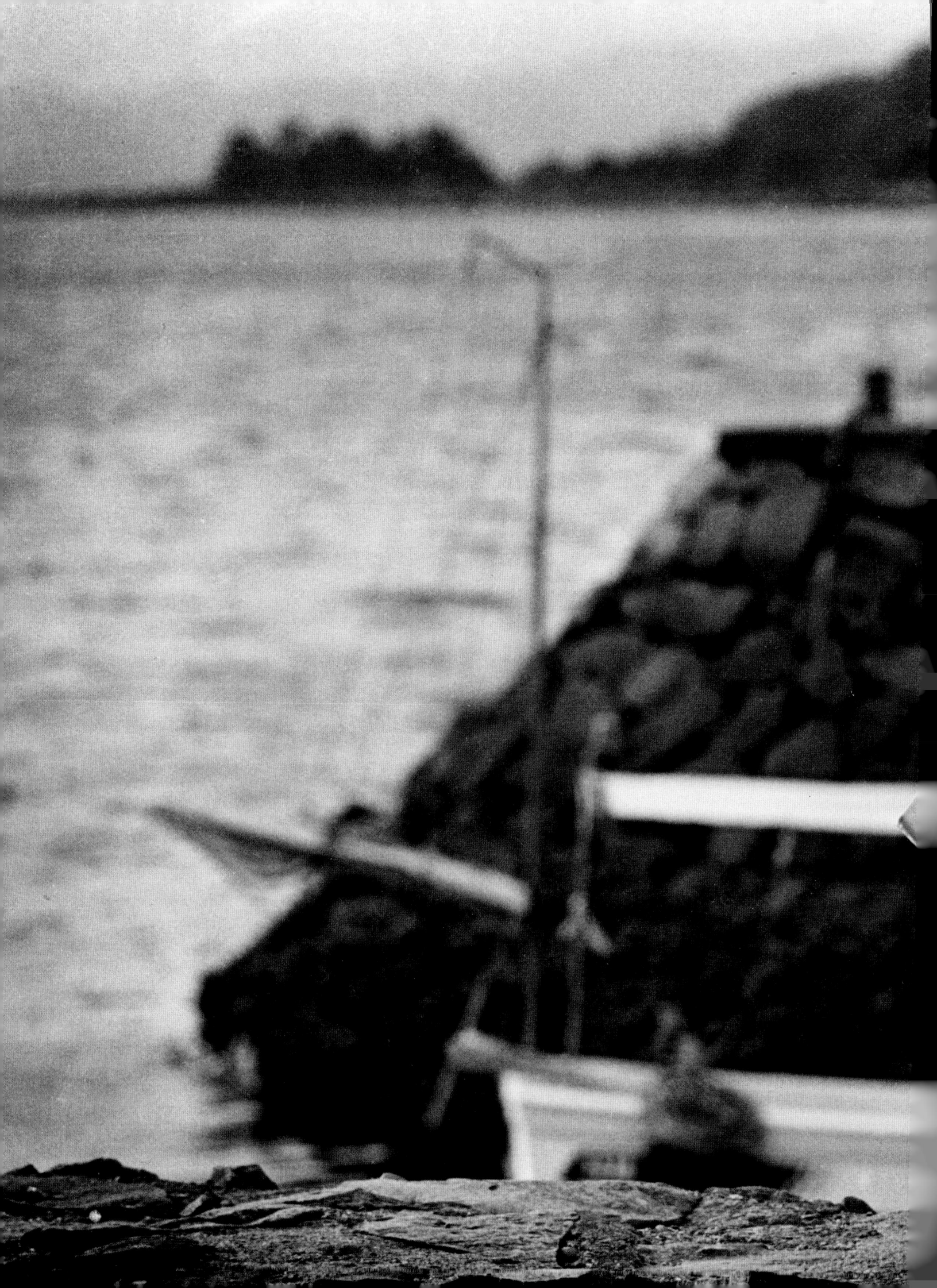

7 中村荒蔵網

水俣の町から離れた集落、袋茂道には、四軒の網元があった。中村荒蔵の網は、ボラ漁で知られた。私はしばしば、荒蔵網の好意を受けた。水俣病禍で漁ができないときでも、漁獲風景を撮れるようにと船を出してくれた。集落全域が受難地である。

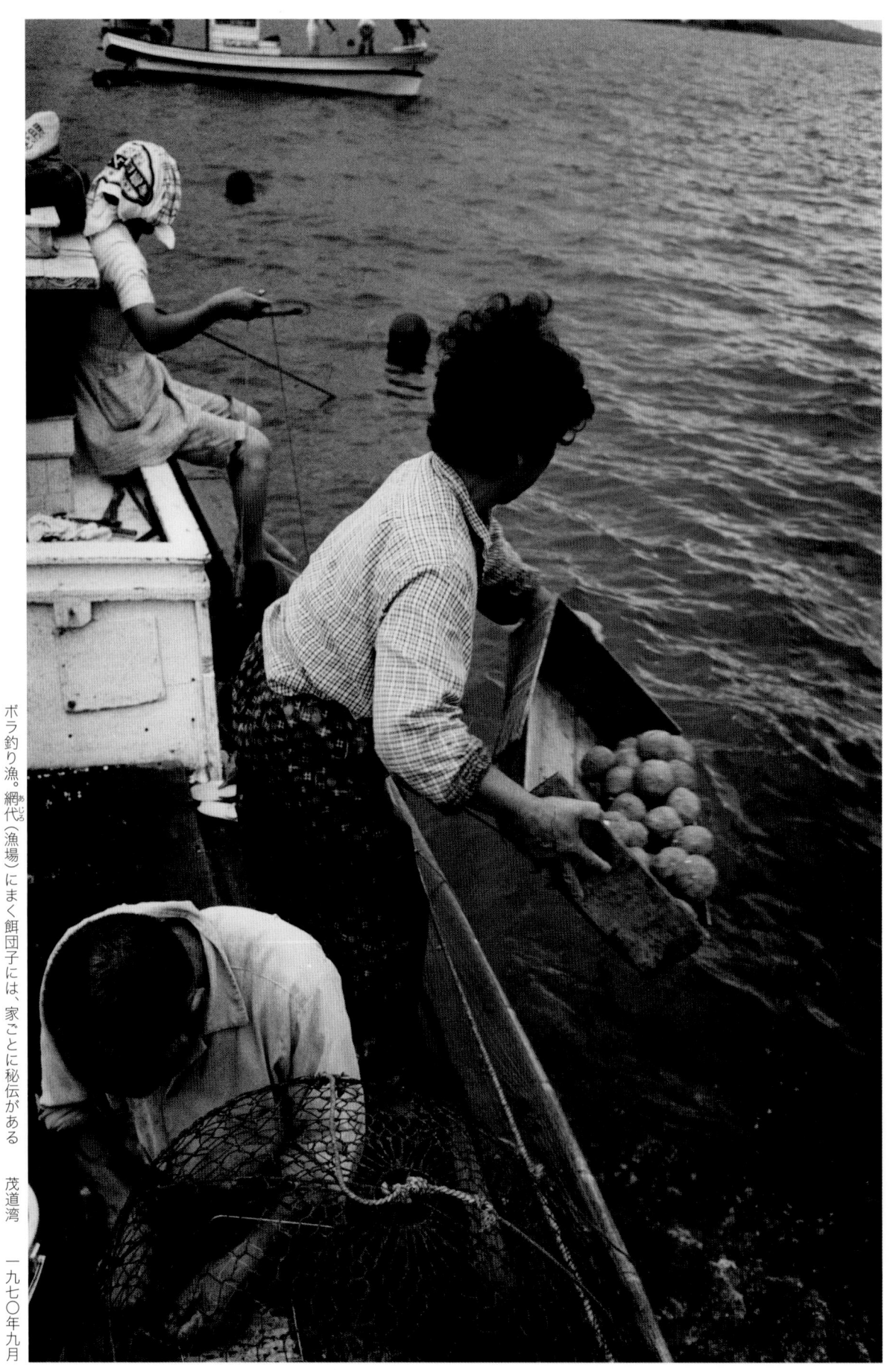

ボラ釣り漁。網代（漁場）にまく餌団子には、家ごとに秘伝がある　茂道湾　一九七〇年九月

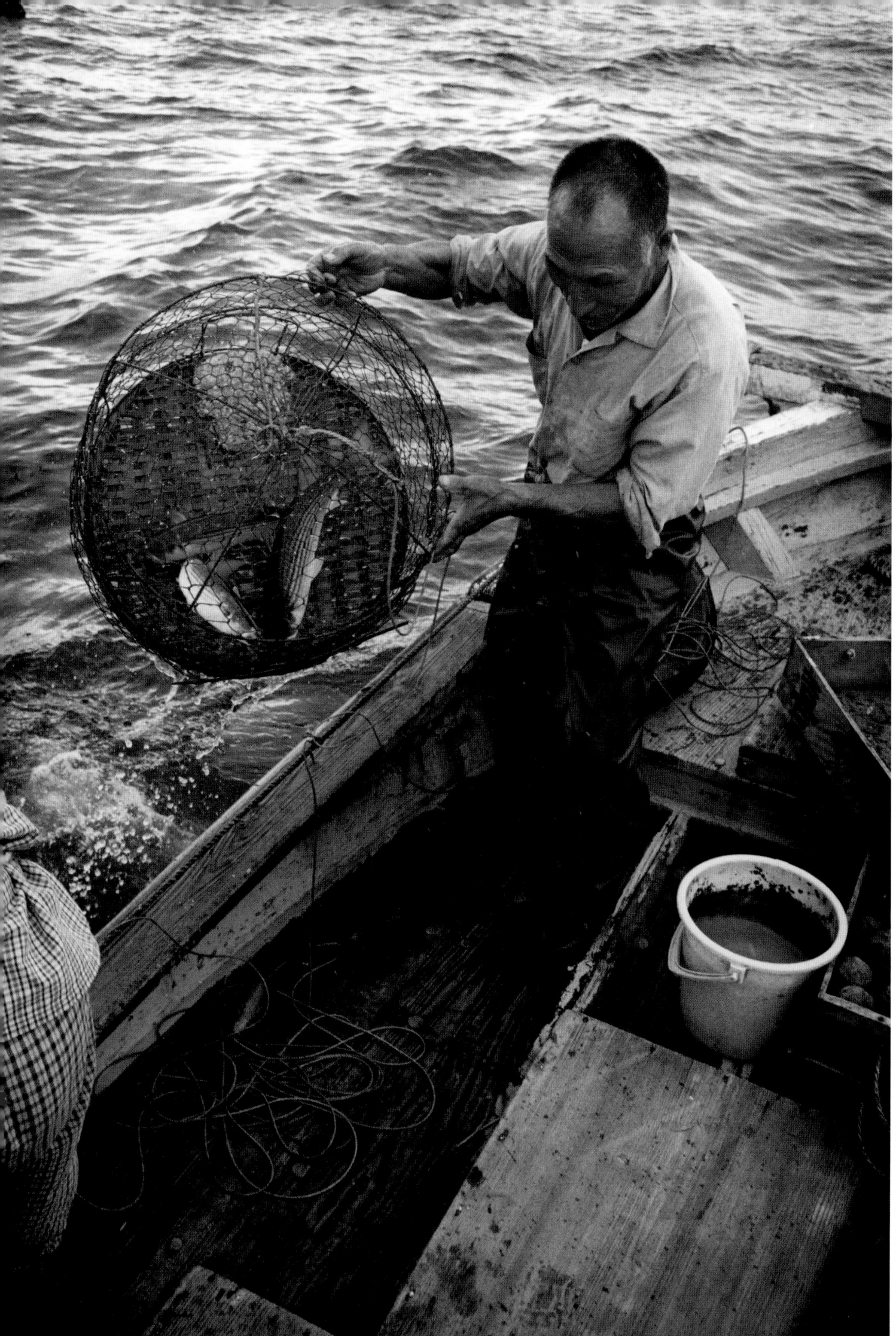

ボラ籠漁の荒蔵58歳。籠に光るのがボラ　茂道湾　一九七〇年九月

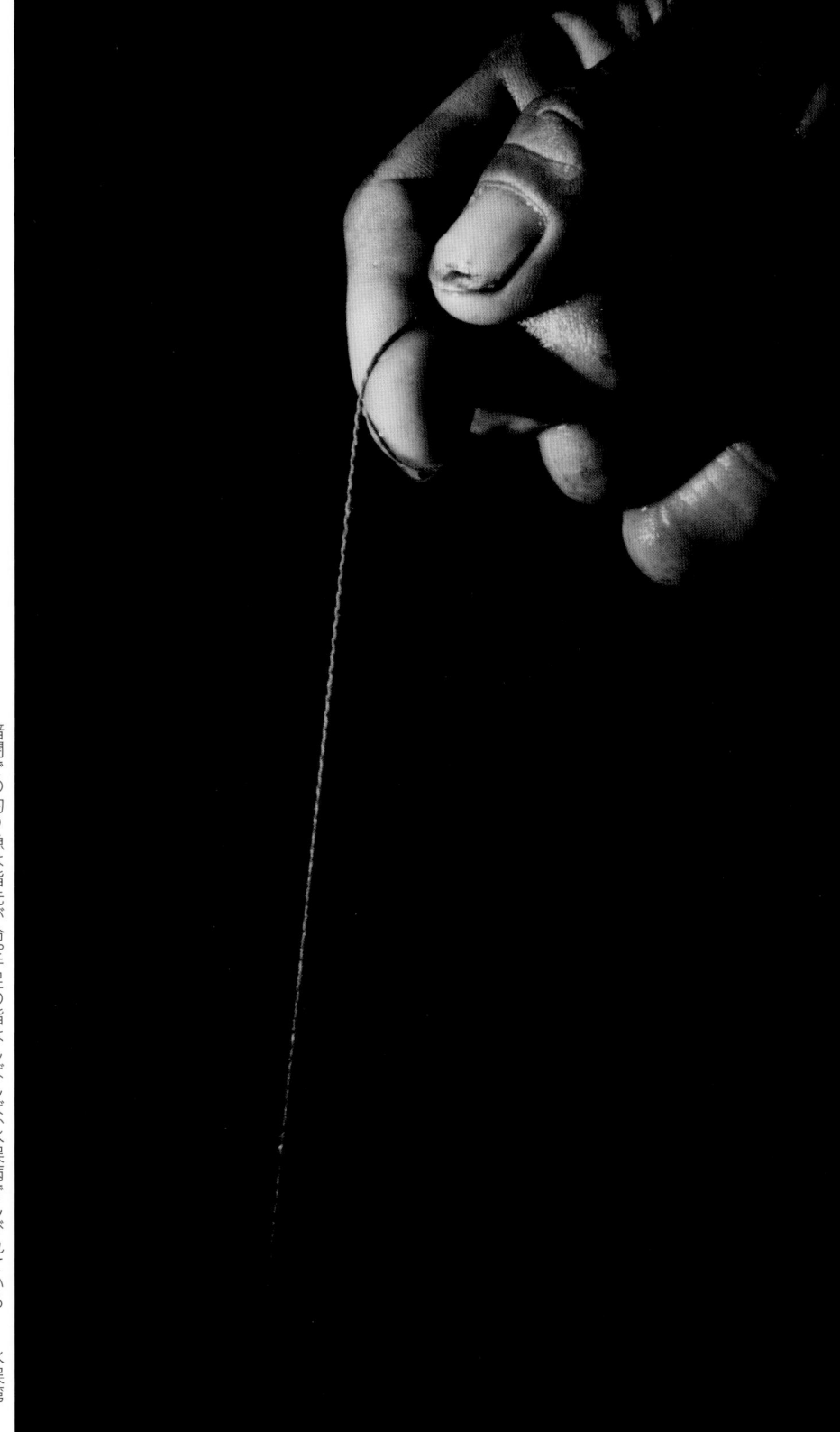

暗闇での釣り漁は指先が命。手足の指はしばしば、水俣病でしびれている　水俣湾　一九六二年八月

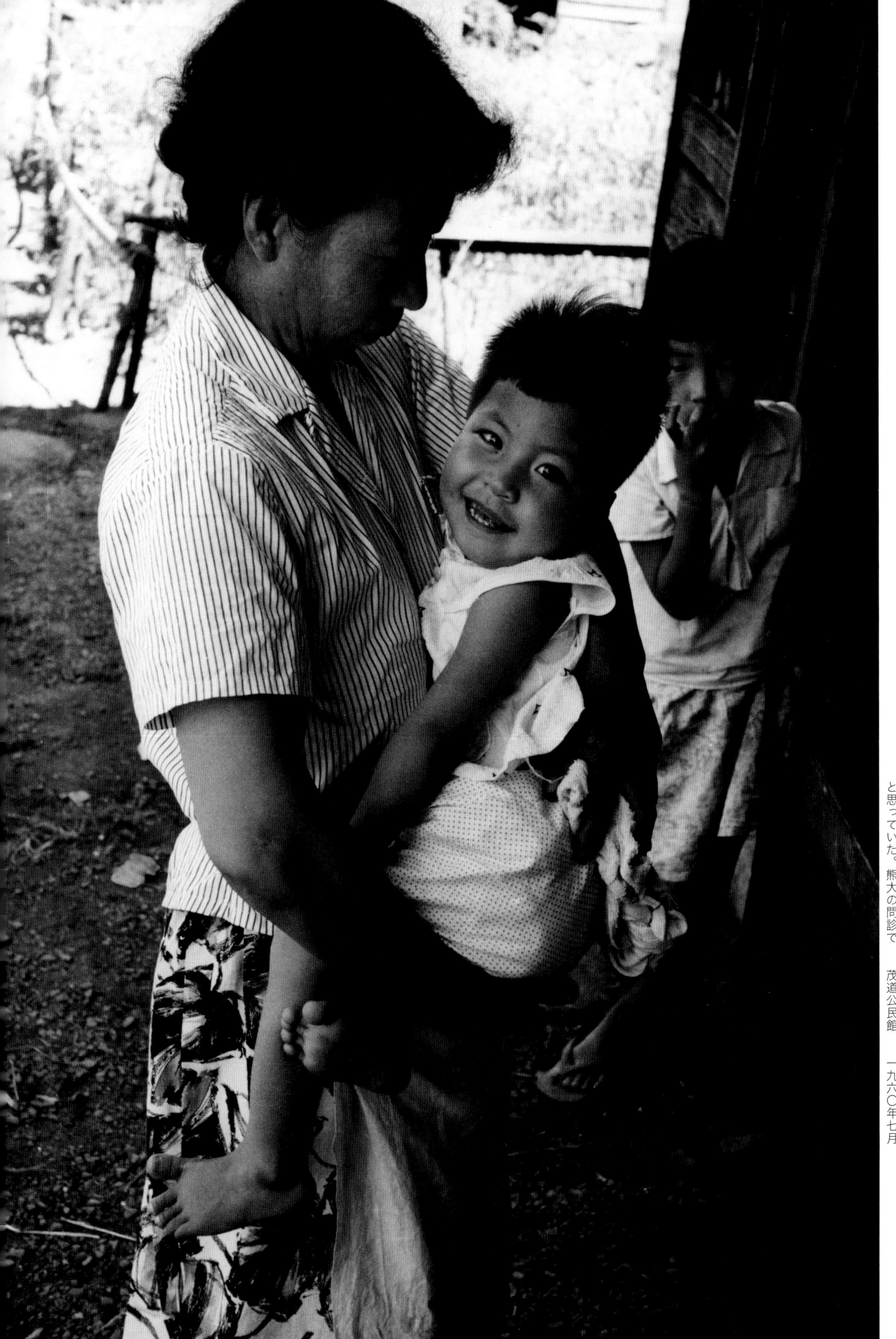

荒蔵48歳とアヤ子44歳の三女千鶴3歳。胎児性患者と認定される二年前だが、私は患者だと思っていた。熊大の問診で　茂道公民館　一九六〇年七月

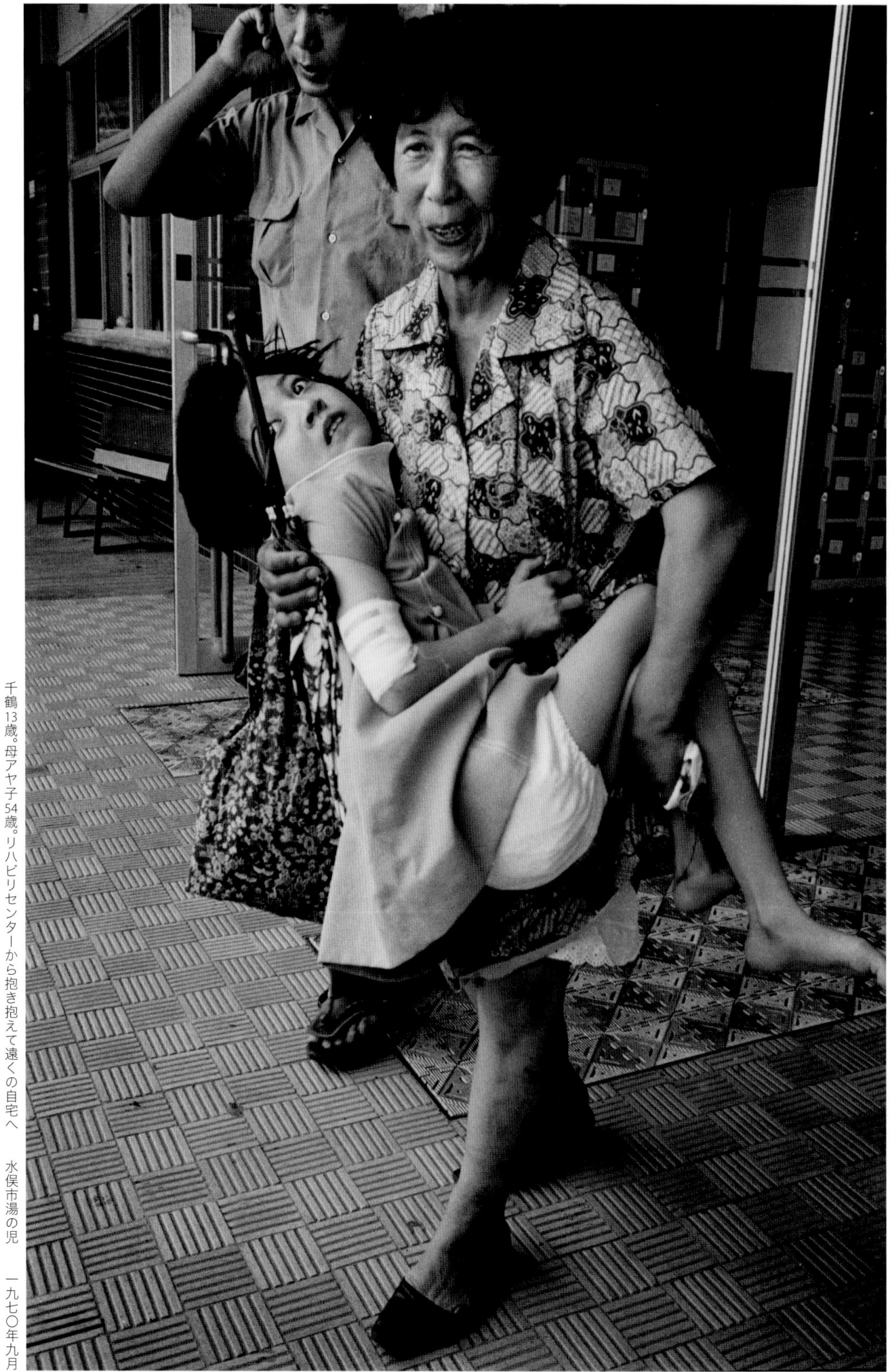

千鶴13歳。母アヤ子54歳。リハビリセンターから抱き抱えて遠くの自宅へ　水俣市湯の児　一九七〇年九月

8 役者をもしのぐ茂道の女網元

初めての女網元になった杉本栄子のよどみない弁舌は、平家琵琶の調べとともに聞きたい、と私は思った。丸出しの水俣弁、嗚咽と感嘆と怒りとを繰り出す語り部は、水俣事件を知らない都会の人たちをうならせた。水俣の人たちは手づくり衣装の田舎芝居も、踊りも、よく楽しんだ。二〇〇八年二月、69歳で没。

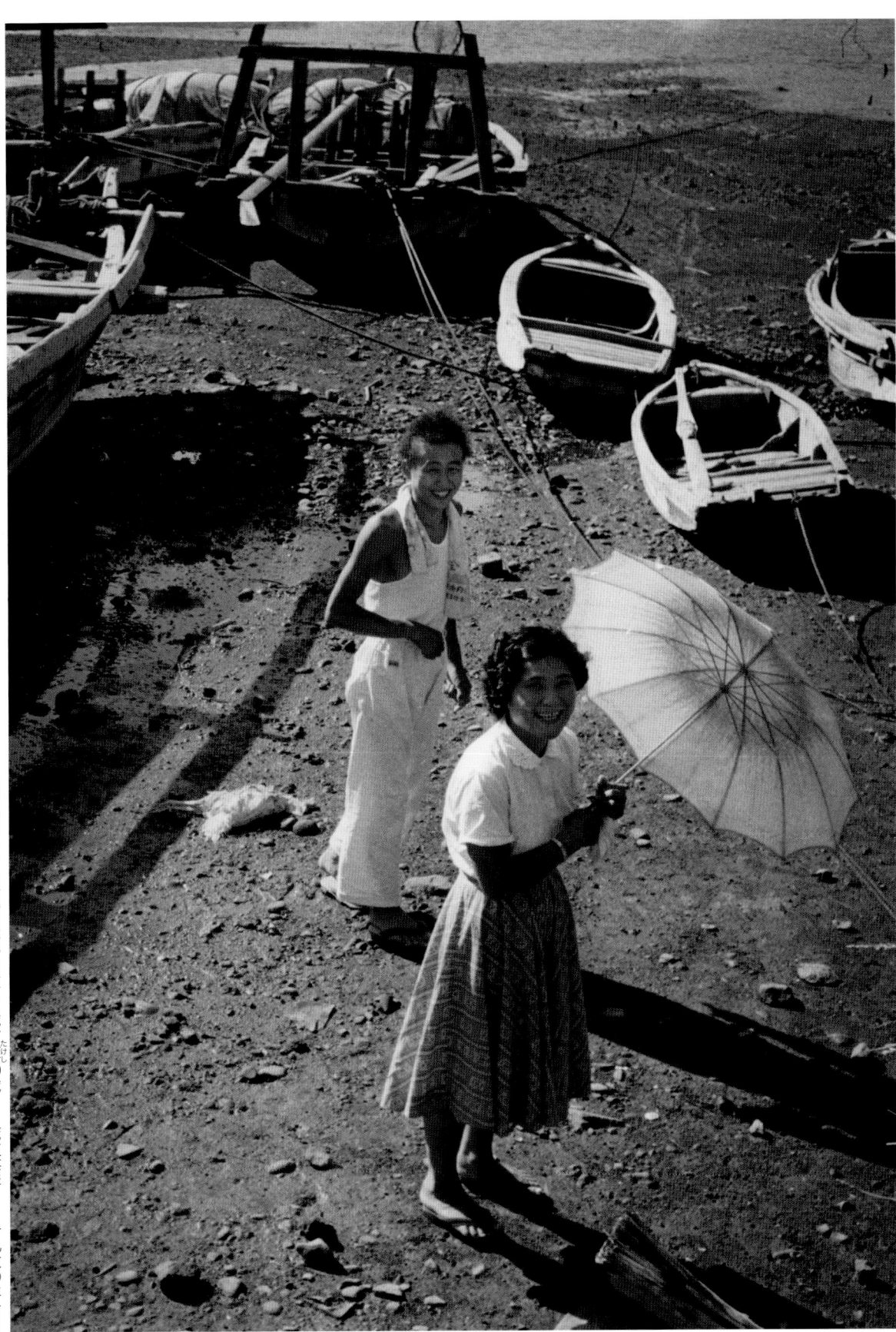

奇病禍の中での新婚生活。栄子21歳、雄20歳　茂道海岸　一九六〇年七月

櫓漕ぎも円熟して。栄子27歳　茂道湾　一九六六年五月

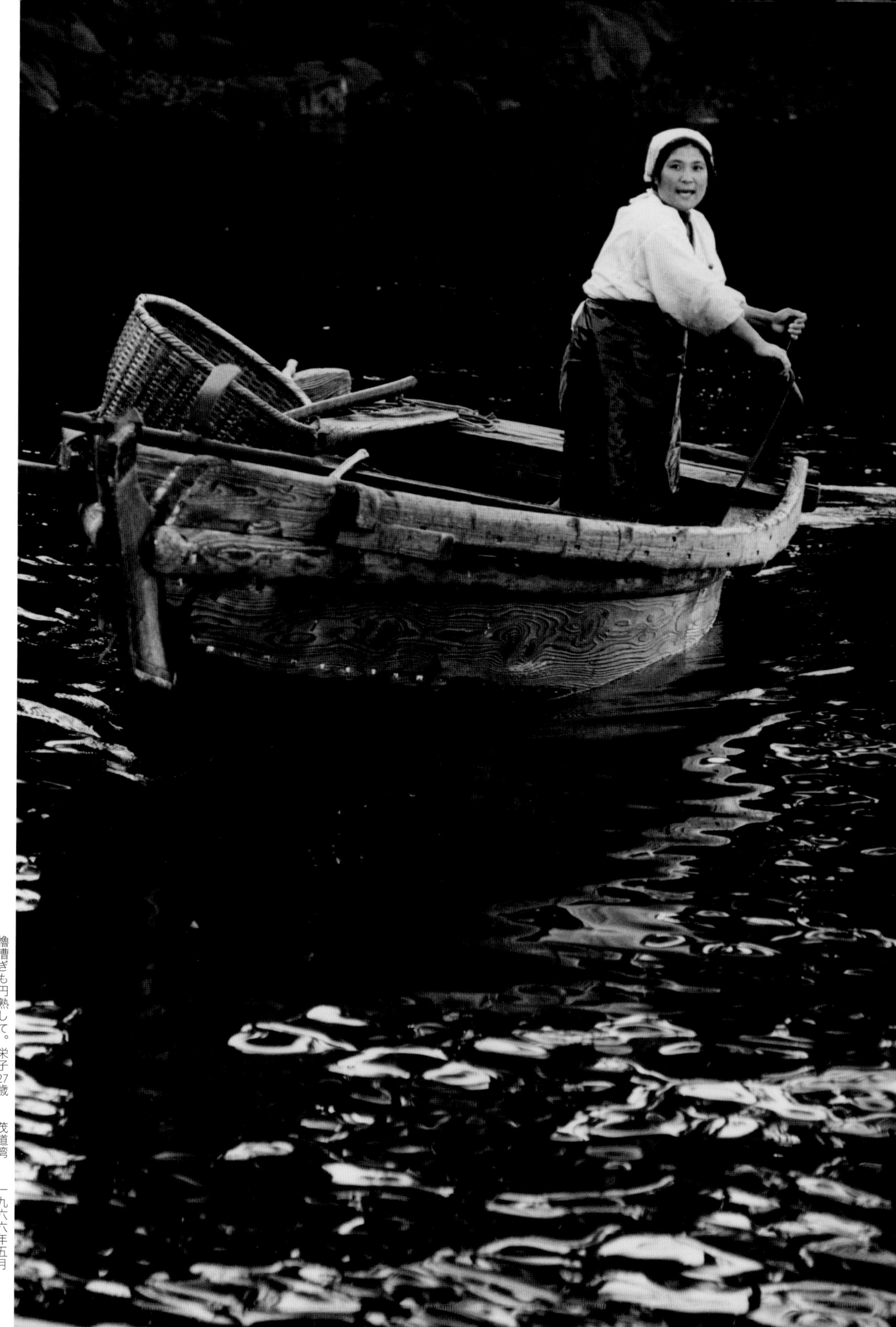

栄子を連れて母トシは網元の杉本進に嫁いだ。進は幼い栄子を女網元に育てた　自宅　一九六〇年八月

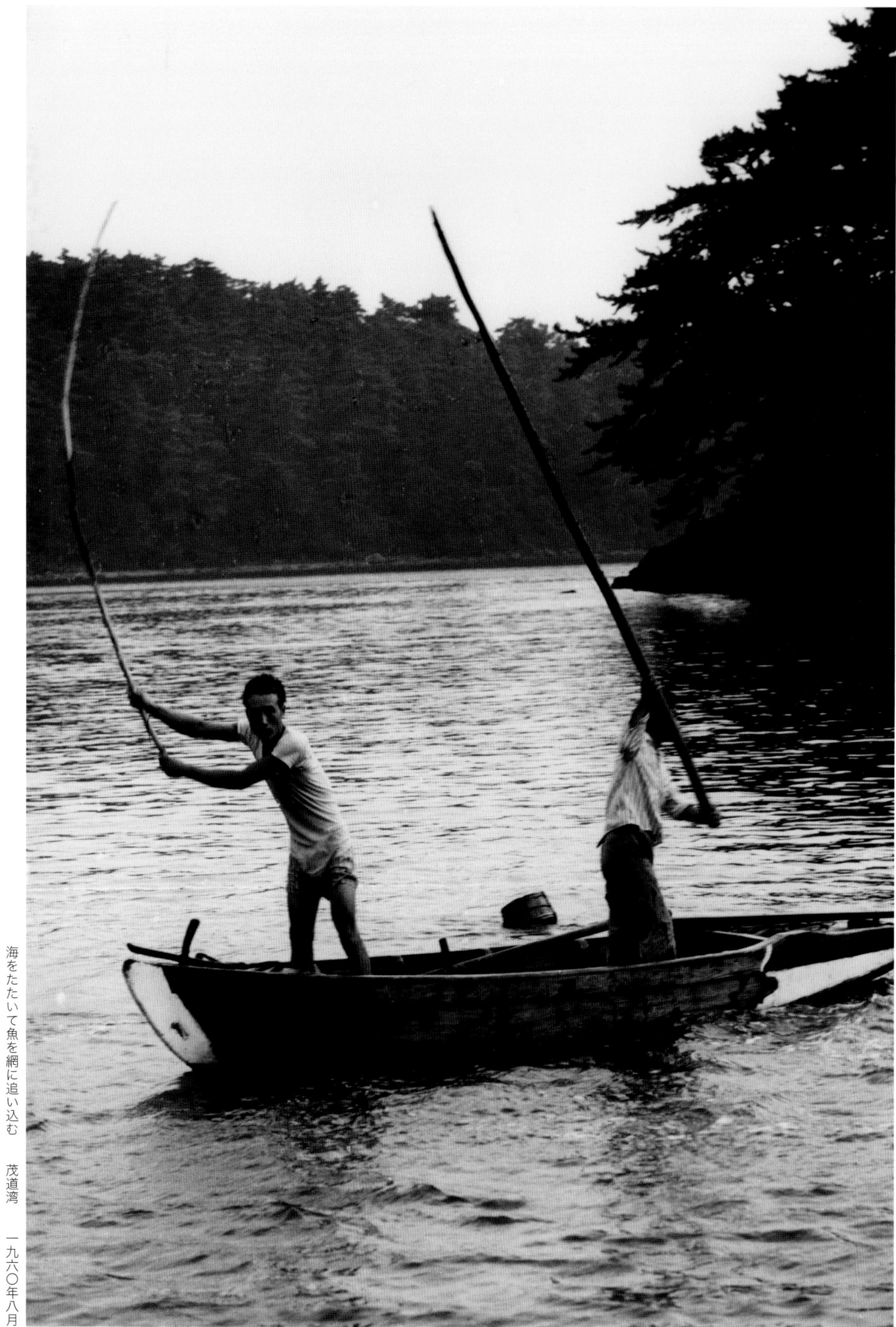

海をたたいて魚を網に追い込む　茂道湾　一九六〇年八月

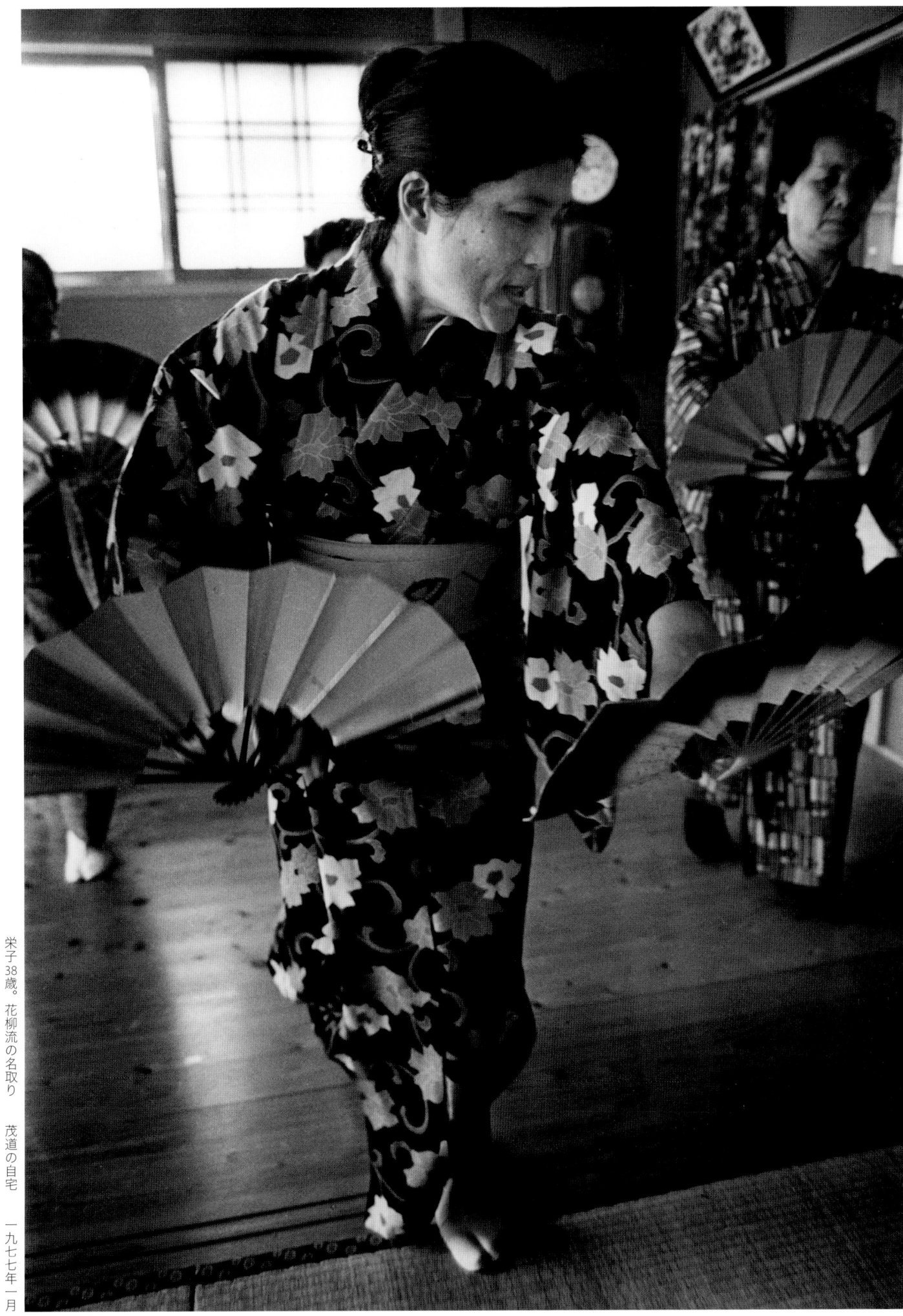

栄子38歳。花柳流の名取り　茂道の自宅　一九七七年一月

9 チッソ水俣工場

一九七〇年代に生産転換と工場縮小がすすみ、現在はJNC水俣製造所。液晶材料の生産などが主力となった。戦後の最大従業員約五〇〇〇人が一桁減った。旧プラントは撤去され、風景は一変した。水俣病を起こした水銀排水を流したとされたのは、一九三二年から一九六八年までの長期にわたった。

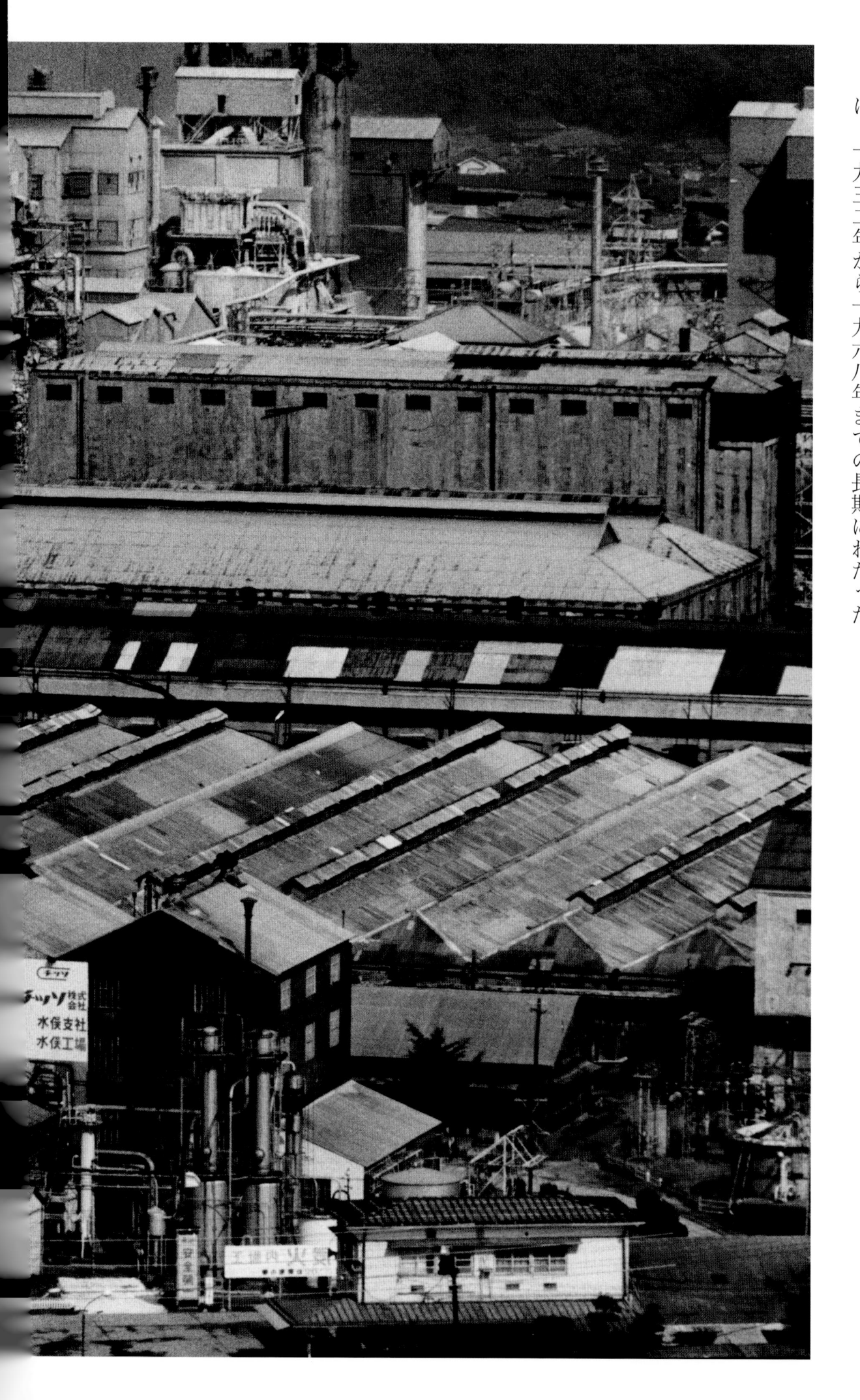

←（次頁）茂道のミカン山からチッソ水俣工場方面を見る　一九七〇年九月

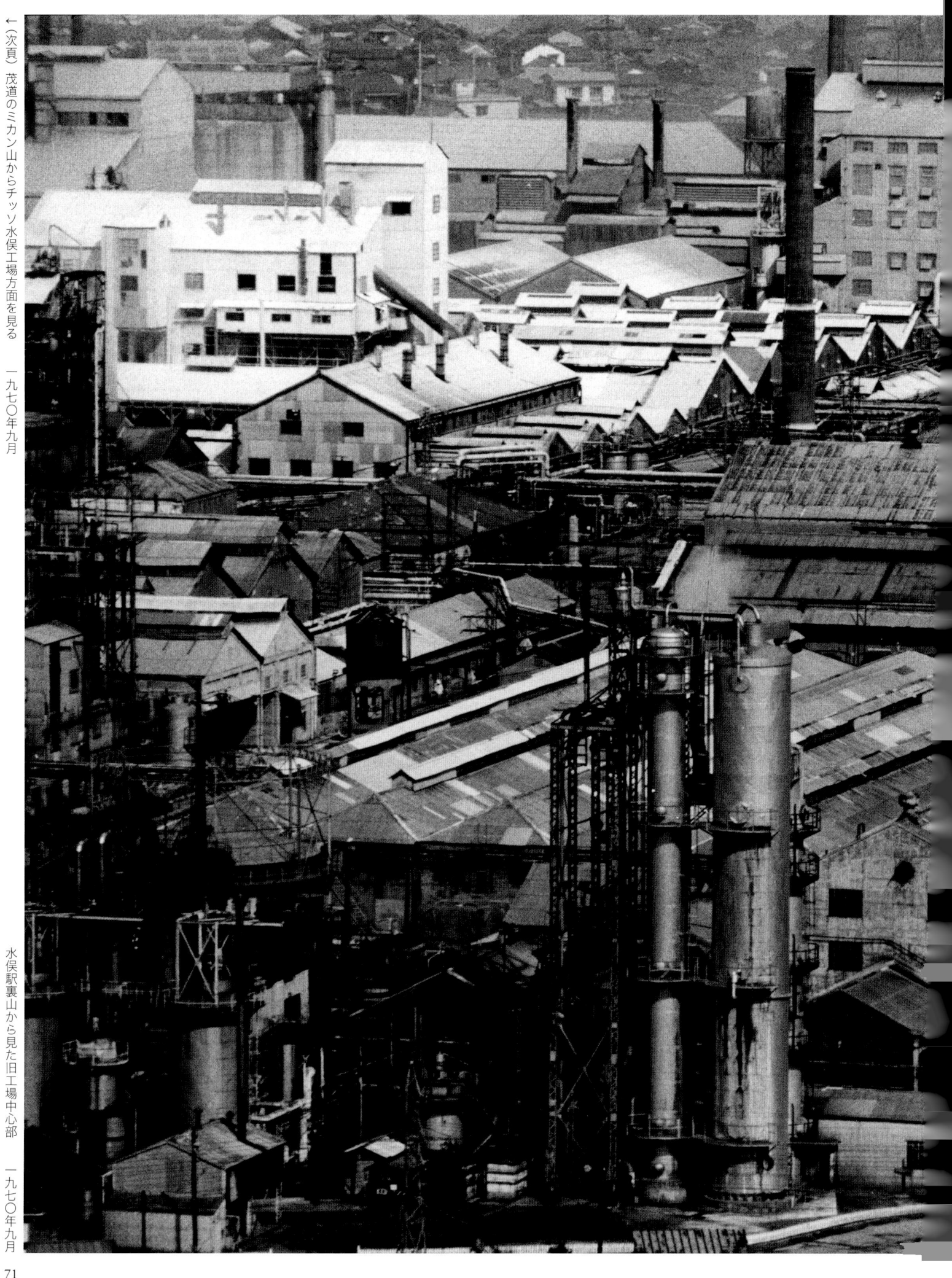

水俣駅裏山から見た旧工場中心部　一九七〇年九月

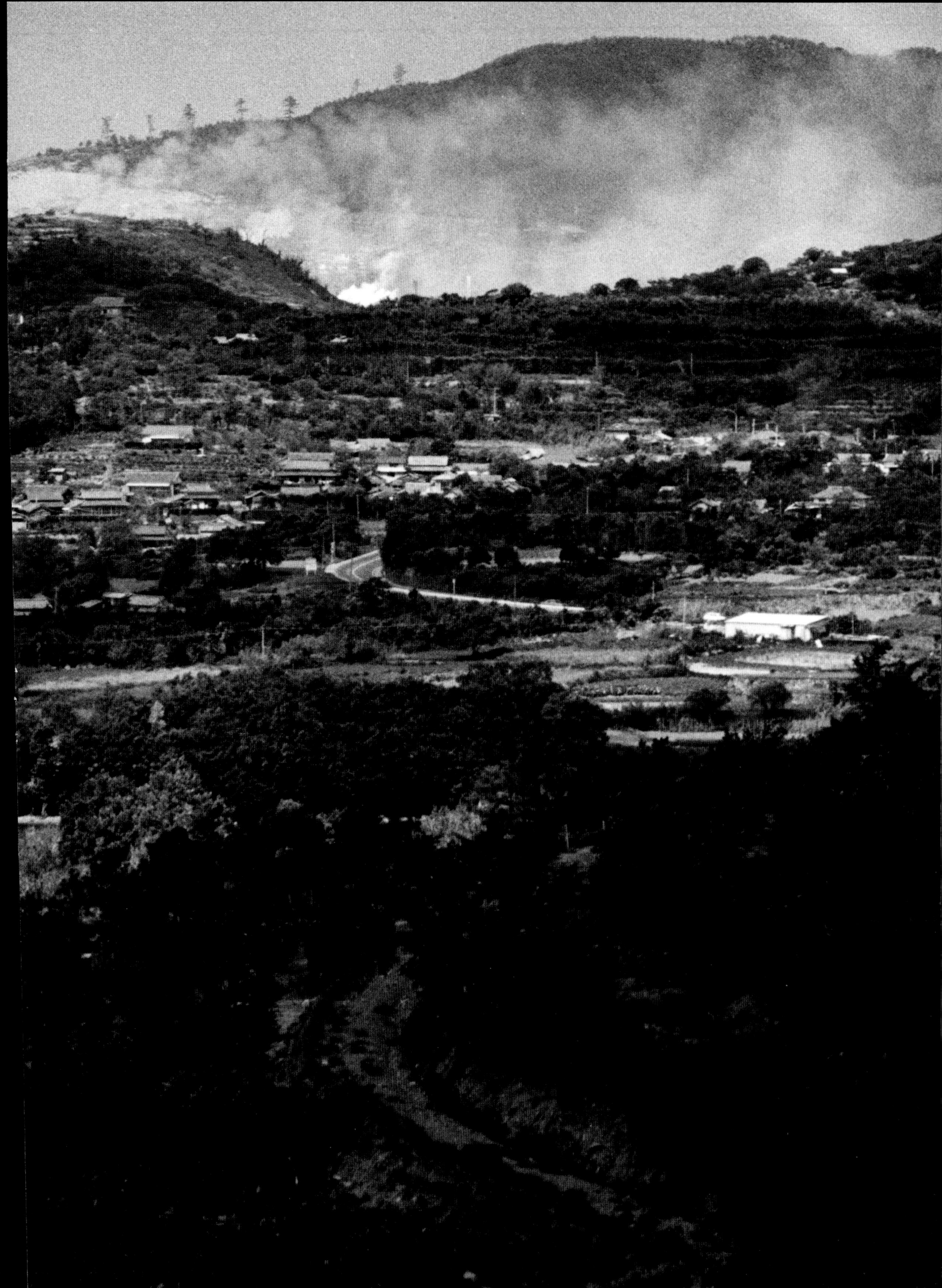

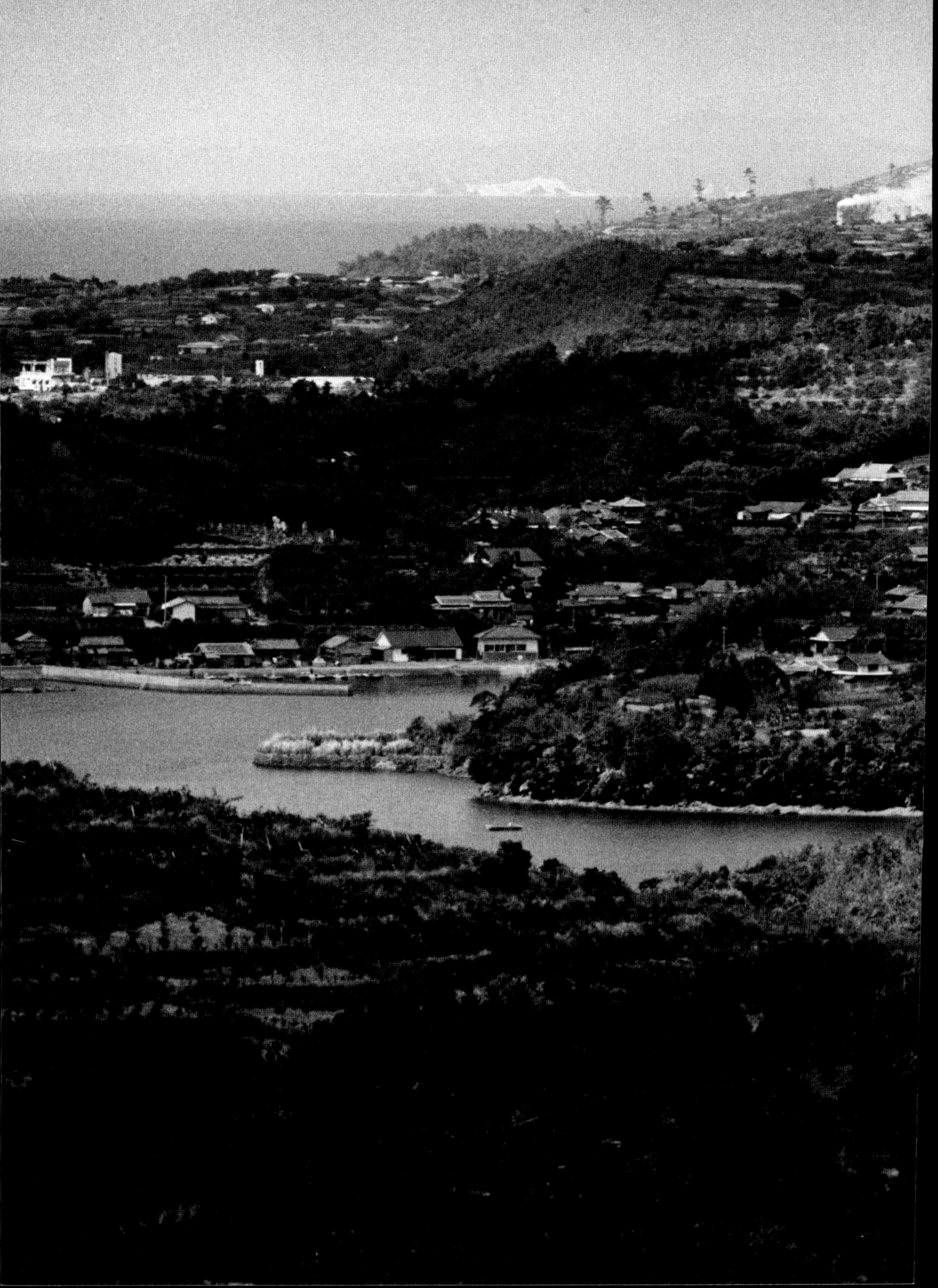

私の水俣病事件

舞台を支える裏方として

久保田好生

最高裁で相次いだ患者勝訴判決

二〇一三年四月一六日、水俣病認定義務付けの溝口訴訟・Fさん訴訟。お壕に近い最高裁判所の南門は判決にむけて上京した患者家族や各地の関係者で賑わった。節目の東京行動に必ず参加される桑原史成さんともども、若者たちの後輩に当たる映画監督の原一男さんとも、写真学校の後輩に当たる映画監督の原一男さんとも、写真学校の後輩に当たる映画監督の原一男さんと記念撮影をせがまれていた。「被写体」の桑原さんは、いつもの笑顔で応じておられる。

私は、上京者の皆に傍聴席を確保しきれるかどうかで頭が一杯だった。最高裁小法廷の一般傍聴席は四八席しかなく、二倍強の倍率の下、東京の支援者総出で並んで抽選券をもらい、当たり券をすぐ回収する。皆が渡してくれた何枚もの当たり券を、抽選に外れた主な上京者にサッと配り、拍手で法廷に送り出してやっと安堵した。判決が二件とも明快な患者勝訴だったので疲れも吹き飛んだ。

九年前、二〇〇四年のチッソ水俣病関西訴訟でも最高裁判決は画期的だった。国と熊本県の水俣病放置責任を認め、水俣病の病像でも新たな見識を示した大阪高裁判決を確定。「終わった」とされかかっていた未認定問題が息を吹き返し、以後新たに水俣病救済を申請する人が六万数千人にも及んだのである。

関西訴訟判決では、今は故人の土本典昭さんや宇井純さんにも当たり券を渡したこと、判決のあと川上敏行関西訴訟団長と一九九五年の第一次政治決着で苦渋の受諾をした患者連合の佐々木清登会長が無言の固い握手をしておられたことを思い出す。

チッソ本社はもとより、三権の牙城そびえる東京は折に触れて水俣病の主要なドラマの舞台になる。のっぴきならぬ闘いを背負って上京した患者・家族の行動

を支えることが、四十数年前からずっと、在京支援者の重要な仕事であり続けている。

「悩める学生」をひきつけた患者の闘い

一九五一年生まれの私は、学園闘争の余燼くすぶる一九七〇年に大学生になった。国家や資本の横溢はもとより、自分の栄達もアジア・第三世界の困窮する人々を踏み台にしているのではないかという問いに答えを見出しかねていた時代。どこかで「身捨つるほどのテーマはありや」と考えていた。一九七一―七三年のチッソ株主総会や、一九七〇年のチッソ本社前自主交渉坐り込みに助っ人で出かけ、水俣ワールドに、はまった。患者さん達には今風に言えば「キャラが立った」人が多く、都会育ちには風土もまるごと魅力的だった。自分の一挙手一投足が、患者の陣地を広げ、時にはそれが報道もされる。親の説教も、水俣支援だと言えば少し緩和された。

チッソ本社座り込みとその後の東京

自主交渉時代は座り込みテントや駅頭で、水俣病の宣伝を毎日行なったが、「怨」の幟旗と患者さんの写真パネルは、必須アイテムだった。新聞紙やその倍サイズのパネルは、支援者にも道行く人々にも事の重大さを深く訴えかけた。写真の多くが桑原史成さんの撮影によるものだと知ったのは後のことで、著作権も肖像権にも鈍感だった。これは大きな反省点である。

一九七三年、全国からチッソ東京本社座り込みに集まった学生たちが補償協定締結をもってテントを畳み、帰郷や水俣移住をする一方で、東京地裁には川本輝夫さんを刑事被告とする裁判が残され、それを支えることが東京在住者の任務となった。同年代の元学生が水俣など不知火海沿岸へ移住した知人友人も一人や二人

ではなかったが、そこまで「身捨つる」覚悟の定まらなかった自分は、東京の支援運動に貼りつく形となった。とはいえ、水俣支援でメシは食えない。運動現場からスーツ姿で採用面接に行ったりもして職業労働にも就く。しかし水俣病のいくさは間歇泉のように何度も中央政治に噴出する。勤めてからは学生時代のように四六時中活動とはいかなくなった。環境庁─環境省交渉、裁判、国会陳情、集会……患者上京は絶えることなく、畢竟、オフタイムは水俣三昧となった。二六歳で就いた教職は昨年還暦で再任用に切り替わりがない。それ以前から関わっていた水俣仕事には終わりがない。

支援の多様な側面

最高裁の隣・国立劇場も歌舞伎の名舞台だが、この春に新装なった歌舞伎座のTVドキュメントを視て舞台を作っている裏方たちに共感した。不知火海沿岸の患者・被害者や水俣市民を中心とする水俣病いくさで、在京支援とは、主役脇役が活躍する舞台を支える大道具や音響照明係に似ているかもしれない。

他方、東京の支援にはツアーコンダクターの要素も欠かせない。その点で東京住民以上に詳しかったのが川本輝夫さん。上京患者が都内観光する際に、浅草にも銀座にも詳しい彼は様々なアドバイスをしていた。東京名所なんて大して興味のなかった私も、以来東京の観光地や土産を見つめなおすようになった。

水俣病が公式確認から半世紀以上を経ても「解決」を見ないのは企業や行政の怠慢に由来する。しかし他方、曖昧な「決着」を拒んできた患者・住民の屹立した闘いがあっての現在とも言える。東京の「出店」暖簾を下ろしてはいられない。

（くぼた・よしお／高校教諭・東京・水俣病を告発する会）

10 胎児性患者たちの成人とその後

水俣病発見の年に生まれた子が、成人の日となった。市役所が営む式典前で、晴れ着の同世代に普段着でビラを渡す胎児性患者もいた。「お金はもらったけど、若い人はなにも救われていません。もう一度、この問題を考え、力をかしてくれないでしょうか」

滝下昌文（右）と鬼塚勇治　水俣市公会堂前　一九七七年一月一五日

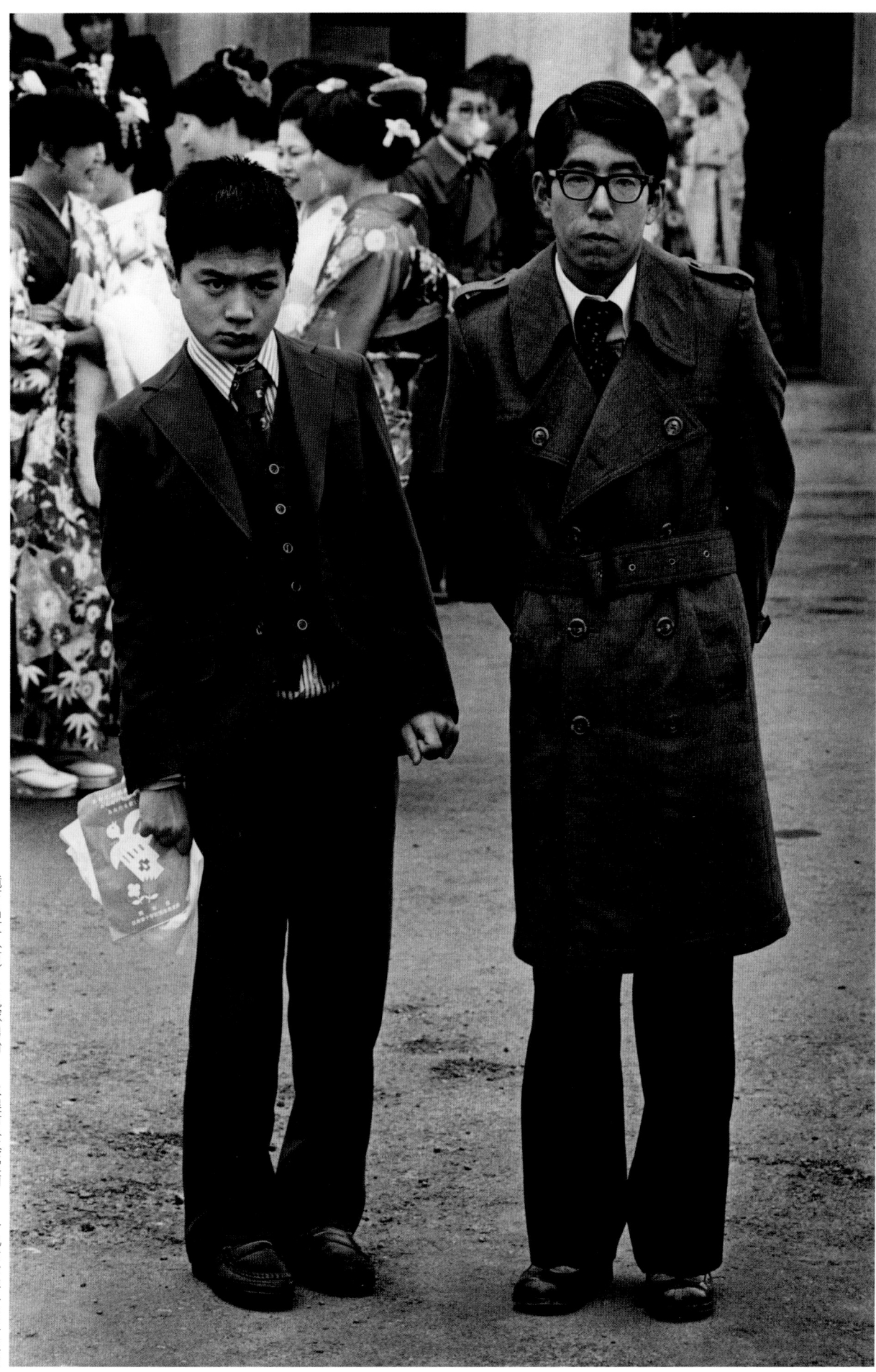

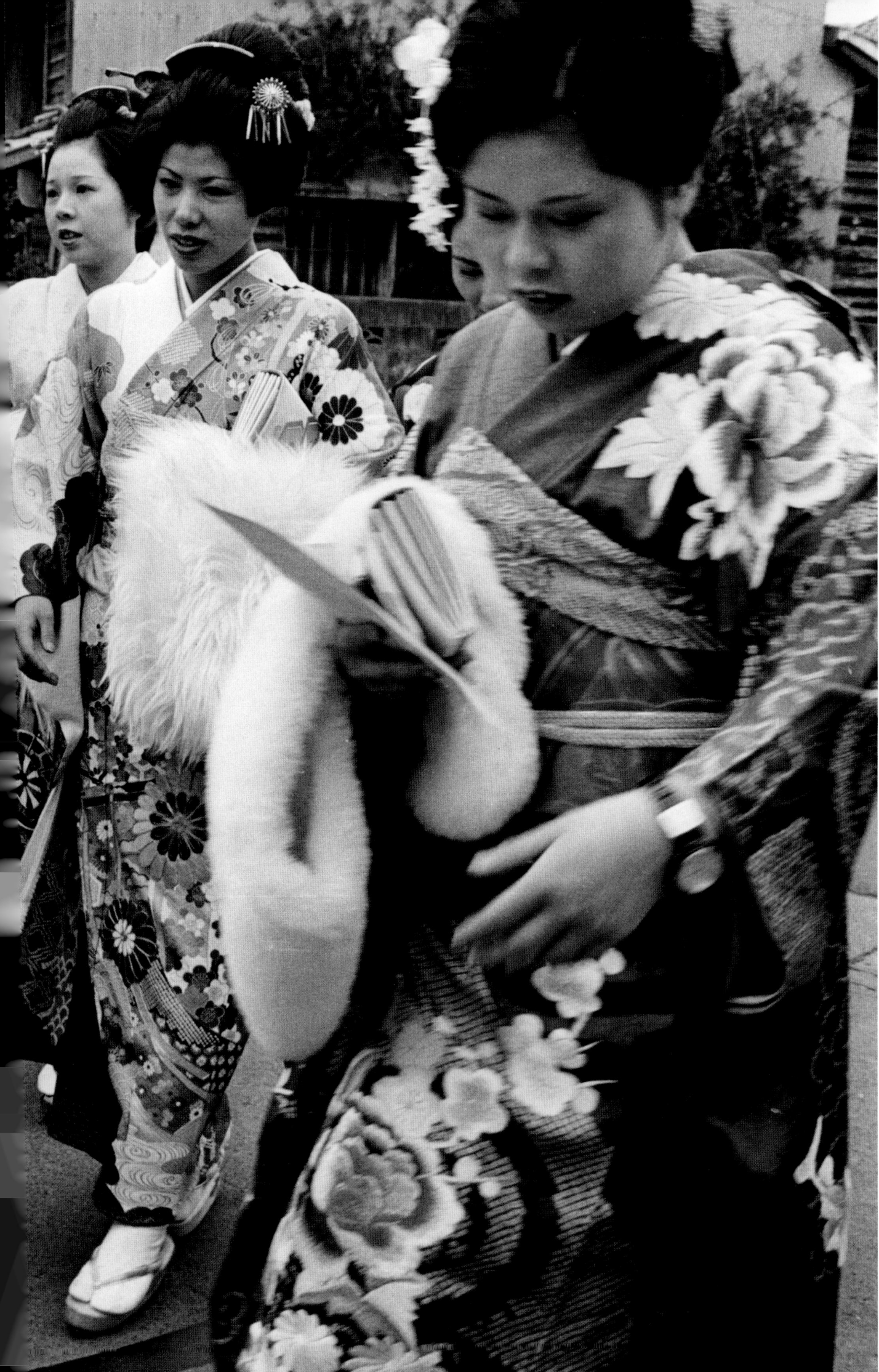

自作のビラを新成人へ。坂本しのぶ（中央）と加賀田清子（左）　水俣市公会堂前　一九七七年一月一五日

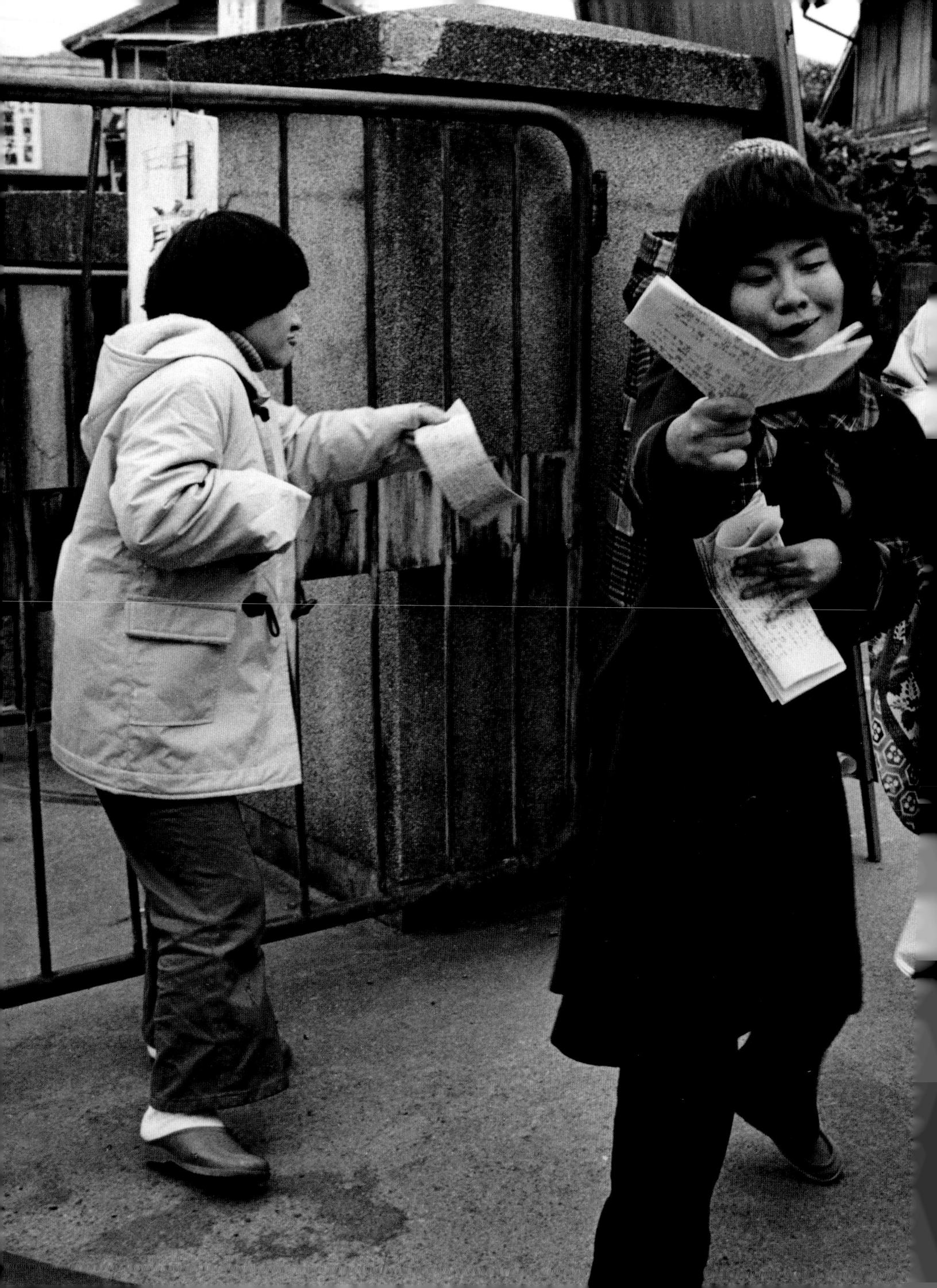

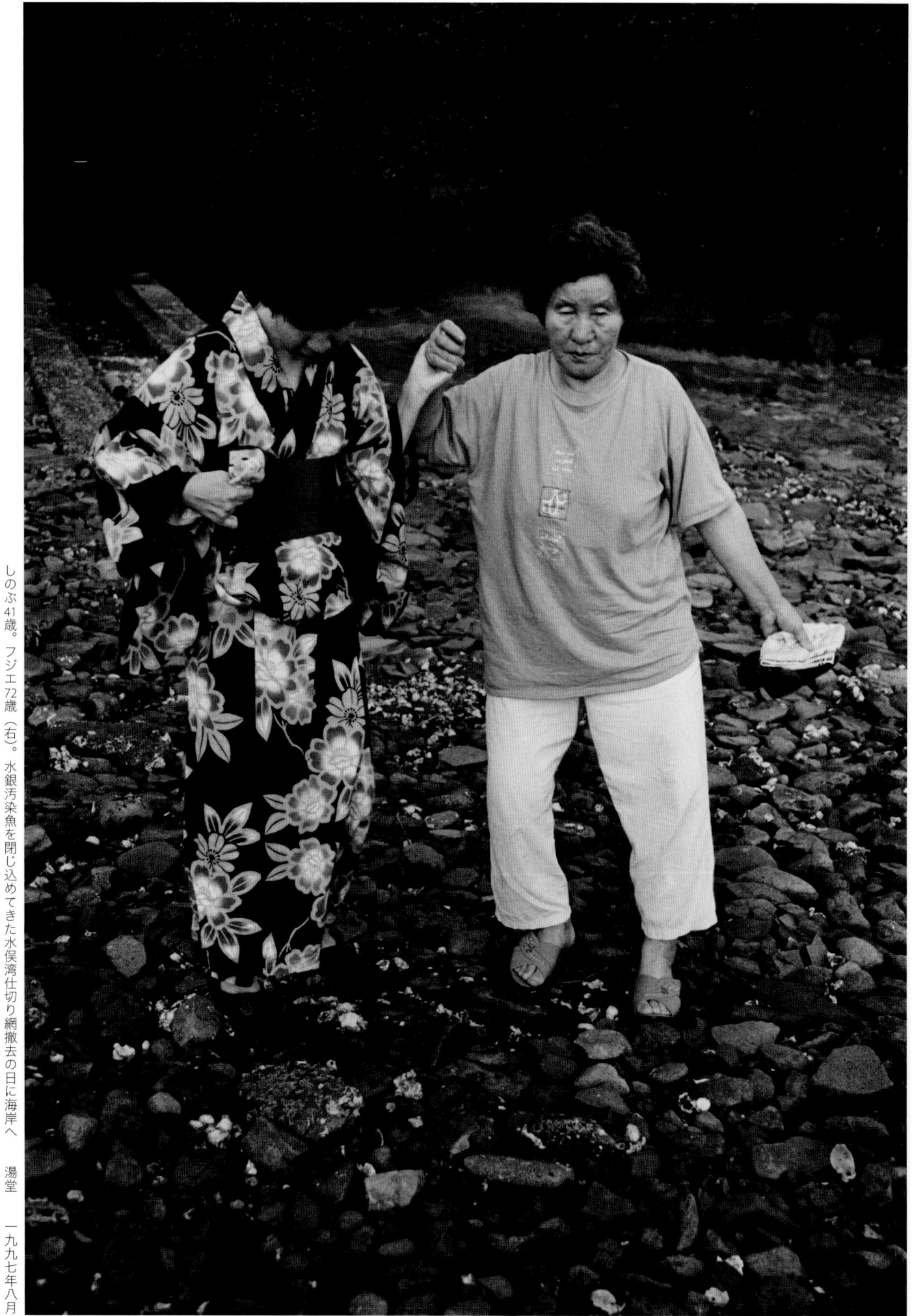

しのぶ41歳。フジエ72歳（右）。水銀汚染魚を閉じ込めてきた水俣湾仕切り網撤去の日に海岸へ　湯堂　一九九七年八月

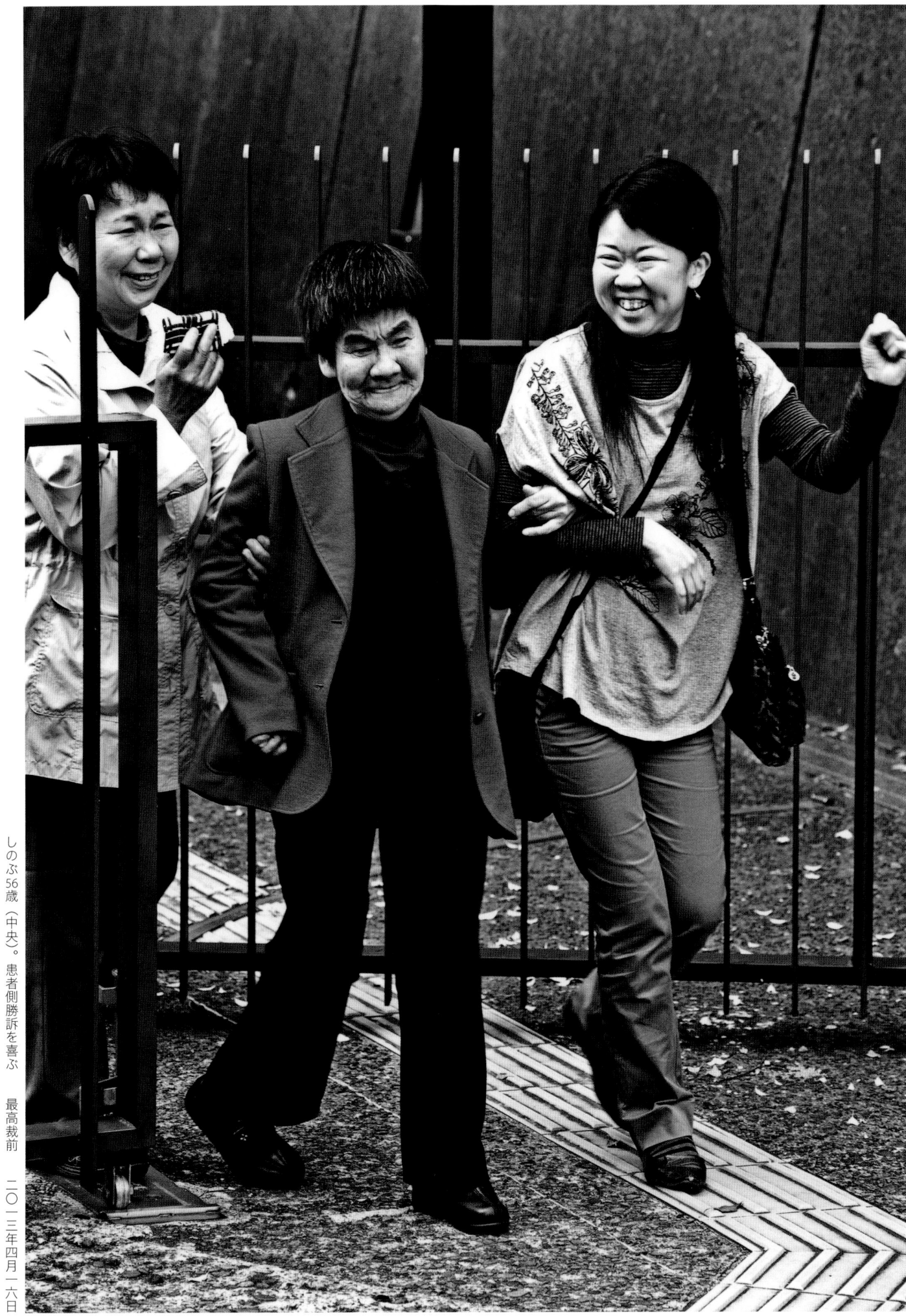

しのぶ56歳（中央）。患者側勝訴を喜ぶ　最高裁前　二〇一三年四月一六日

私の水俣病事件

水俣病の底辺 ― 慢性微量汚染の取り組み ―

藤野 糺

停止後も水俣病発生が続いていたことから「慢性微量」中毒と、対照とした有明海の水俣病類似患者の存在年変化を比較したが、やはり同様の結果であった。二〇〇五～一〇年にアセトアルデヒド工場操業停止後の出生者（六八年五月～八六年五月）一一七人を検診した。手足の末梢優位の感覚障害を八九％に確認し、一七人の臍帯メチル水銀濃度は非汚染地域の二倍を超えていた。〇九、一二年には全国各地から一四〇名を超える医師の参加で不知火海全域の一〇〇名検診を実施し、国の救済対象地域・年（六九年一一月までの出生）外にも多くの患者が存在することを明らかにした。

これまでに被害者として名乗り出た者は行政認定の二二七五人を含め八万二千人以上を数える。しかし被害者は天草や山間部、転出先にまだ数万人単位で潜在すると予測でき、全汚染地域の健康調査が不可欠である。

水俣病の発生防止と予見可能性について考える。アセトアルデヒド工程で有機水銀化合物が副生されることを報告したフォクトとニューランドの論文をチッソが保有していたことは、七一年水俣病訴訟において馬奈木昭雄弁護士によって明らかにされたが、本年二月入口紀男はこの文献が熊大医学部図書館においても八〇（昭和五）年に受け入れられ、開架されていることを報告した。入口紀男はチッソのアセトアルデヒド工場操業開始の三二（昭和七）年にはメチル水銀中毒症の恐るべき病態を含めてこれらの事実は当時の化学者や当業者の間で広く知られていたと述べている。

被害は広範囲に及んでいた

水俣病は一九五六（昭和三一）年細川一博士により「原因不明の中枢神経疾患」として発見され、熊本大学水俣病研究班により五九年「原因はある種の有機水銀中毒」、六三年「毒物はメチル水銀化合物」と結論づけられた。原因究明で功績のある徳臣晴比古、岡嶋透らは六〇（昭和三五）年患者多発地区住民検診により「水俣病は五三年に始まり六〇年で終焉」と報告したが、それは急性劇症など重篤例のみのチェックであった。その後確認した胎児性水俣病を加え「患者総数一一一人」で過去の病気とされていた。

六五（昭和四〇）年新潟で第二の水俣病が発生し、六八年国は水俣病を公害病と初めて認定する。翌年水俣病患者・家族がチッソを相手に提訴し、私も七〇年より水俣病の底辺を明らかにする取り組みを開始した。

私は旧認定の原告患者やその家族、隣人を診察し水俣病像を掴んでいった。どの地域でも認定の重症患者と変わらぬ人々を多数発見した。七二年より多発地区内の精神科病院に勤務し、治療と患者発掘を進めた。私たちの掘り起こしで七三年七月までに申請者二二〇人中二〇二人（九六％）が認定となる。

また、七〇（昭和四五）年夏より、胎児性水俣病の多発地域であり、多発年の出生者が在籍している袋中学の全員を対象とした健康調査を行った。生徒の一八％に水俣病にみられる神経症状を伴った知的障害を確認し、それらをメチル水銀の影響と考えた。

七三（昭和四八）年、熊大第二次水俣病研究班長　武内忠男は濃厚汚染地区の悉皆調査で、生存認定患者三七人の八・五倍の患者（全人口比三二・一％）が存在すると発表。同時にアセトアルデヒド生産停止後も水俣病発生が続いていたことから「慢性微量中毒」と、対照とした有明海の水俣病類似患者中毒」と、対照とした有明海の水俣病類似患者中毒」の問題を提起した。後者は稼働中の水銀電解法苛性ソーダ全国四九工場の安全性を確認する必要性を示唆し、その直後原田正純がその工場のある大牟田市で、私がその生産高第一、二位の二工場が立地する徳山湾で類似患者を発見した。

七一（昭和四六）年の過去棄却者の行政不服審査請求事件で、熊本県の厳しい認定基準を否定していた環境庁は立場を変え、新潟水俣病で功績のあった椿忠雄を班長とする健康調査部会を発足させ、類似患者をすべて「シロ」判定した。第三水俣病を認めれば、ソーダ工場は操業停止を余儀なくされるからである。そして七七（昭和五二）年には「感覚障害を基礎に運動失調、視野狭窄などの組み合わせを要する判断条件」を作り、水俣病患者の切り捨て政策に転じてきた。

この政策に対し、私たちは七四（昭和四九）年に水俣診療所（後に水俣協立病院）を開設して患者の治療や訪問看護を進めるとともに、汚染の実態解明に取り組んだ。七四年から六年がかりで全住民を精査し「魚介類の多食と手足の末梢優位の感覚障害があれば水俣病」という診断基準を確立した。桂島検診で、汚染源操業停止後出生した女児一人に手足の末梢優位の感覚障害を認め、微量の汚染の影響と考えた。

数万人の潜在患者の存在

七七～七八年御所浦町住民で過去の熊大二次研究班受診者三〇四人を六～六・五年後に検診し、自覚症状と感覚障害、運動失調、難聴、視野狭窄などの神経症状の増加と、新たな水俣病の発生を確認した。この調

（注）Richard R. Vogt and Julius A. Nieuwland : THE ROLE OF MERCURY SOLTS IN THE CATALYTIC TRANSFORMATION OF ACETYREN INTO ACETALDEHYDE, AND A NEW COMMERCIAL PROCESS FOR THE MANUFACTURE OF PARALDEHYDE, J. American Chemical Society, 43, 7, 2071-2081, 1921

（ふじの・ただし／水俣協立病院名誉院長）

11 水俣病専用病棟や自宅の患者たち

　私が現地撮影に入った一九六〇年七月、専用病棟入院中は一八人だったと記憶する。同年末までの認定患者八七人のうち三四人は劇症で死亡。私が撮って間もなく死んだ人もいた。他の在宅患者はひっそりと孤立無援に近く、胎児性患者は未認定だった。

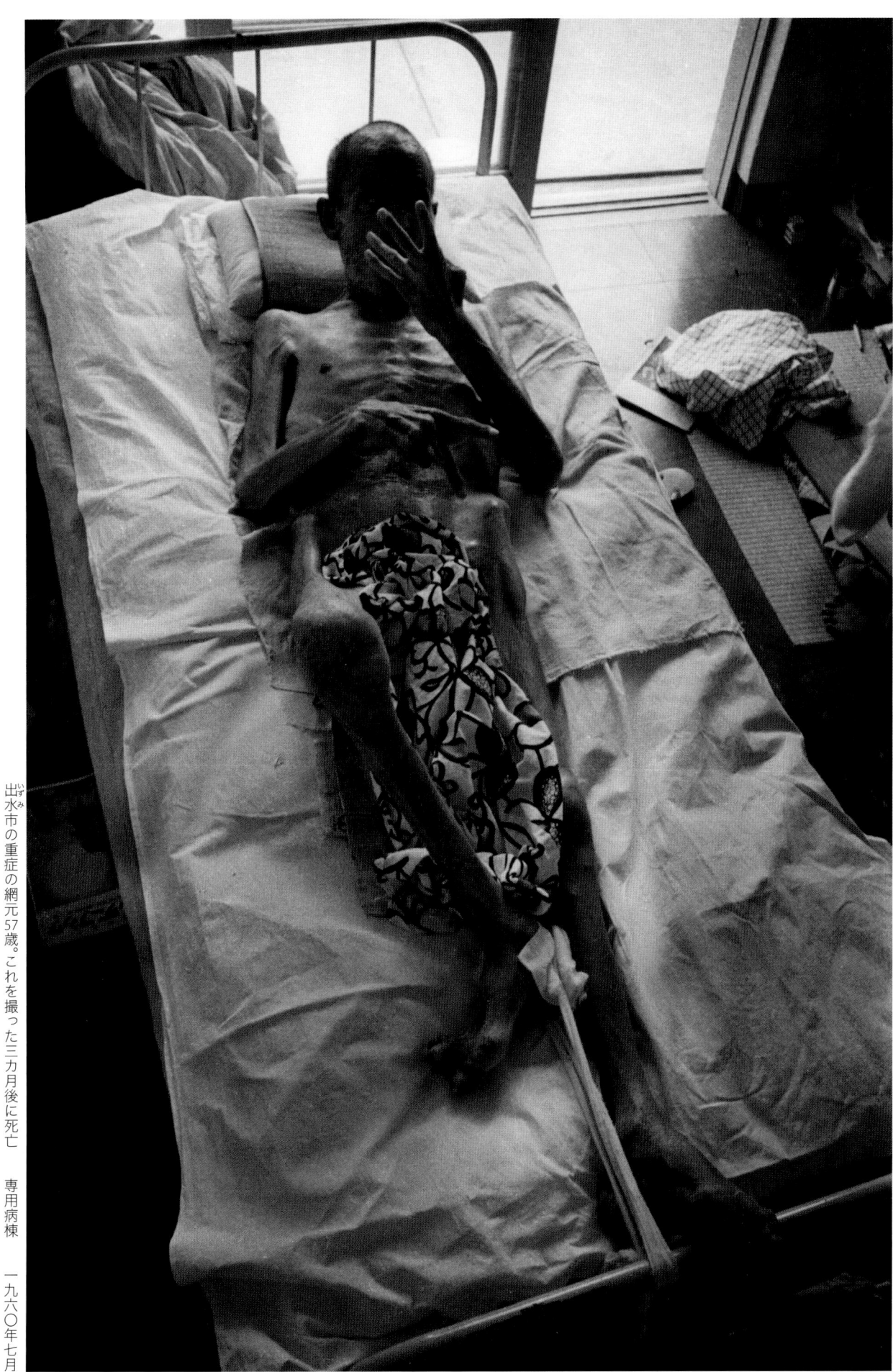

出水市の重症の網元57歳。これを撮った三カ月後に死亡　専用病棟　一九六〇年七月

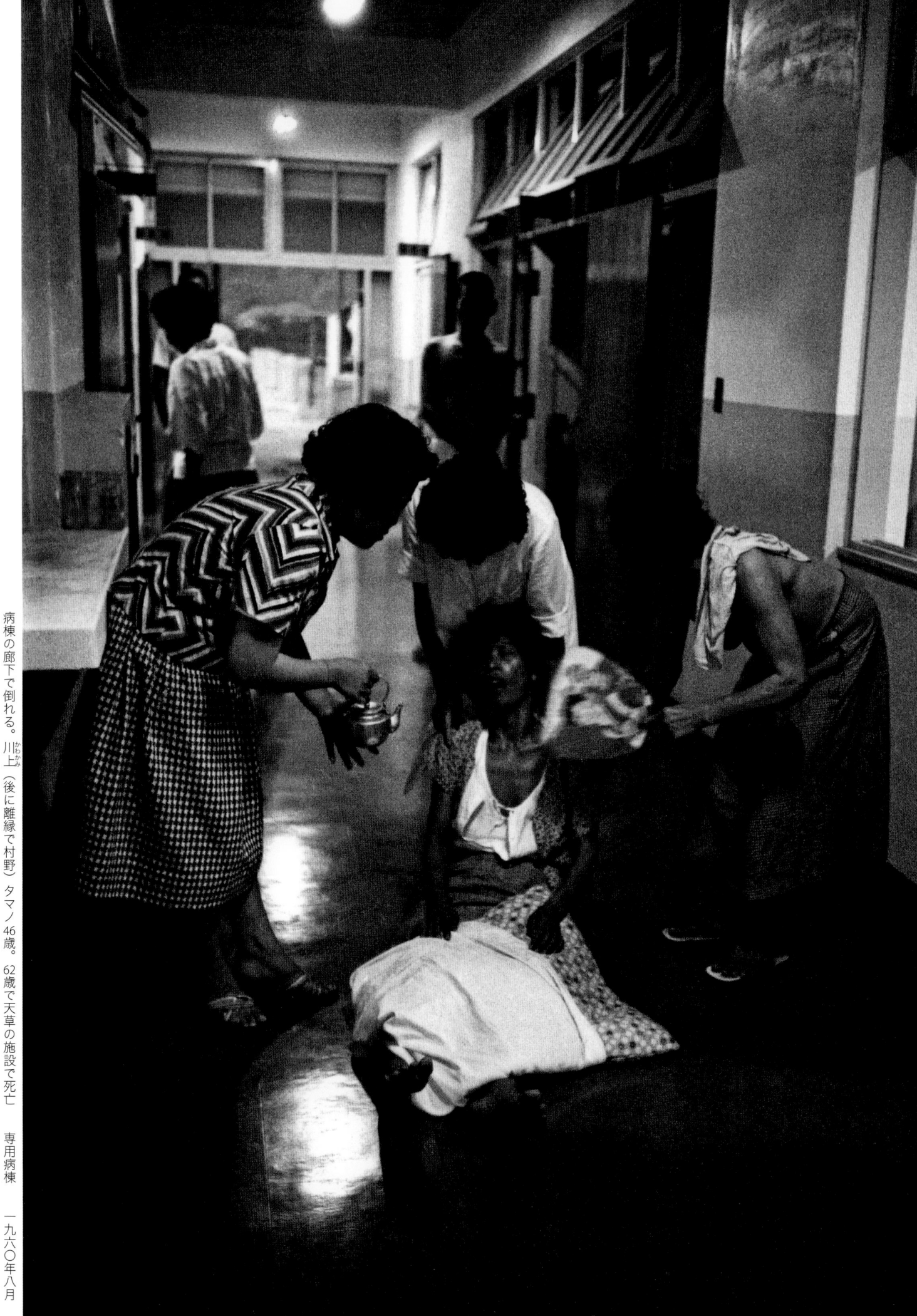

病棟の廊下で倒れる。川上(後に離縁で村野)タマノ46歳。62歳で天草の施設で死亡　専用病棟　一九六〇年八月

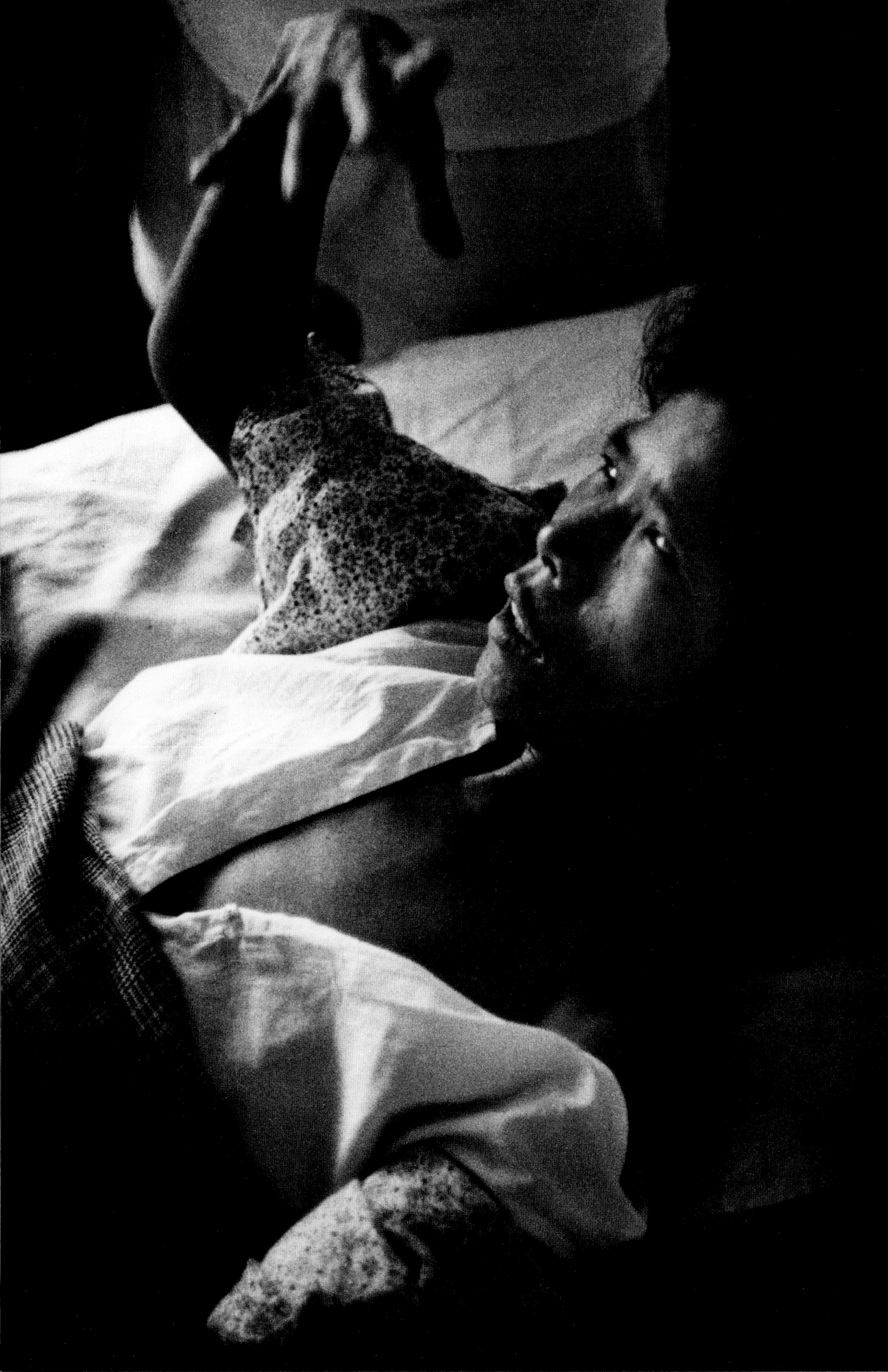

寝ていても発作　専用病棟　一九六〇年八月

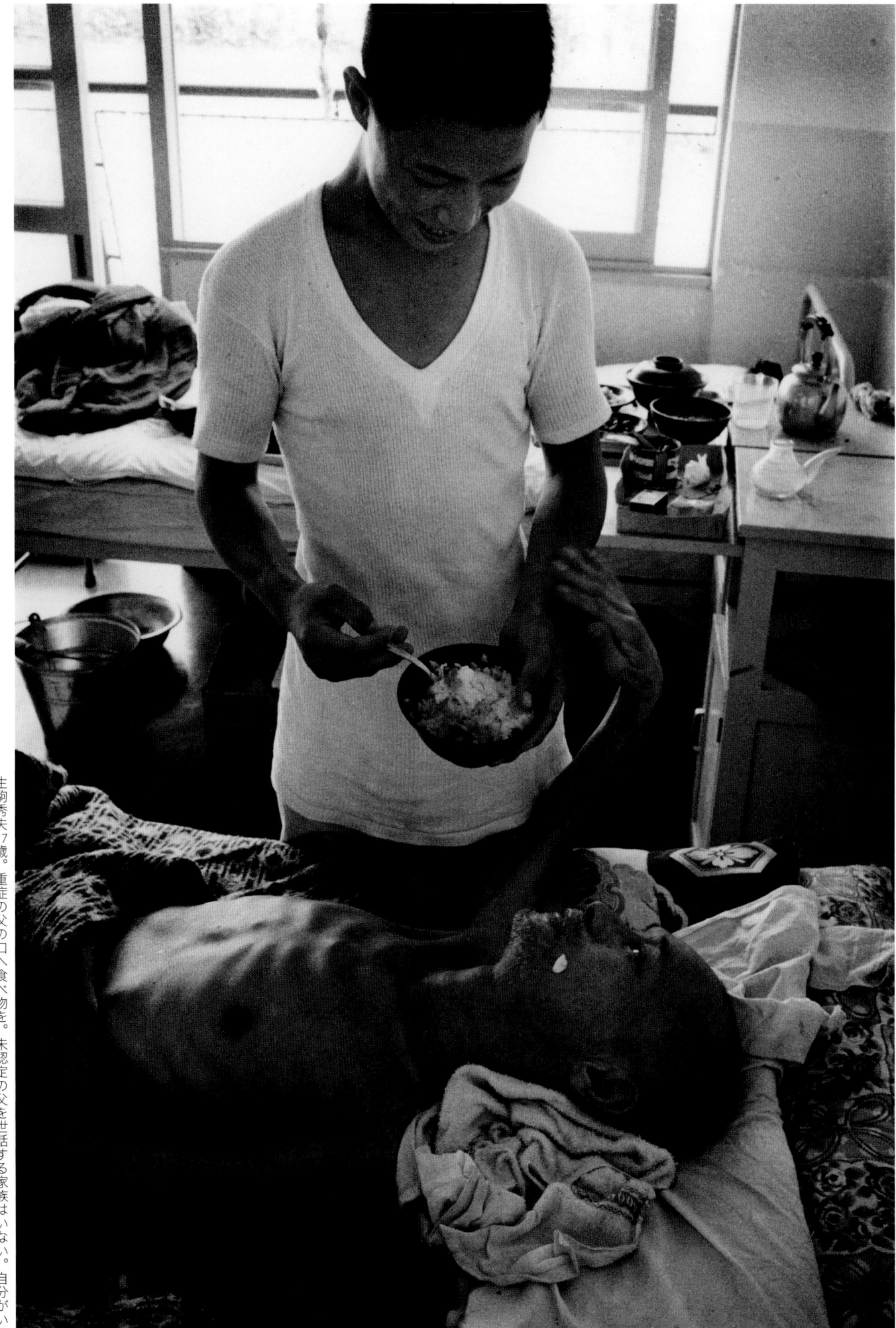

生駒秀夫17歳。重症の父の口へ食べ物を。未認定の父を世話する家族はいない。自分がいる専用病棟へ父のベッドを移動してもらう　一九六〇年八月

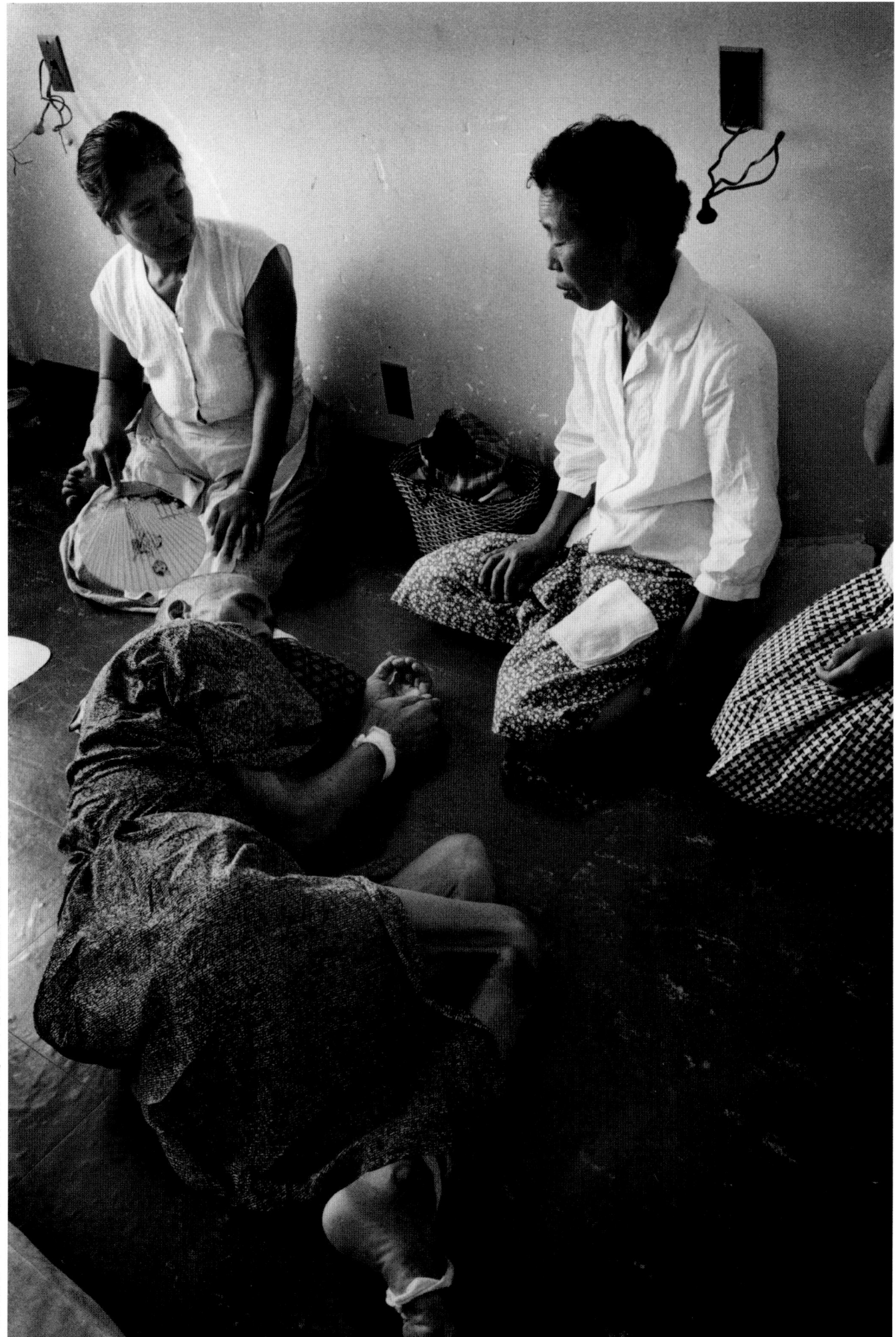

ベッドに上がれず床に寝る重症患者、67歳。一年九カ月後に全身衰弱で死亡　一九六〇年七月

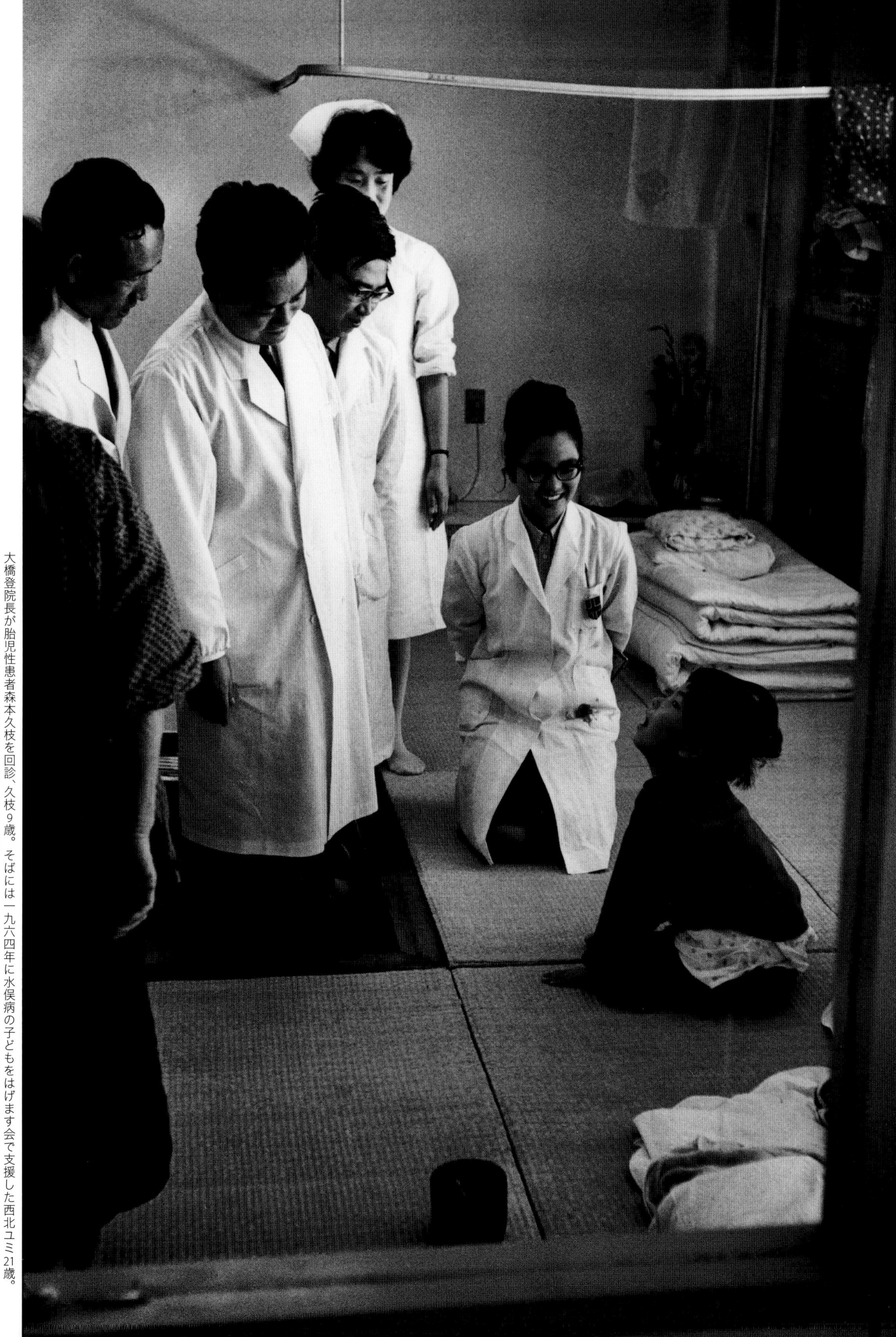

大橋登院長が胎児性患者森本久枝を回診、久枝9歳。そばには一九六四年に水俣病の子どもをはげます会で支援した西北ユミ21歳。湯之児リハビリセンターが全国初のリハビリ専門病院として一九六五年開院、専用病棟の患者全員が転院した 一九六六年五月

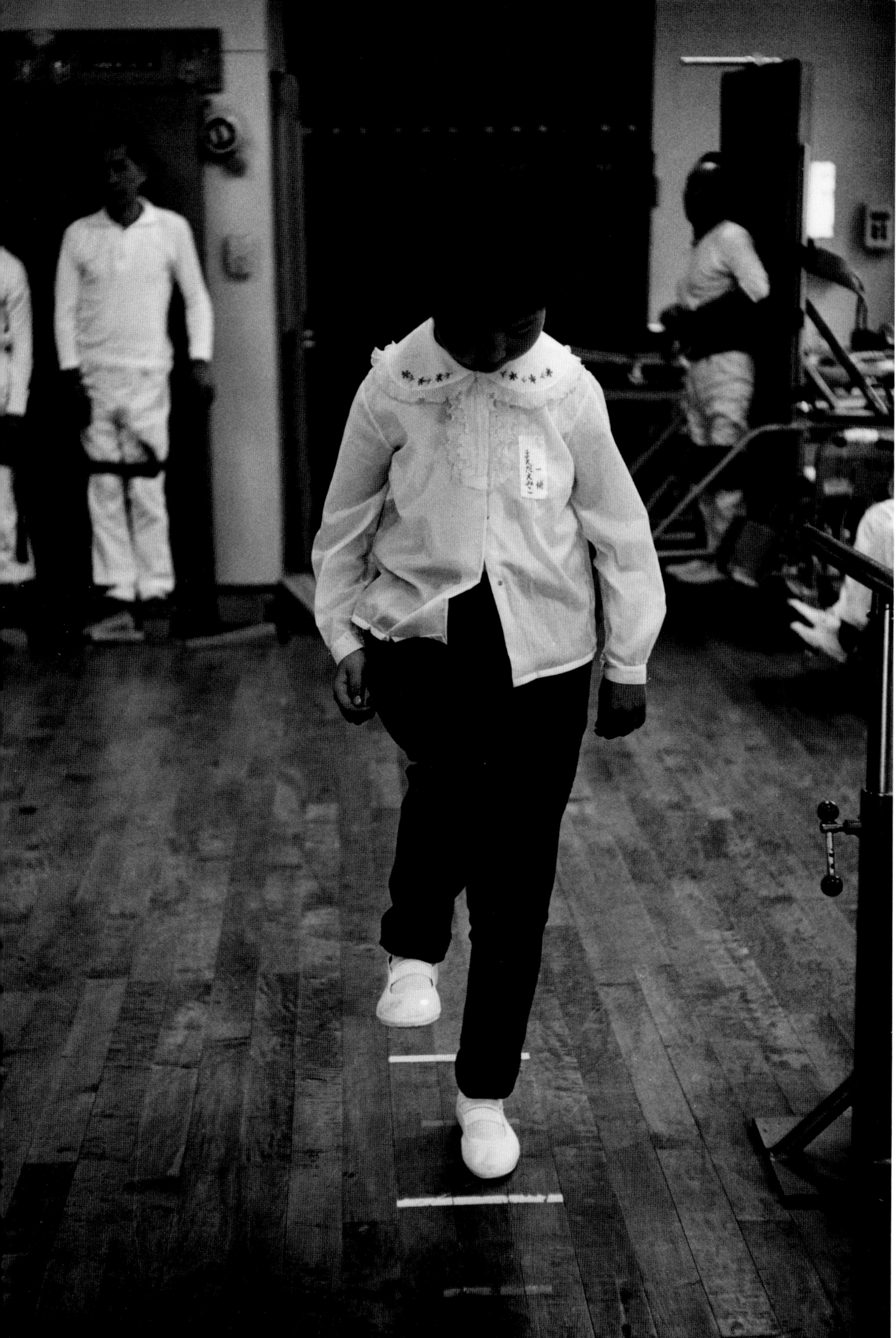

歩行訓練。小児性患者の前田恵美子12歳　リハビリセンター　一九六六年五月

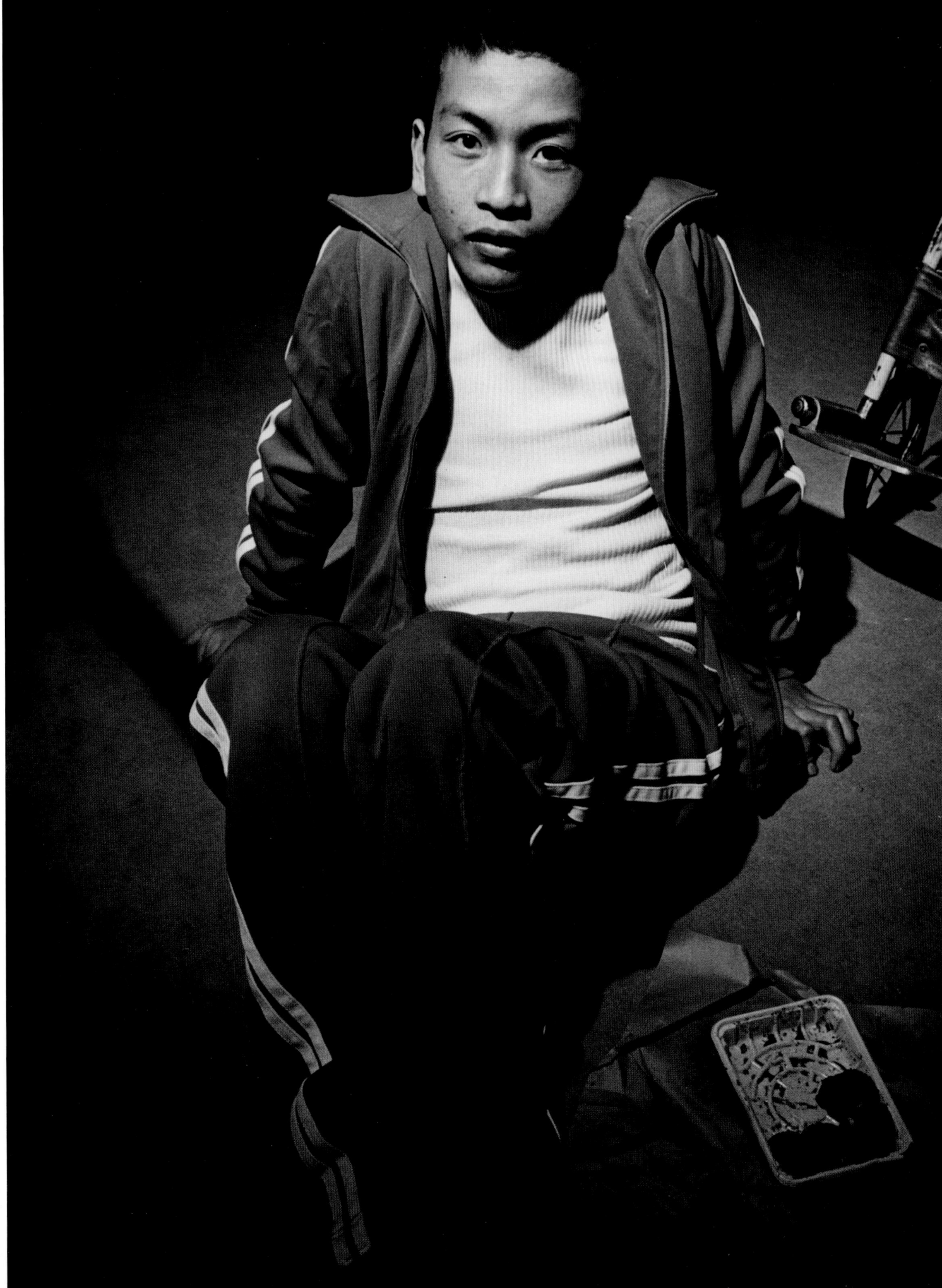

胎児性患者の長井勇19歳　患者の入る施設の明水園　一九七七年一月

尾上光雄53歳　百間町の自宅　一九七〇年九月

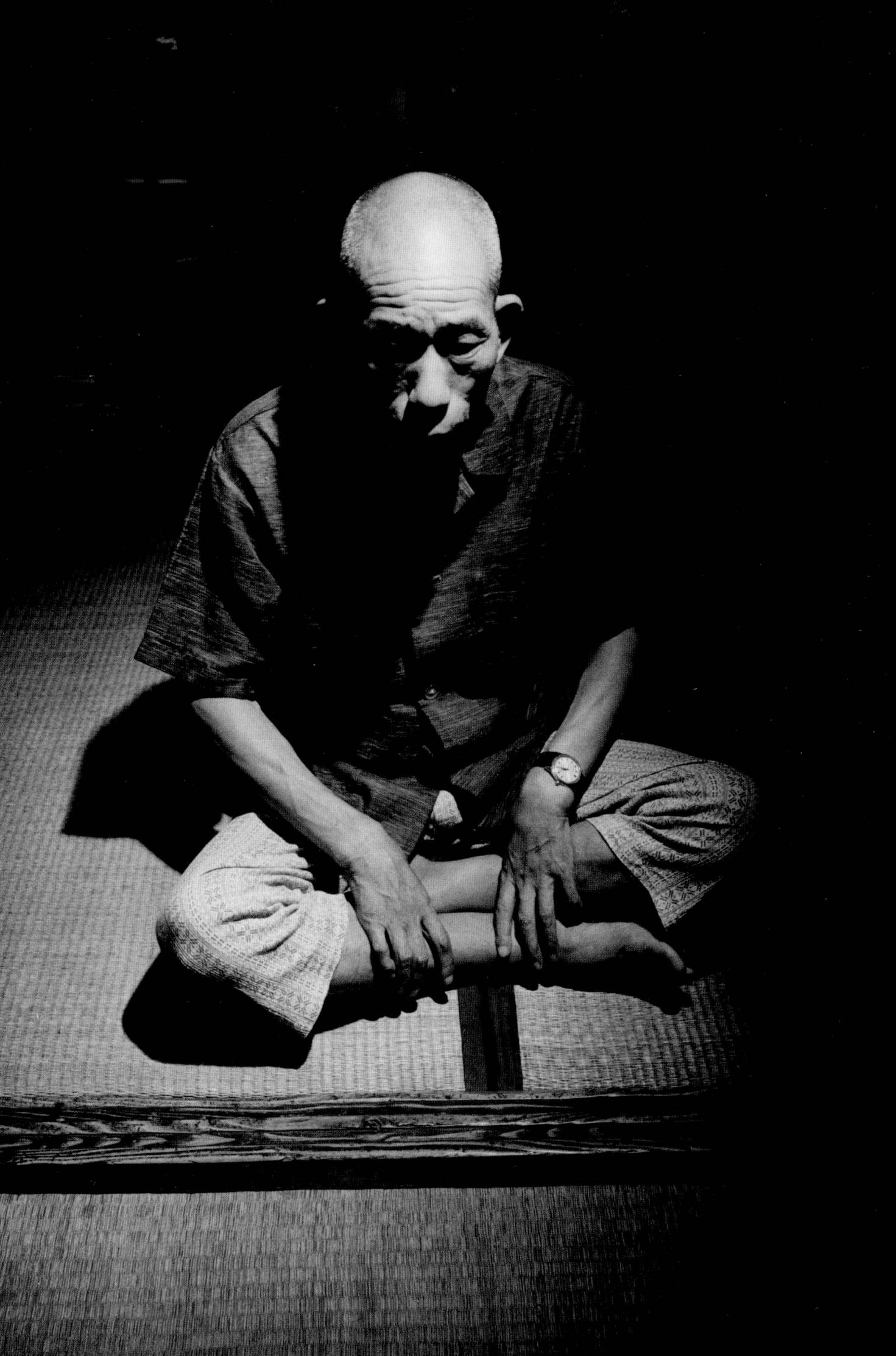

私の水俣病事件

磁力ということ

高峰 武

今も続く水俣病の構造

時折、潜り込む会社の部屋がある。

水俣病三次訴訟第一陣の現地検証。胎児性患者が入る施設「明水園」の検証を終えた裁判官の声を直接とばどんどん書いて下さい」。磁力は、個々ではあったが、「官」の責任者の一人だった。

水俣市の資料室。熊本日日新聞の創刊——一九四二（昭和一七）年四月一日——からの新聞が綴じられている。ここでセピア色に変色した生の新聞をめくり、立ち止まる記事がある。

一つは一九五四年八月一日付。「猫てんかんで全滅 水俣市茂道部落 ねずみの激増に悲鳴」。初めて水俣病の被害を伝えた記事だ。百二十戸の漁村で百余匹の猫が全滅、よそからもらってきてもすぐ死ぬため、増えたねずみの駆除を住民が水俣市に申し入れた、という。水俣病の前兆として貴重な自然界のサインだったが、生かされることはなかった。次に記事が出るのは一九五六年五月の公式確認。二年も後のことだ。

もう一つは一九五九年一一月八日付。「水俣工場排水停止は困る 市民の生活に響く——各種団体が知事に陳情」。市長、市議会議長、商工会議所会頭、地区労議長など水俣市の二十八団体の代表が熊本県知事に陳情した。チッソ依存の生活を守るために、排水を止めずに工場の操業を継続してほしい……。「オール水俣」の代表。いないのはただ一つ、漁民である。大を生かすために小を犠牲にする構図。

二つの記事の前で、時間が止まる。私たちは水俣病を本当に克服したのか、この構造は今も生きてはいないか、と。

「現場」の力

水俣病は多面体で、見る人の角度によってさまざまな姿を見せる。そして、取材の現場では、言葉が突然、降りてくることがある。

水俣病一次訴訟で患者勝訴の熊本地裁判決（一九七三年）を言い渡した斎藤次郎裁判長は、判決文とは別にコメントを出した。異例のことだ。そこで、裁判には限界がある、企業、政治、行政の誠意ある努力なしに公害は解決しない、と訴えた。斎藤裁判長はその後、待たせ賃訴訟の控訴審（一九八五年判決）も担当するという、不思議な巡り合わせを持った。裁判官が肉声を漏らすことはそうない。しかし、こちらは何とかしてあれこれ手を尽くし、斎藤裁判長と接触した。一次訴訟の判決から約十年もたっている。にもかかわらず、認定制度をめぐる裁判が続いていること自体が意外だったようだ。私が、当時の原告の名前を挙げると、「お元気ですか。みなさん僕のこと、悪く言っていないでしょう」と答えた。その言葉が実に温かった。患者の勝訴を確信したものだ。

水俣病一次訴訟の控訴審（一九八五年判決）……国と熊本県の責任を全面的に認めた画期的なものだったが、心証という点で決定的だったのは、あの現地検証だった。「現場」が放つ強力な磁力が、裁判官も包み込んだ。

一九八七年の熊本地裁判決は、国と熊本県の責任を全面的に認めた画期的なものだったが、心証という点で決定的だったのは、あの現地検証だった。「現場」が放つ強力な磁力が、裁判官も包み込んだ。

「工事中のヘドロの埋め立て地でたまたま見かけた」という説明だったが、ヘドロ処理をめぐる役所内部の会議録などめったにお目にかかれない文書の束。川本さんが言う「たまたま見つけた」とは到底信じ難いものだった。何らかのルートで川本さんのところに渡ったのだろう。こうした見えないルートにも「官」の素顔を感じたりもした。

磁力は記者個々にも届いた。「水俣病を告発する会」や「水俣病研究会」などがあったが、ここには、新聞、テレビの記者や関係者の姿があった。仕事として取材、報道するという地点とは立場を異にし、いわば「個」として加わったものだ。その活動は今も継続されている。自分は何をすべきかという自問への一つの答えだが、こうしたことも水俣病の運動の内面を豊かにしていることの一つだろう。

新聞に戻って紹介したい記事がある。水俣病の公害認定を伝える一九六八年九月二七日付熊本日日新聞朝刊に、写真家・桑原史成氏がこんなコメントを寄せている。「できれば水俣という地を世界の人々が知らないまま過ごす歴史であってほしかった。そして一人のカメラマンなども出現しなくてよかったのである」。レンズを通して水俣病を見続けた一人の人間の心優しいコメントである。

自分は何をすべきか

「官」も、業務の時の無機質な表情とは別の顔を見せることがあった。水俣湾のヘドロ処理（一九九〇年終了）に関してのこと。「実は正直、自分たちも分か

（たかみね・たけし／熊本日日新聞社取締役）

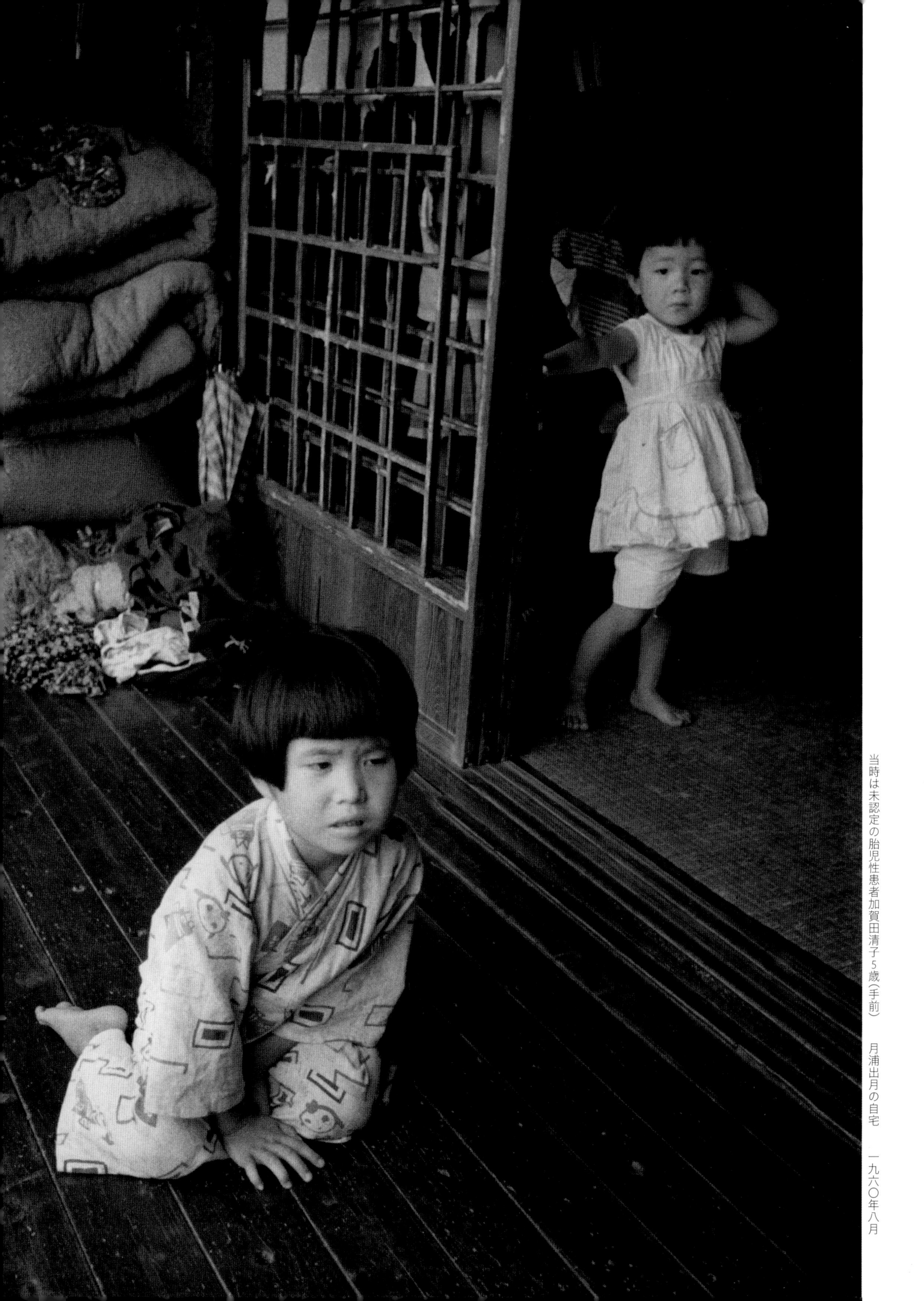

当時は未認定の胎児性患者加賀田清子5歳(手前)　月浦出月の自宅　一九六〇年八月

92

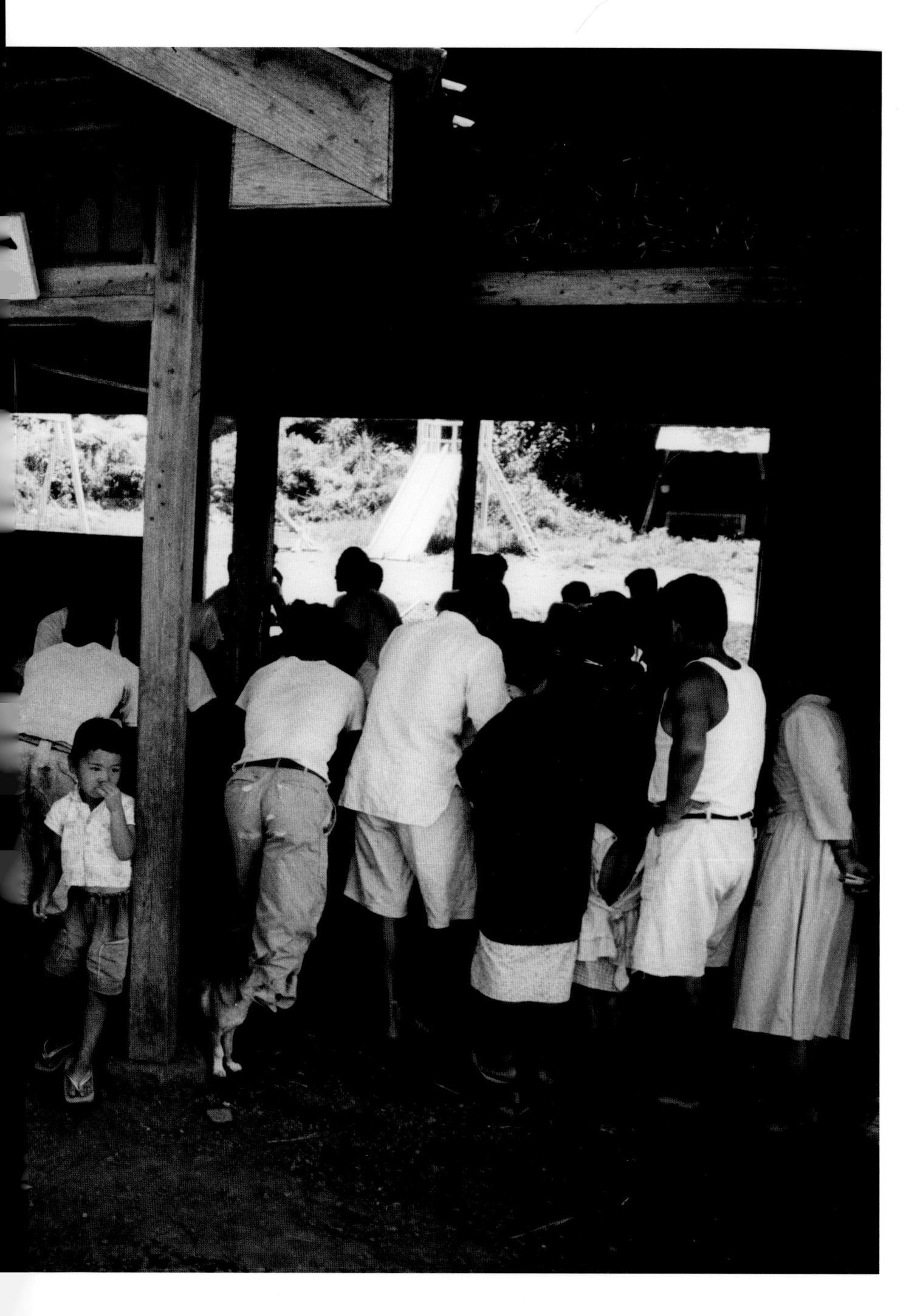

熊大第一内科の現地問診につめかけた住民　茂道公民館　一九六〇年七月

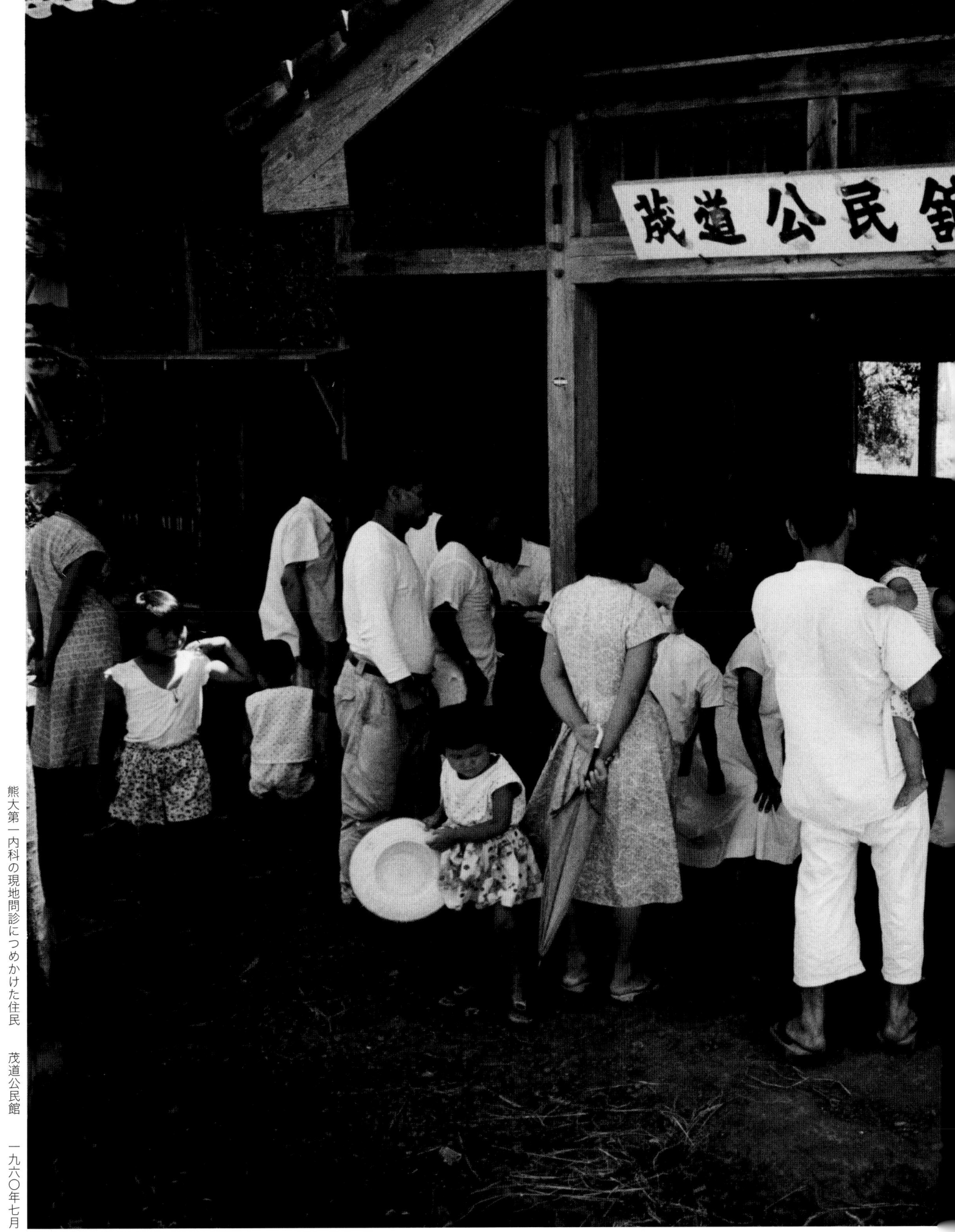

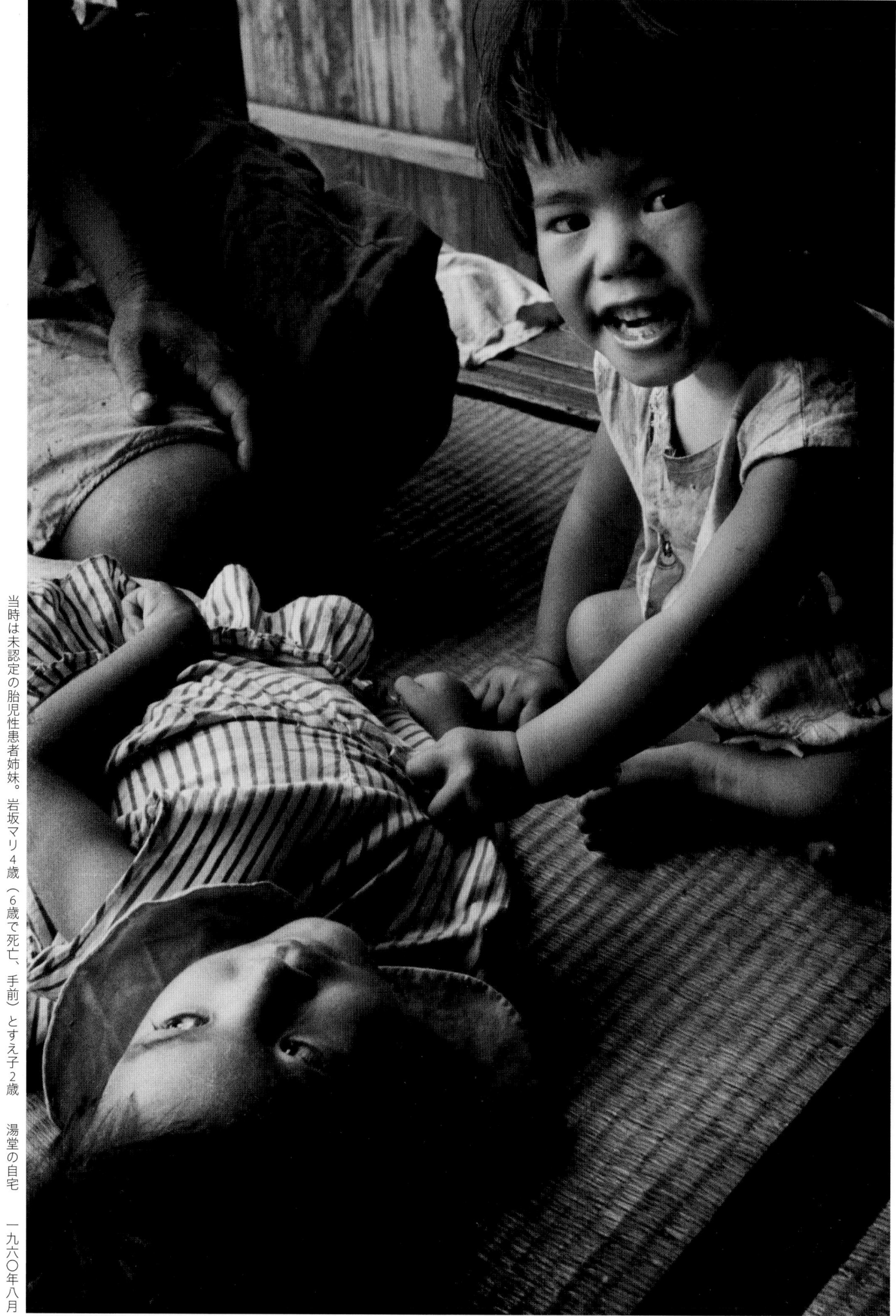

当時は未認定の胎児性患者姉妹。岩坂マリ4歳（6歳で死亡、手前）とすえ子2歳　湯堂の自宅　一九六〇年八月

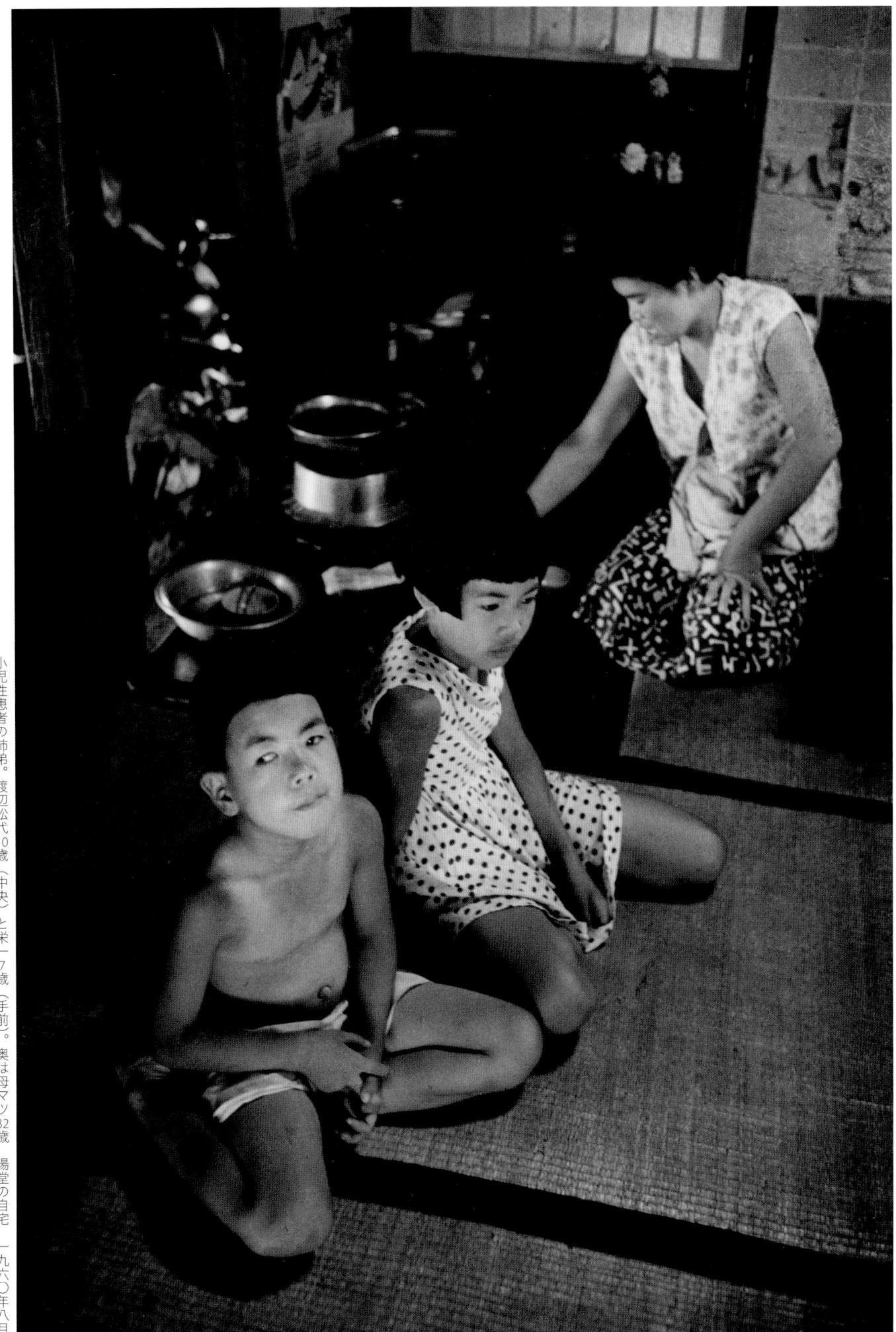

小児性患者の姉弟。渡辺松代10歳（中央）と栄一7歳（手前）。奥は母マツ32歳　湯堂の自宅　一九六〇年八月

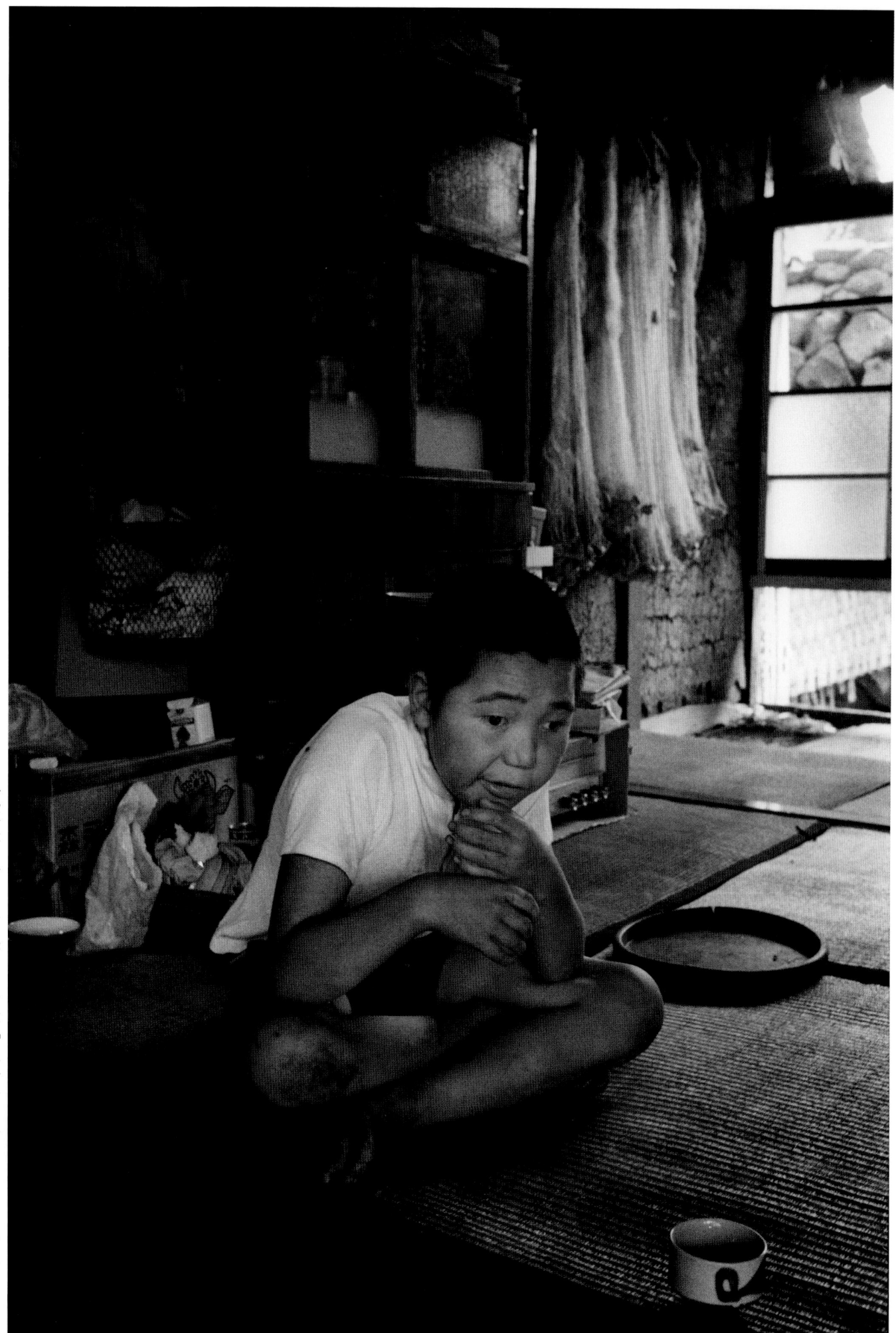

小児性患者の松田富次11歳。石牟礼道子『苦海浄土』冒頭に描かれた山中九平少年のモデル。目がみえずラジオで楽しむ野球と相撲では解説の"名人" 湯堂の自宅 一九六〇年八月

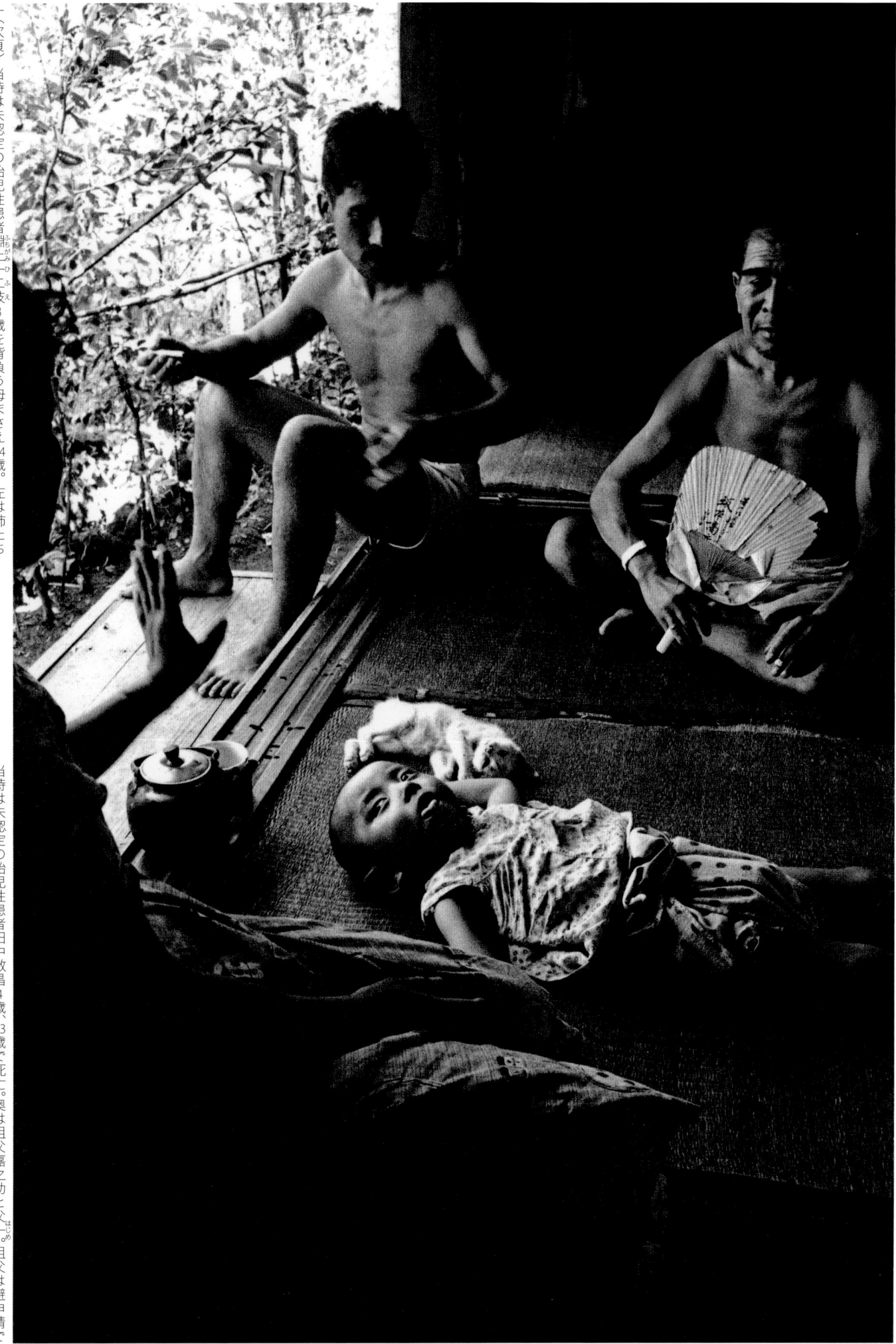

←〈次頁〉当時は未認定の胎児性患者淵上二二枝3歳を背負う母まさえ44歳。左は姉たち 茂道の旧海軍弾薬庫跡に住み着いた自宅 一九六〇年八月

当時は未認定の胎児性患者田中敏昌4歳、13歳で死亡。奥は祖父嘉之助と父一。祖父は避申請で死亡、祖母と父母は一〇年以上後に認定。猫も発病か 湯堂の自宅 一九六〇年七月

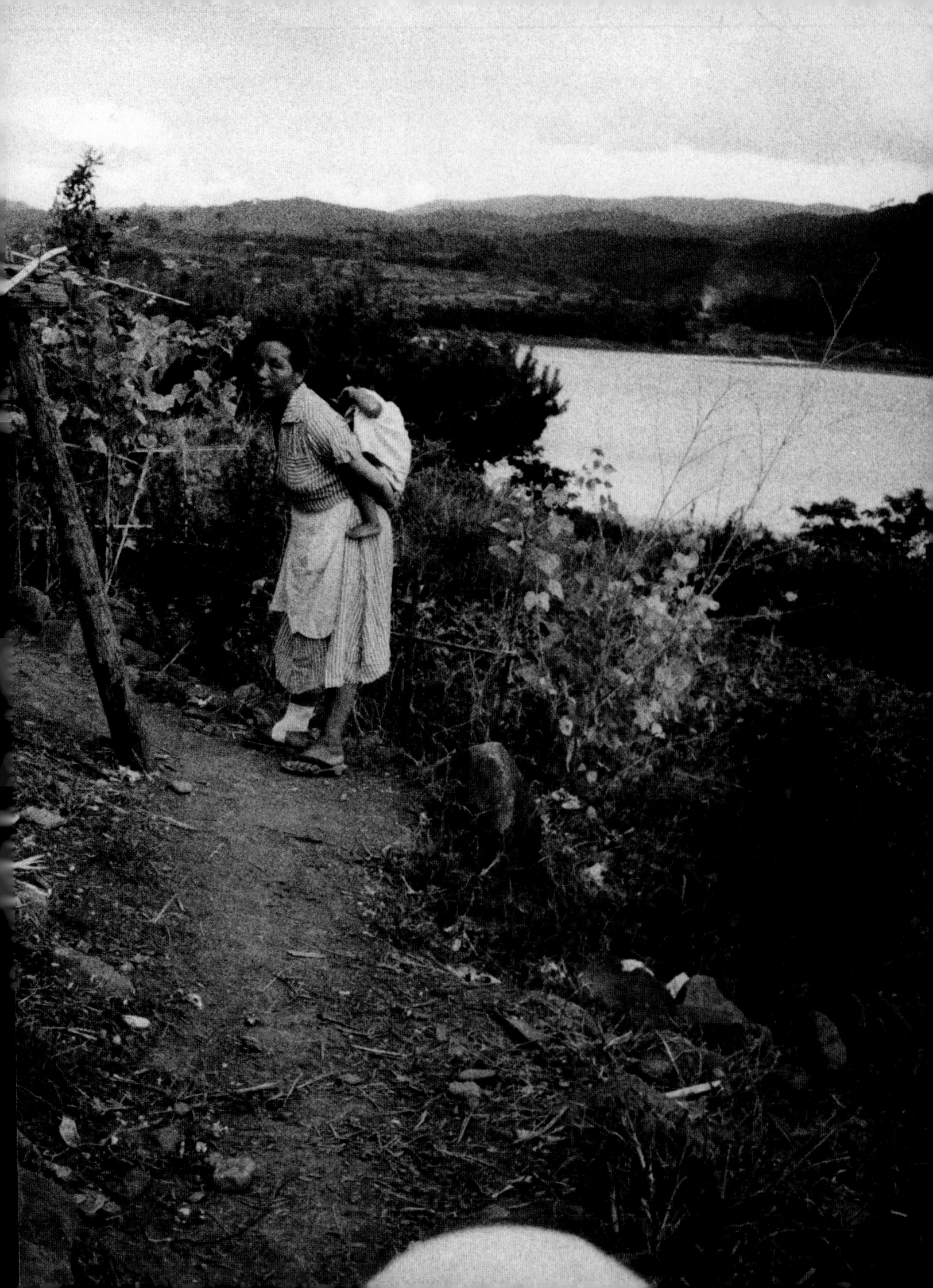

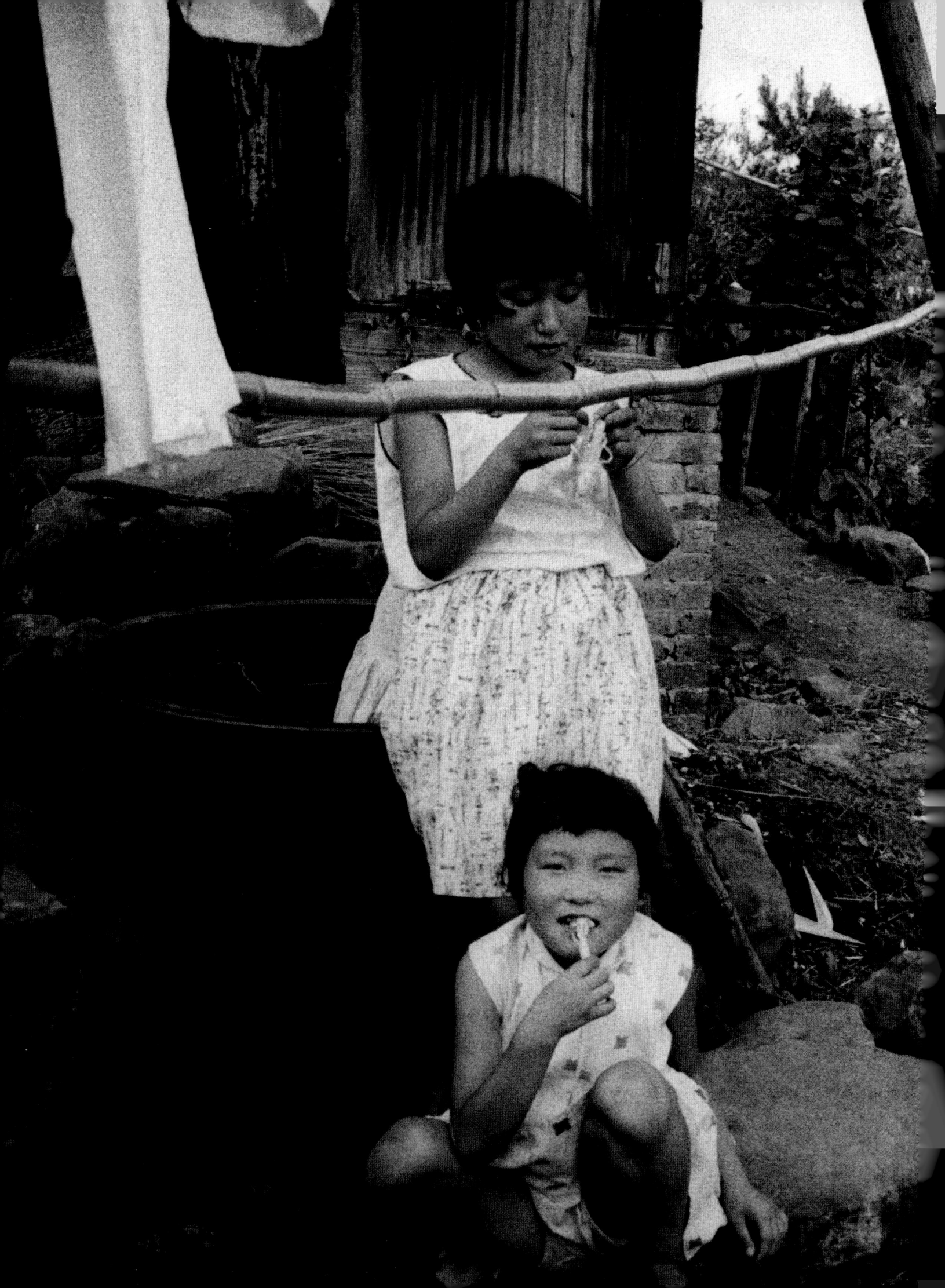

私の水俣病事件

「水俣病にはなってしまったが生きていて良かった」冥土連・設立宣言

旗野秀人

映画「阿賀に生きる」のつながり

私の本業は親の代から家を建てること。生まれ育ったところは河口から約三〇キロ上流の阿賀野川のほとりで、阿賀野市（旧安田町）は半世紀も同じ保守地盤の土建屋王国。水俣病事件があっても原発事故があってもそれは変わらない。この町で本業と水俣病に関わり続けて四〇年余りになる。

映画「阿賀に生きる」（一九九二年）は水俣病患者である以前に阿賀の川筋に暮らす人生の達人たちの日常をそのまま撮ってほしいと、酒の勢いで故佐藤真監督に語ったことが始まりだった。二〇年経った去年、三〇〇人余りからのカンパでニュープリントが完成し、全国の劇場でリバイバル上映中だ。出演してくれた患者さんが亡くなって始めた追悼集会も二一回を数える。毎年五月四日には親戚の法事みたいに全国から一〇〇人余りの老若男女が集い、こんなに楽しく笑っていいのかと不思議がる。幾組ものカップルがこの場で誕生し、子連れで里帰りもしてくれる。集いの途中で「冥土のみやげ全国連合」事務局長を名乗るHさんが突然、怪しげなTシャツを着てプログラムにはない、その設立を宣言した。「水俣病にはなってしまったが生きていて良かったと、患者さんに喜んで貰える冥土のみやげをつくろう！」

Tシャツの背中には「阿賀に生きる」のタイトル文字と同じ小山素雲さん揮毫の「冥土連」の太文字、胸には絵本「阿賀のお地蔵さん」の作者WAKKUNの若芽を持った少年。あの世の患者さんが次世代の肥やしとなって新しい芽が出る、そのキャラクターデザインを「輪廻」と理解した。フィナーレには早速、患者会の長老九六歳の参治さんがTシャツを着て歌い、大阪網かけ一座の皆さんが踊る。この集いこそがあの世とこの世を結ぶ「冥土のみやげ」だと思った。

「冥土のみやげ」をつくろう

「安田患者の会」は新潟水俣病第二次訴訟の元原告である。九五年の政治決着後に一番の望みを尋ねたら、温泉に泊まりがけで行きたいとのこと。当日は何度も温泉に浸かり、カラオケを皆で歌って大満足する。翌朝「ありがとね、冥土のみやげが出来たよ。生きていて良かった！」と感謝された。家族や支援者の手前、温泉やカラオケは我慢してきたという。

二〇〇人余りいた高齢の患者会はすでに十分の一に減っていた。裁判のため、運動のためと言いながら一番大事なことを忘れていた。高齢で残された僅かな時間ではあるが、とにかく楽しく喜んで貰える仕掛けをと「冥土のみやげ企画」を立ちあげる。春にはお花見会、会津コロリ三観音巡りにお地蔵さん石を探しに水俣へ。北は北海道から南は沖縄まで「冥土に生きる」のフィルムと「安田患者の会」の全国行脚が始まる。その主役は「阿賀のみやげツアー」の全国行脚が始まる。その主役は「阿賀のみやげ治さん。しかし、毎年のように同志は欠けて逝き、今はたったの六人となった。

民謡が大好きな参治さんの米寿のお祝いでは「唄は百薬の長」というCDアルバムをつくってプレゼントした。子どもの頃から盆踊りの櫓の上で太鼓を叩き、三度の飯より唄を好きなことは町中に知られ、しかも川漁師でも船頭でもない、屋根葺き職人でニセ患者代表のように陰口された。正直言って私も出会った頃

その元気さに驚き、もう少し「水俣病患者らしく」してほしいと思った。一五年ほど前、病院に行く途中で転倒し大腿骨を骨折、やむなくケアハウスに入居。まず始めたことは自慢の喉で「おはようございます」とあいさつ運動、食事の配膳の手伝い。車椅子競争では応援歌をつくり選手宣誓もやった。運動会ではいつも一等賞。「唄は薬だ」と朝一番で誰もいない食堂で歌い、夕食を終えてベットに入ってもまだ歌っている。ついには隣室から「老人らしくしてほしい」と事務所に通報される。ありのままの参治さんを私はようやく承知できて自分自身も解放された。

常に患者さんの傍に

思えば一九七一年の暮れにチッソ本社前での故川本輝夫さんとの出会いが、水俣病事件に関わったきっかけだった。初めて訪ねた患者さんに門前払いされ、ようやく家族のようにつきあい始めたG家の四二歳のアキさんが四人の子どもを遺して自死する場面に遭遇し、あまりのショックで為す術もない私に「すぐに行ってやれ、傍に居てやることが大事だ」と亡き母は教えてくれた。

その後、未認定問題から行政不服や第二次訴訟そして和解といろいろあったが、常に患者さんの傍にいて大事さを自覚する。そしていま、「冥土連」の立ち上げをJA職員やガソリンスタンドマンにパチンコ屋の若者たちが面白がって手伝ってくれている。私は新しい同志を迎え、なんだかワクワクして落ちつかないでいる。

（はたの・ひでと／建築大工・新潟水俣病安田患者の会事務局）

12 新潟水俣病事件

同じ原因で二度も惨禍が起きた。今度は新潟県の川魚を食べる人がやられた。水俣事件を調べた宇井純は述べる。「私と桑原氏が、会社側の秘密実験の結果を知ったにもかかわらず、公表しないために第二の水俣病が阿賀野川で発生した責任のある部分を、私は負わなければならない」（自著『水俣病』）

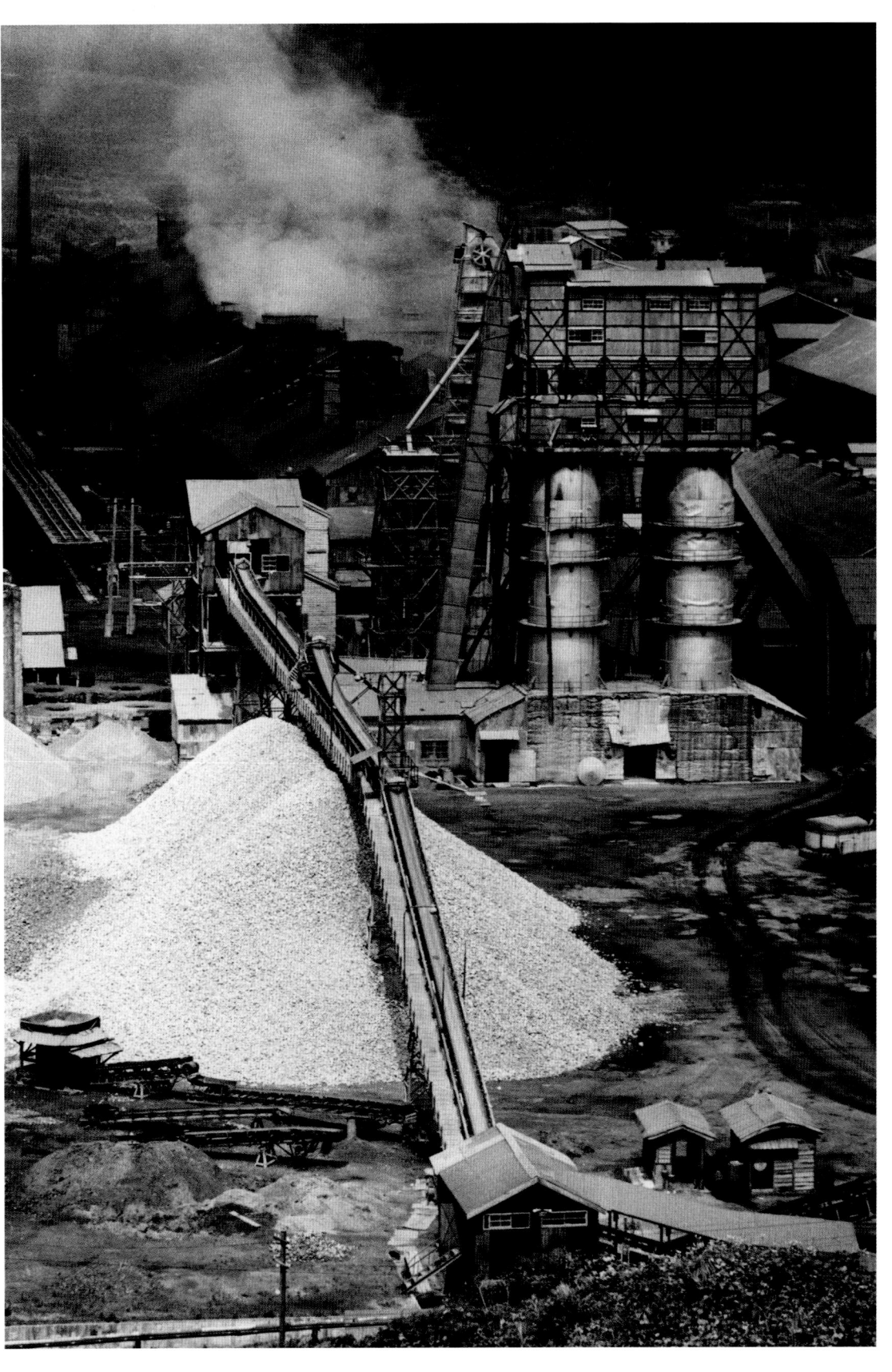

加害企業は昭和電工鹿瀬工場。第一の水俣事件と同類の有機水銀排水たれ流しのアセトアルデヒド工程があった。一九六五年に事件が表面化した工程の生産停止へ向かっていた　新潟県鹿瀬町　一九六七年八月

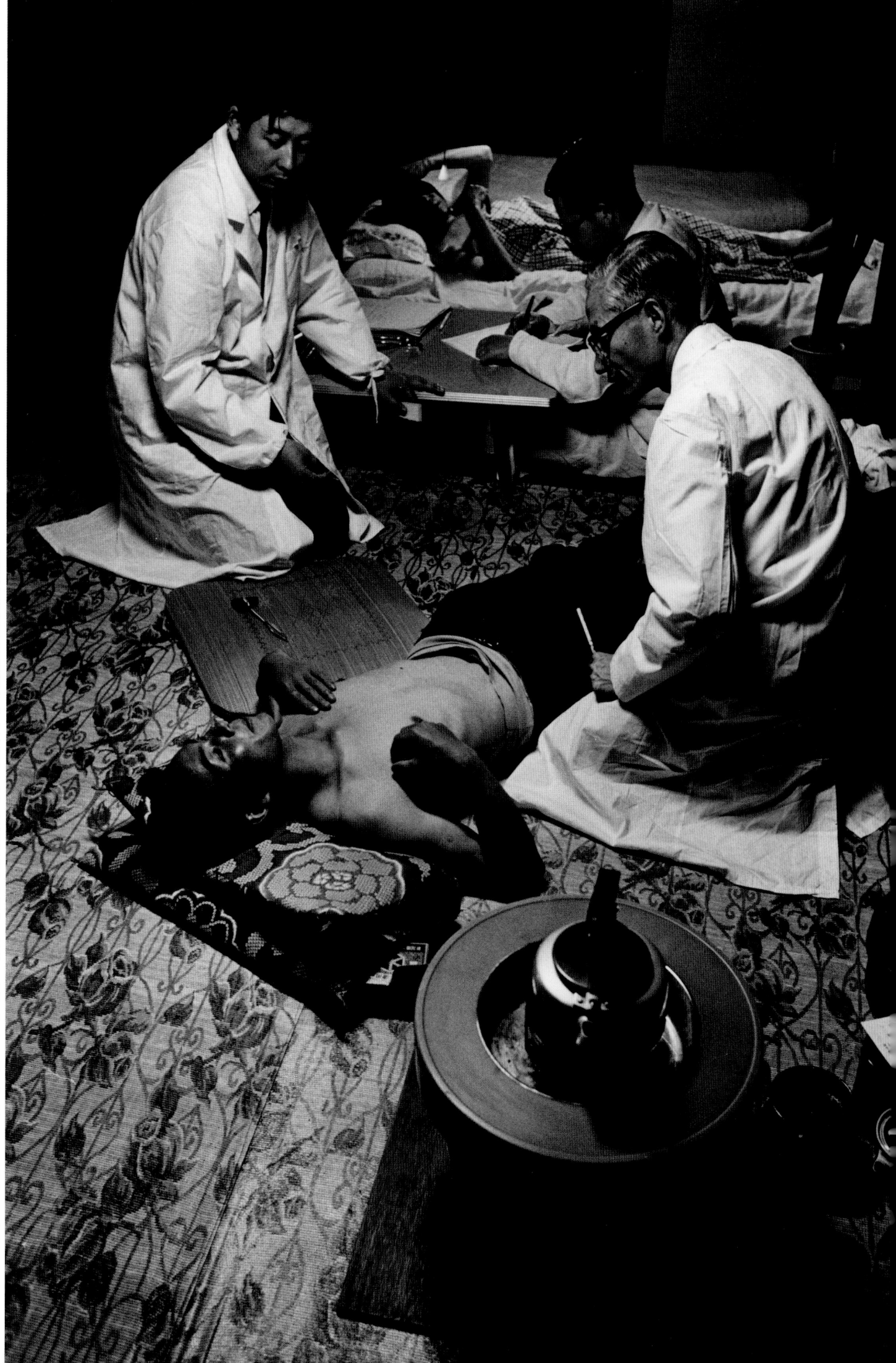

阿賀野川流域の住民検診。一九六〇年にあった水俣事件での問診とは違う風景だった　新潟市大川など三会場　一九六七年六月

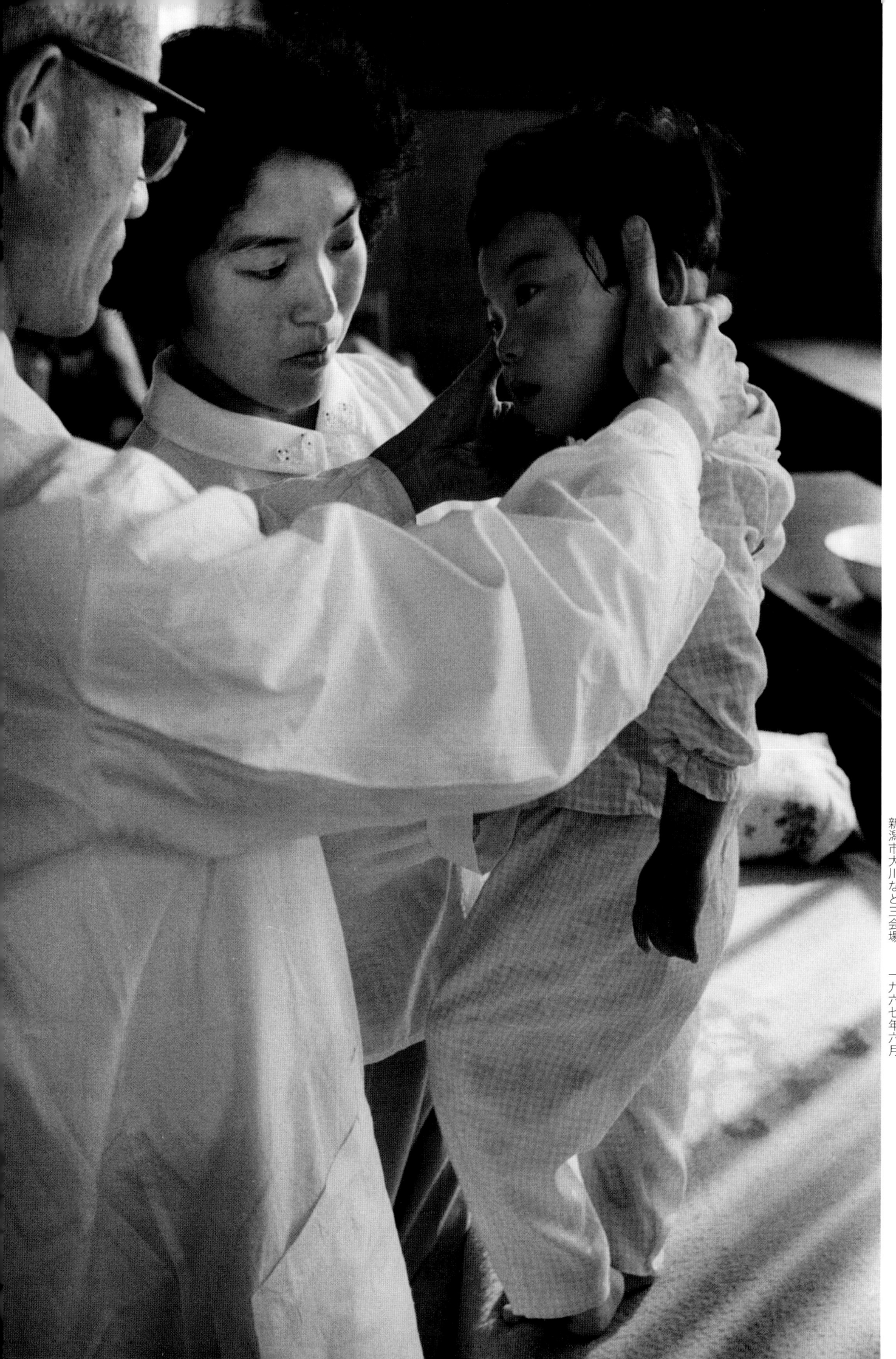

当時は未認定の胎児性患者、古山知恵子を診察する新潟大教授椿忠雄。認定は三年後 新潟市大川など三会場 一九六七年六月

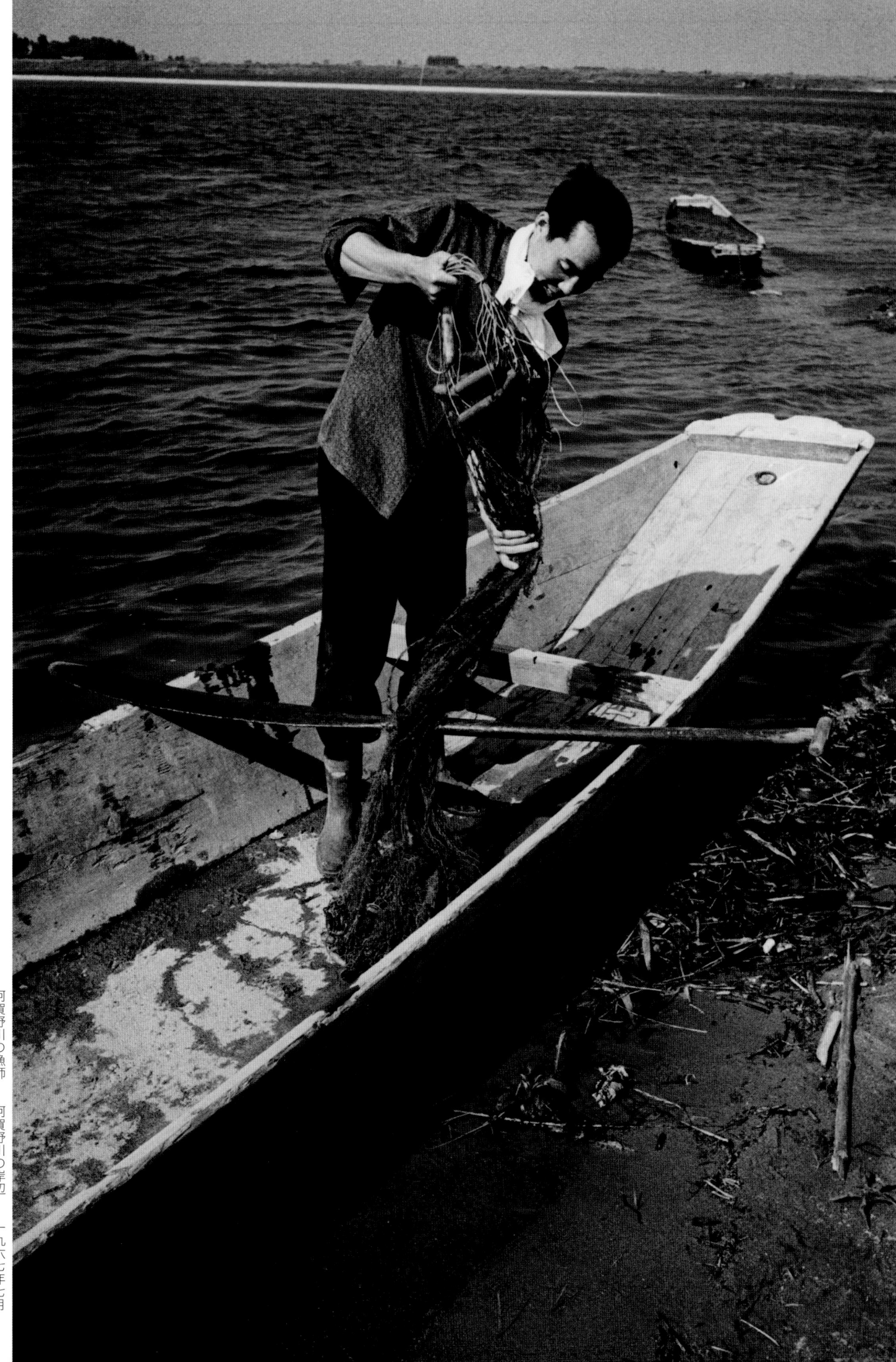

阿賀野川の漁師　阿賀野川の岸辺　一九六七年七月

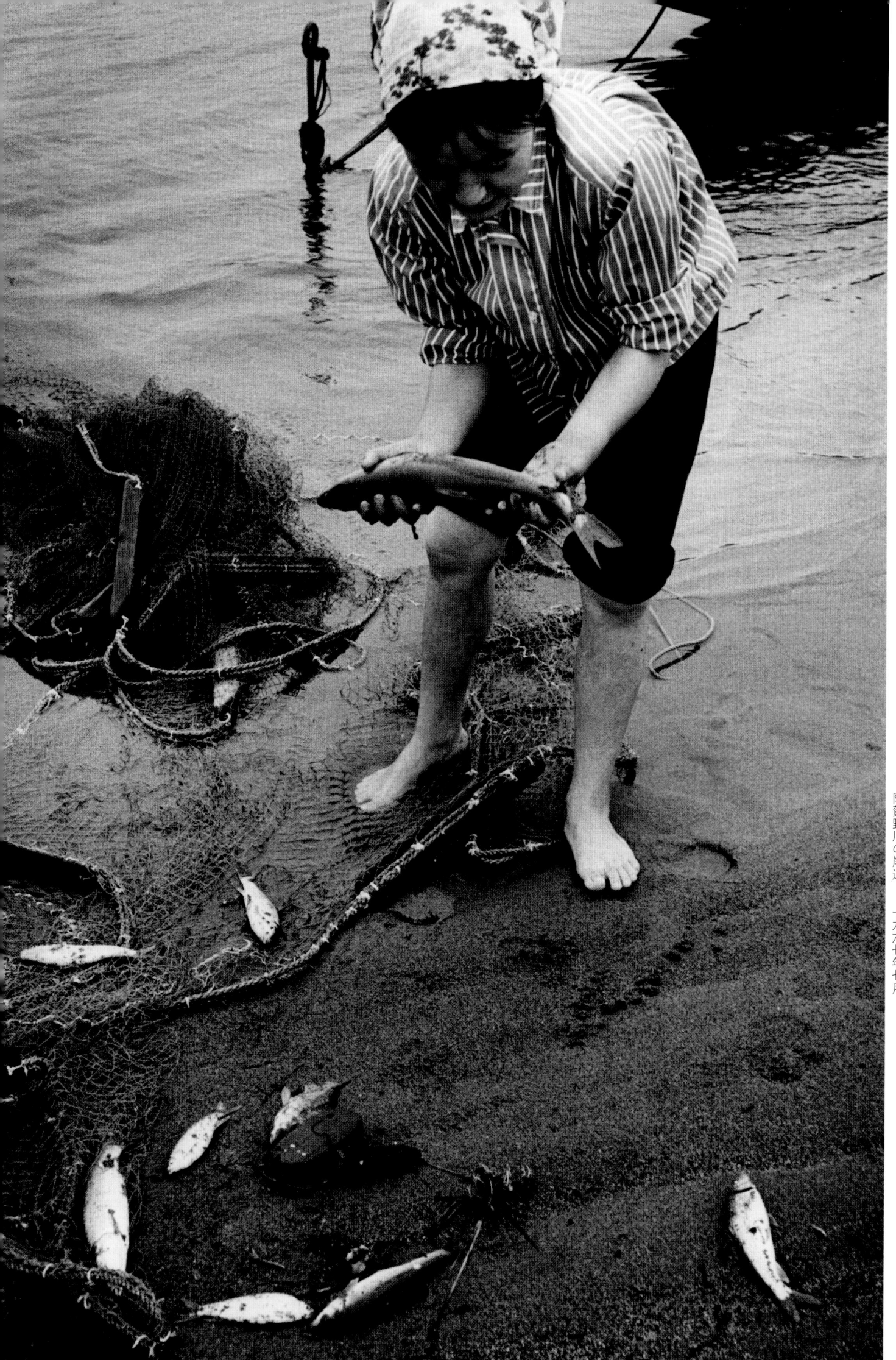

下流部の水流量は日本最大級。川の魚はでかい。魚をつかむのは重症患者だった桑野忠吾の娘　阿賀野川の岸辺　一九六七年七月

私の水俣病事件

見舞金契約と細川証言

坂東克彦

桑原史成さんの最初の写真集は、新潟水俣病第一次訴訟の書証としても提出された。彼の写真が訴訟運動に与えた影響も大きく、私にとっても忘れ得ぬ人の一人である。この事件で欠かせぬ重要部分の事実を以下列記して、本書への記録としたい。

見舞金契約

昭和三一年五月一日、水俣病患者の発見が新日窒水俣工場の排水所へ届けられた。水俣病の原因が工場排水にあることは早くから疑われていた。

昭和三四年八月、熊本大学医学部研究班が、「原因はある種の有機水銀である」と発表したことによって水俣病の原因が工場排水にあることが確定的になった。工場技術部では、アセトアルデヒド合成中に有機水銀が生成されることをモデルプラントを使った実験によって確認していた。また、同工場附属病院細川一院長がアセトアルデヒド排水を直接投与していたネコ四〇〇号が昭和三四年一〇月に水俣病症状を呈していることを確認し、同年一一月三〇日の社内研究班会議の席上、細川が工場幹部に四〇〇号ネコ発症の事実を報告していた。

これら二つの事実は、水俣工場の排水が水俣病の原因であることを示す重要な事実であったが、チッソはこの事実を秘匿し続けていた。

昭和三四年一二月三〇日、水俣病患者家庭互助会とチッソとの間で、いわゆる「見舞金契約」が締結された。見舞金契約は、チッソが死者一人に対する三〇万円の見舞金と生存患者に対する年金を主な内容とするものであったが、契約書には「将来水俣病が工場排水に起因しないことが決定した場合において」はその月をもって見舞金の交付を打ち切る。（第四条）」、「水俣病が工場排水に起因することが決定した場合においても新たな補償金の要求は一切行わない。（第五条）」とする条項が入れられていた。

見舞金契約の締結を契機に、会社はアセトアルデヒドの生産設備を増設し、有機水銀を含む排水を以前にも増して大量に不知火海に排出し続け、これによって水俣病の被害は不知火海全域に広がり、水俣病被害を一層深刻なものにしていった。

細川ノート

昭和四四年四月二九日、坂東は水俣病市民会議の要請をうけて、細川が保管しているネコ四〇〇号に関する記録の存在とその内容を確認するため伊予大洲の細川宅を訪ねた。細川が坂東に示したノートには次のように書かれていた。

○34醋酸係排水を直接猫に投与した実験

【病理組織学的所見】（九大遠城寺）猫No.四〇〇（中略）

【実験方法】
醋酸係の排水を毎日二〇cc宛基礎食にかけて経口投与した

（動物猫）当院で二回とりに行った。
7/21-10/7-10/24　昭三四　病状発現　衰弱のため屠殺した。

【註】
（1）この実験は切望したが出来なかった。西氏が排水をとりに行ったが拒まれた。
（2）病理所見は大島君から九大にたのんだ。
（3）工場長転勤の際許可を得て再び開始す。之がH・I液である。H・I実験は東大へ依頼したが（斎藤氏渡米前）紛失した。

（4）社内研究班会議（技術部側—徳江、市川、上妻、川崎、病院側—細川、久保田、小島、大島出席）。
昭三四・一一・三〇
病院側から係排水の研究（本実験）を強調したが徳江氏等にけられた。

坂東は、このノートが工場排水でネコが発症していたという動かしがたい証拠であると考え、カメラに収めた。

細川証言

昭和四五年七月四日、東京 大塚の癌研究所附属病院において細川の臨床尋問が行われた。坂東は、予め準備していたノートの写真を細川に示して尋問した。細川は、社内研究班会議における猫四〇〇号発症の報告を中心に詳細な証言を行った。

地裁判決

昭和四八年三月二〇日、熊本地裁は熊本水俣病第一次訴訟の判決を言い渡した。判決は見舞金契約について次のように述べている。

本件見舞金契約は、加害者である被告が、いたずらに損害賠償義務を否定して、患者らの正当な損害賠償請求に応じようとせず、被害者である患者ないしその近親者の無知と経済的急迫状態に乗じて、生命、身体の侵害に対する補償額としては極端に低額の見舞金を支払い、そのかわりに、損害賠償請求権を一切放棄させるものであるから、民法第九〇条にいわゆる公序良俗に違反するものと認めるのが相当であり、したがって無効である。（原文のまま）

（ばんどう・かつひこ／弁護士）

13 労働争議の町と化した水俣

三井三池炭鉱争議の二年後、一九六二年に総資本と総労働の対決が町を巻き込む。「安定的に賃上げを約束する間、ストは一切しない」との協定を迫る経団連路線の新日窒提案に、労働基本権剥奪だと総評と合化労連。引くに引けぬ長期ロックアウトとストで、現地の労組も商店街も家庭も分裂した。

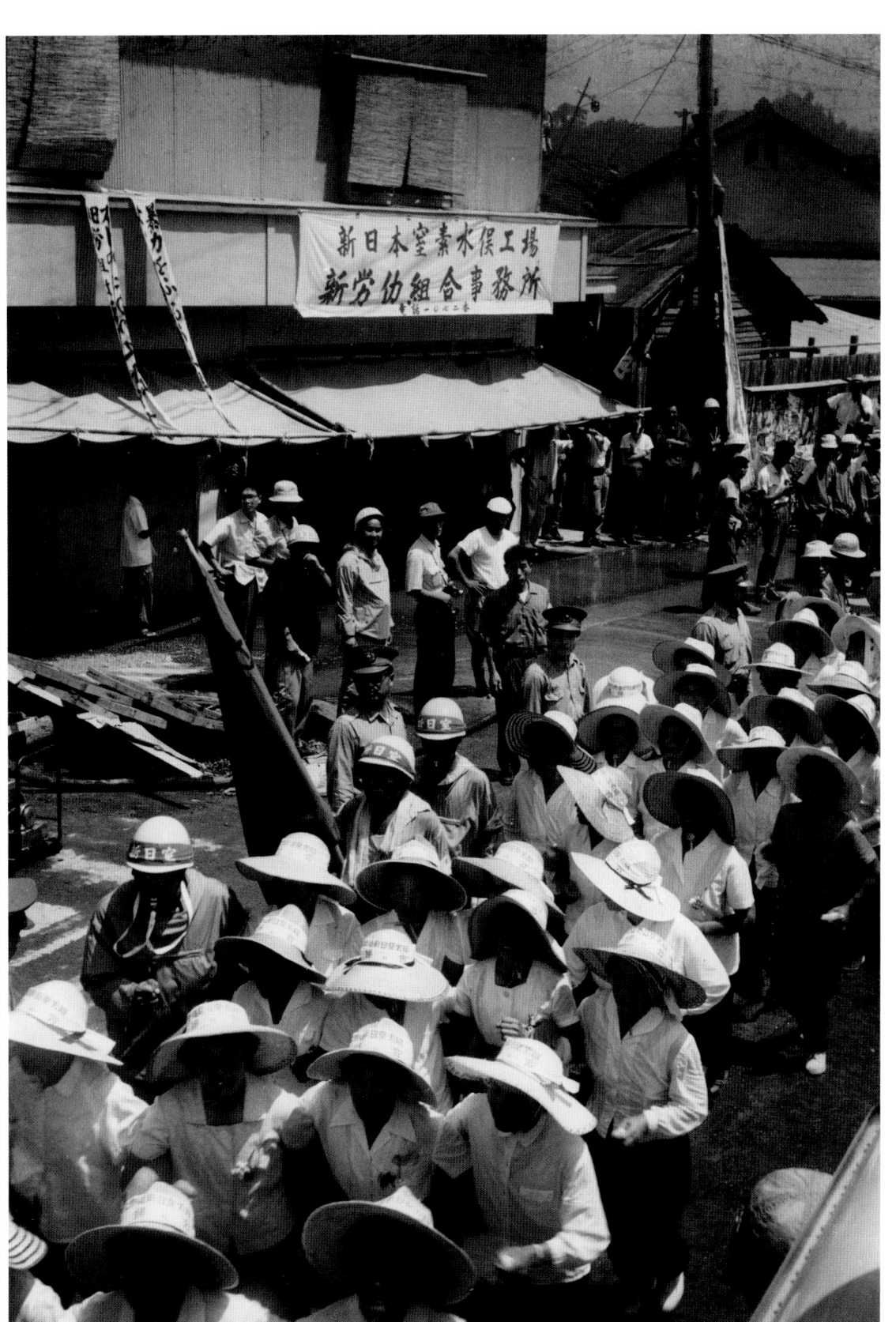

第二労組（新労）の事務所前に、第一労組が主婦を先頭にデモ。会社の第一労組差別に対抗する一〇年闘争で、後に水俣病患者の裁判闘争を支援する労働者も生まれた　水俣市中心街　一九六二年八月

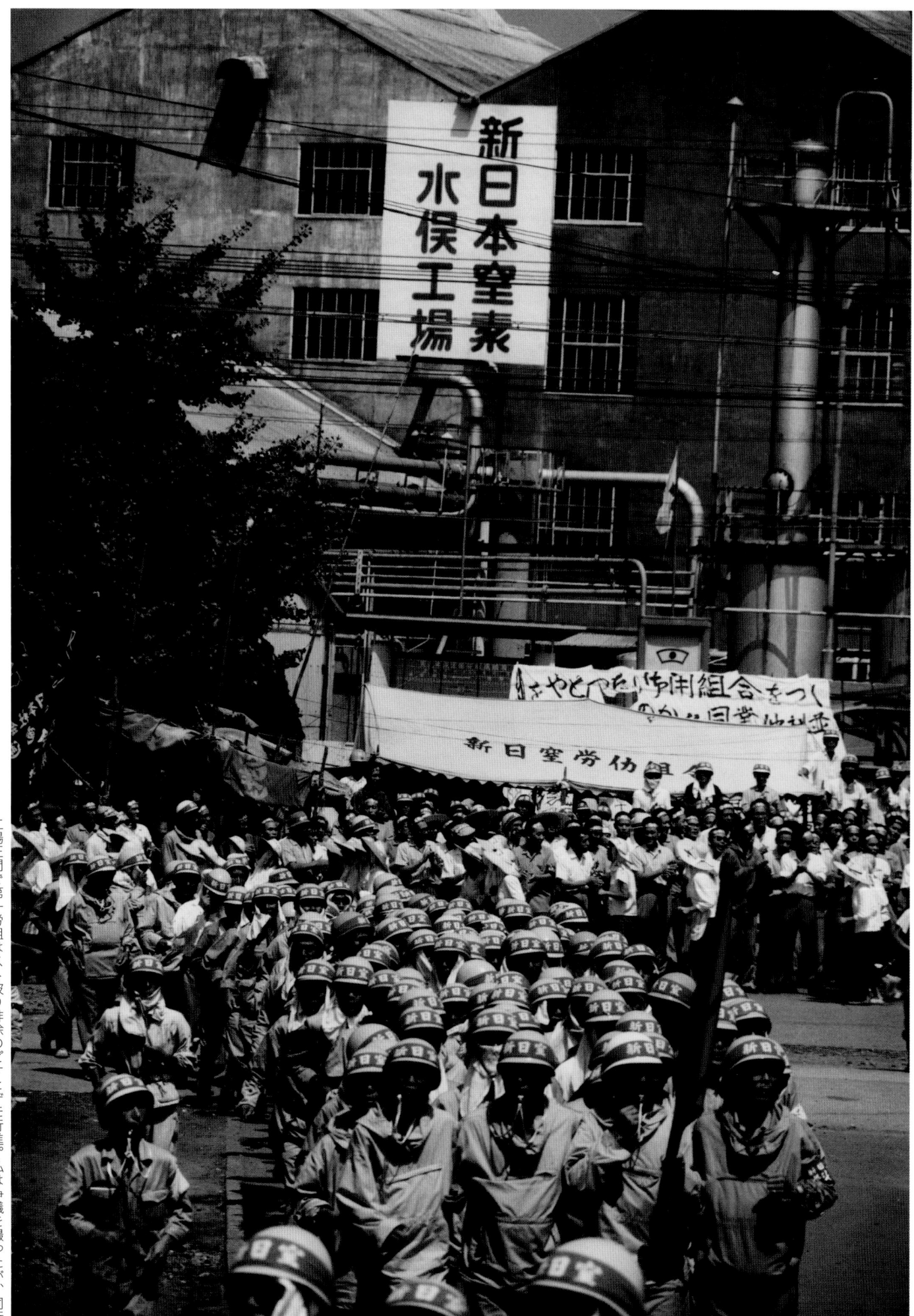

工場正門で第一労組はスト破り排除のピケとデモ行進。私は争議を撮ったが、同行の宇井純は争議には見向きもせず、水俣病事件を調べていた　一九六二年八月

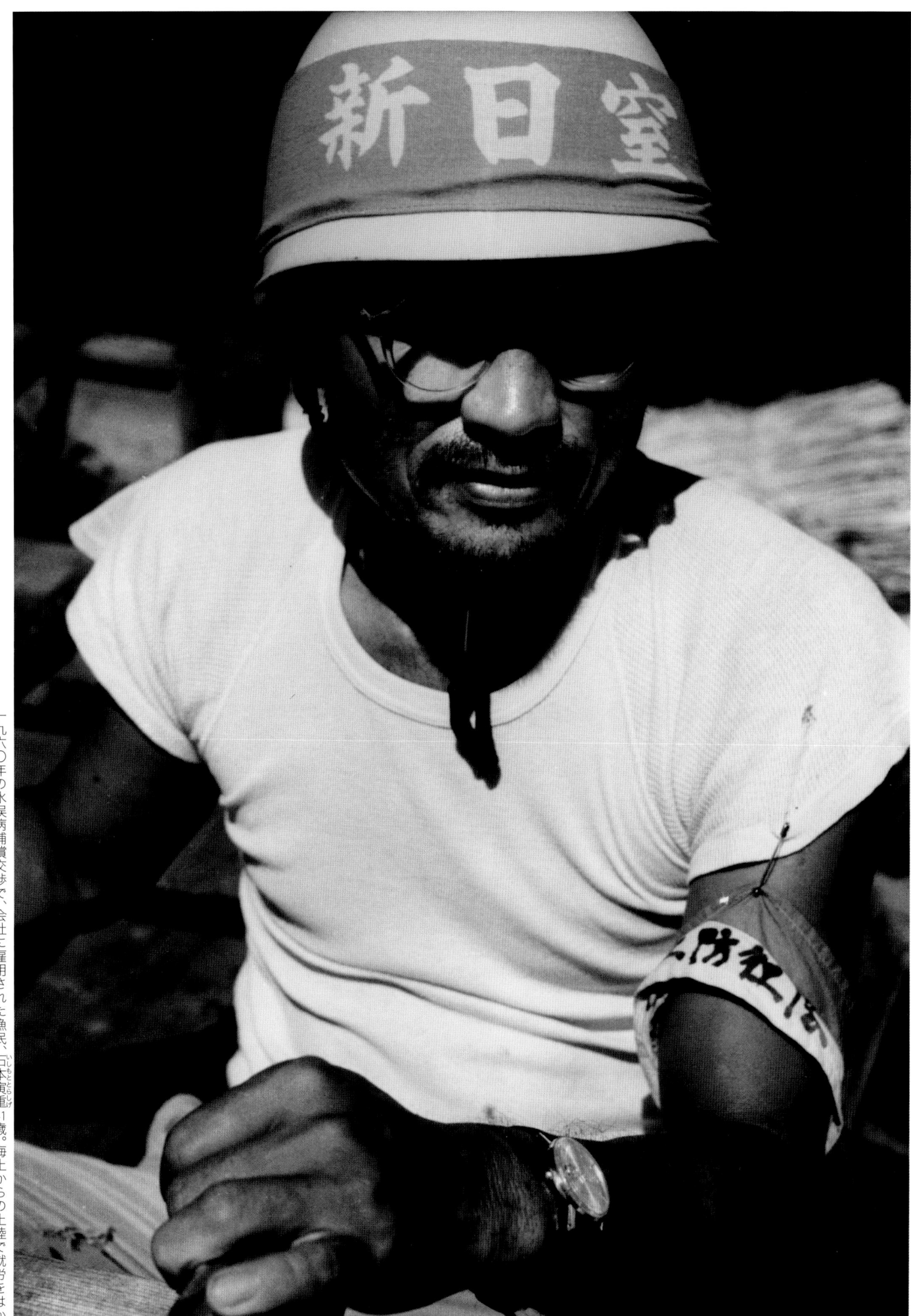

一九六〇年の水俣病補償交渉で、会社に雇用された漁民、石本寅重41歳。海上からの上陸で就労をはかる第二労組側を漁船で監視した。隠れ患者だったが、七三年六月認定　水俣湾　一九六二年八月

14 熊本水俣病一次訴訟

患者への支援活動の始まりは、一九六八年一月に、宇井純らの呼びかけで新潟の患者らが水俣を訪問してからだった。水俣病対策市民会議の発足、同年九月の政府による水俣病の公害病認定を経て、患者の訴訟派が翌年補償を求めて提訴、支援運動は全国へ。

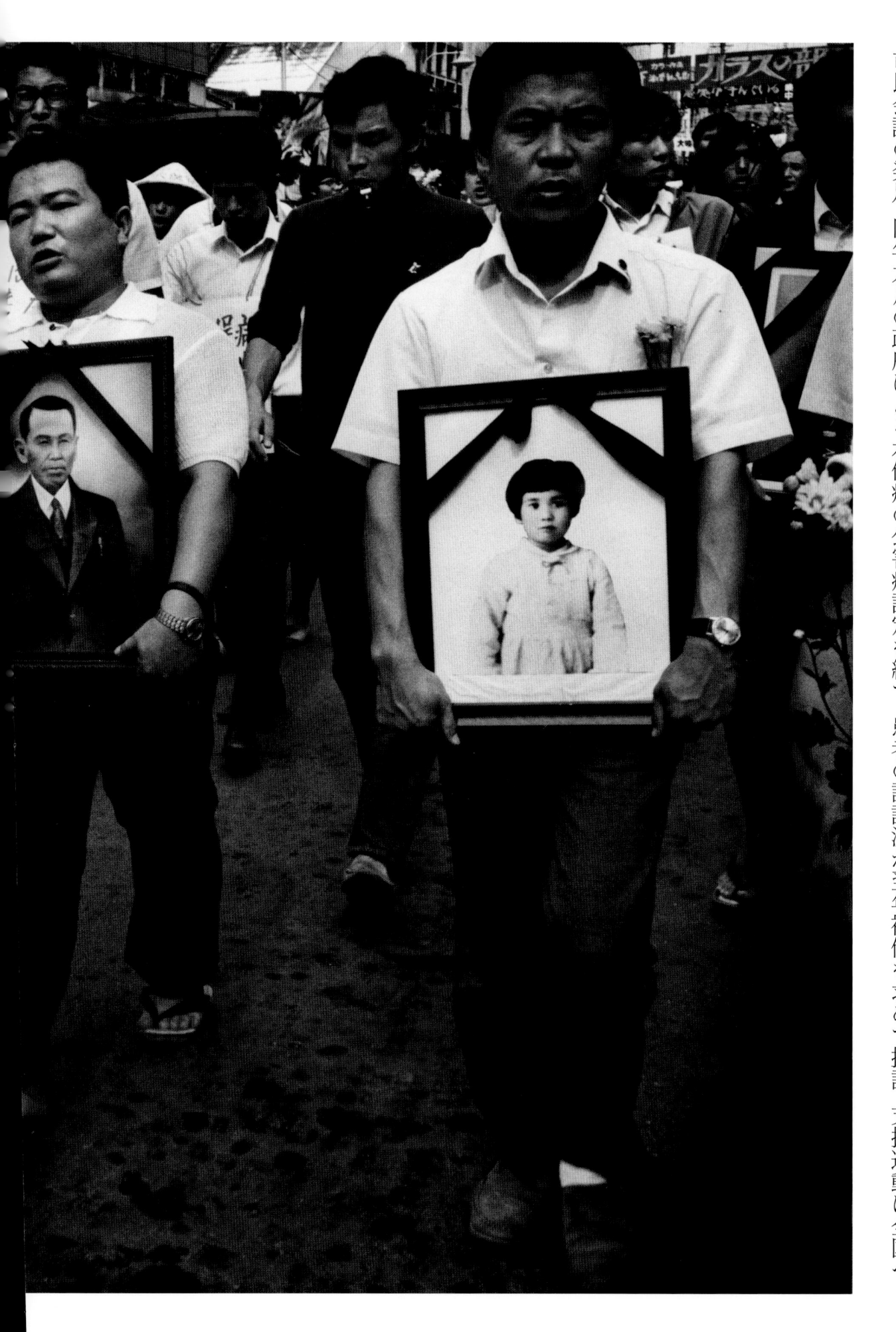

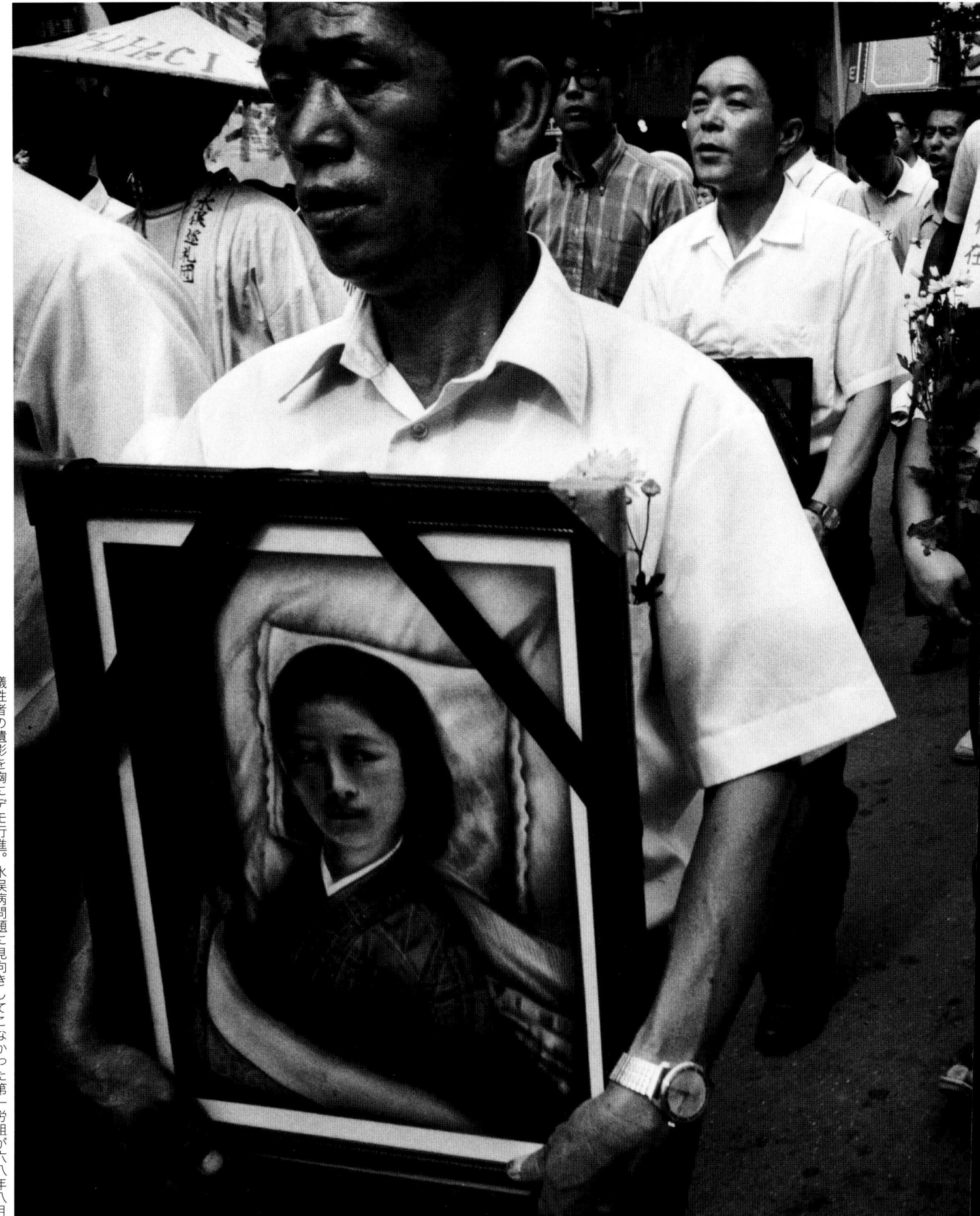

犠牲者の遺影を胸にデモ行進。水俣病問題に見向きもしてこなかった第一労組が六八年八月に「恥宣言」を出し、デモに参加する労働者も　熊本市の中心街　一九七〇年七月

患者支援デモの先頭に私の作品が無断で掲げられる。東京・水俣病を告発する会の発足日　都内　一九七〇年六月

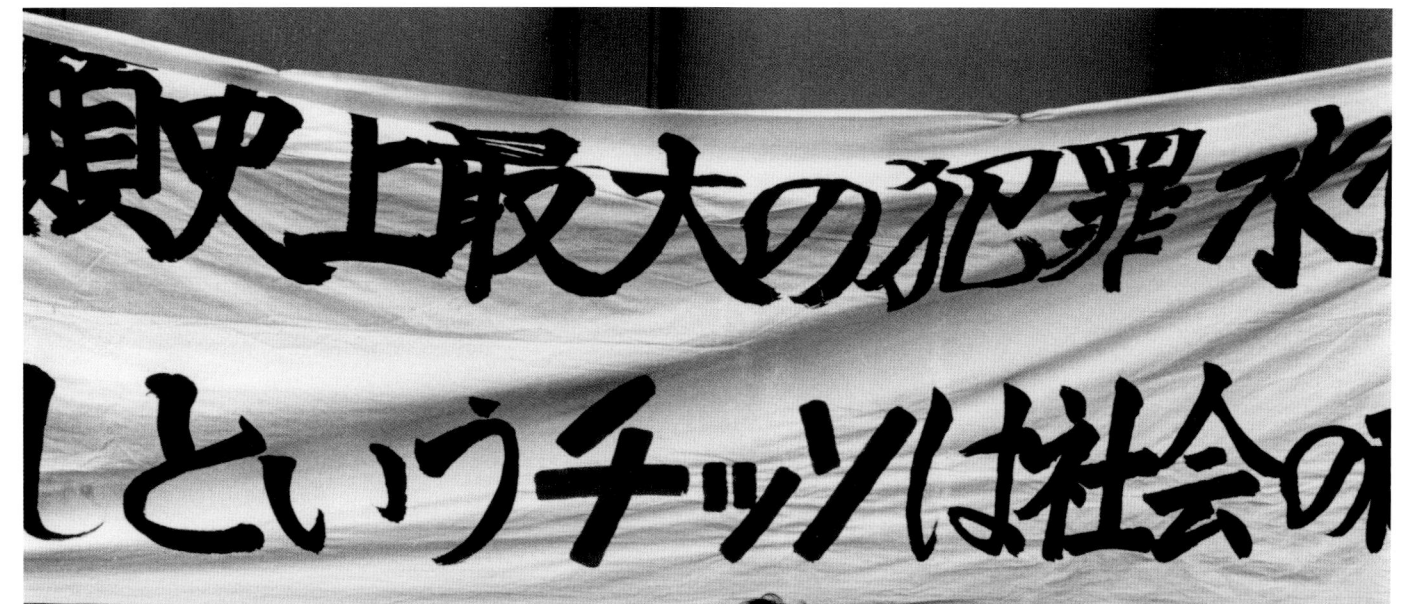

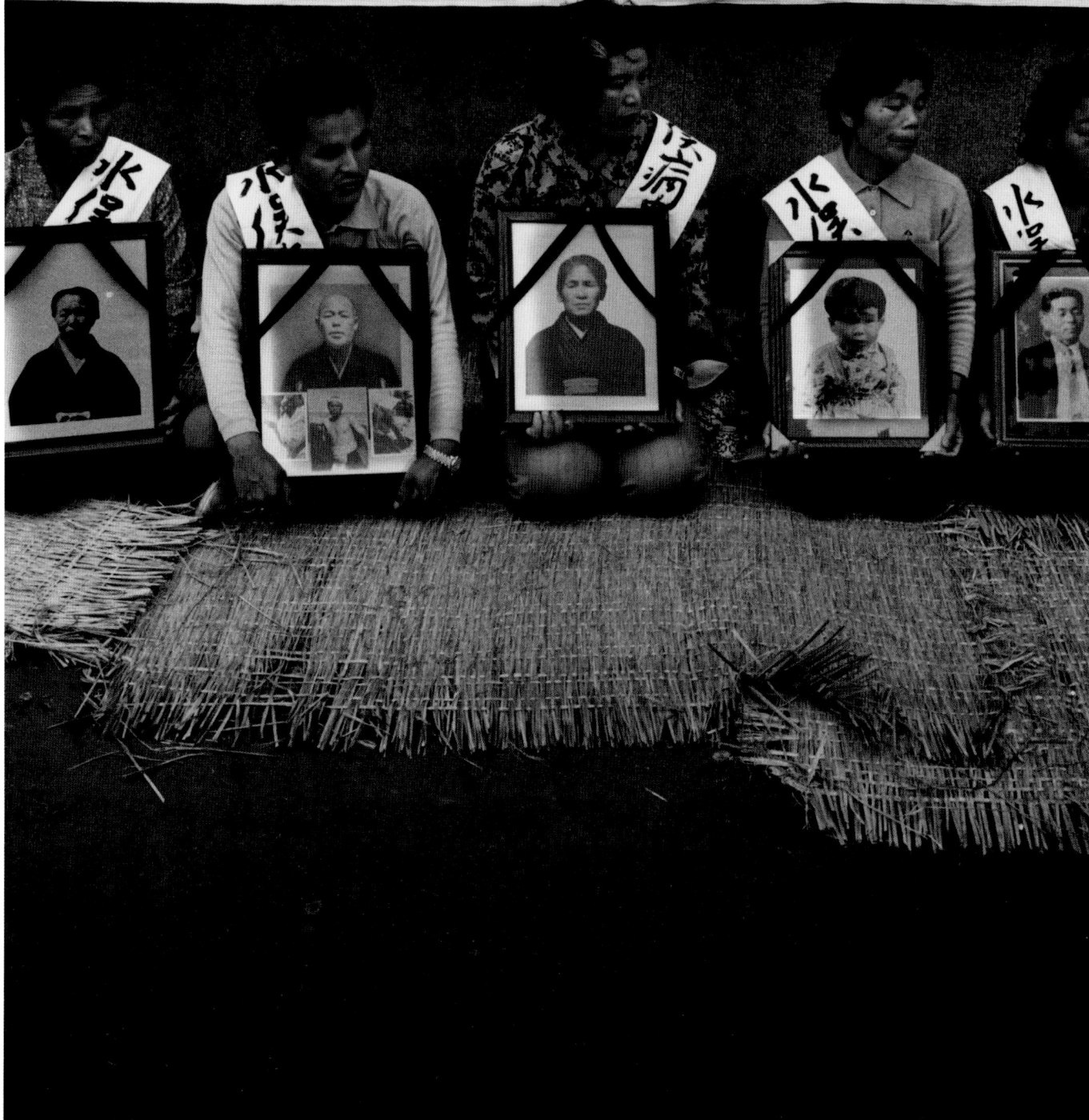

患者が上京して初の座り込み。厚生省に補償額をまかせる一任派への低額補償に訴訟派が抗議　東京駅近くのチッソ東京本社前　一九七〇年五月

15 苦海地獄

「俺っどもにはな、地獄も地獄。だれも助けてはくれんじゃったぞ」。会社との見舞金契約（一九五九年末）で得た金は、生活保護費から差し引かれた。漁獲高は、一九五〇―五三年平均で年四六〇トン。年々ガタ減りで五八年は四一トン。五九年には、魚の買い手がなくなった。

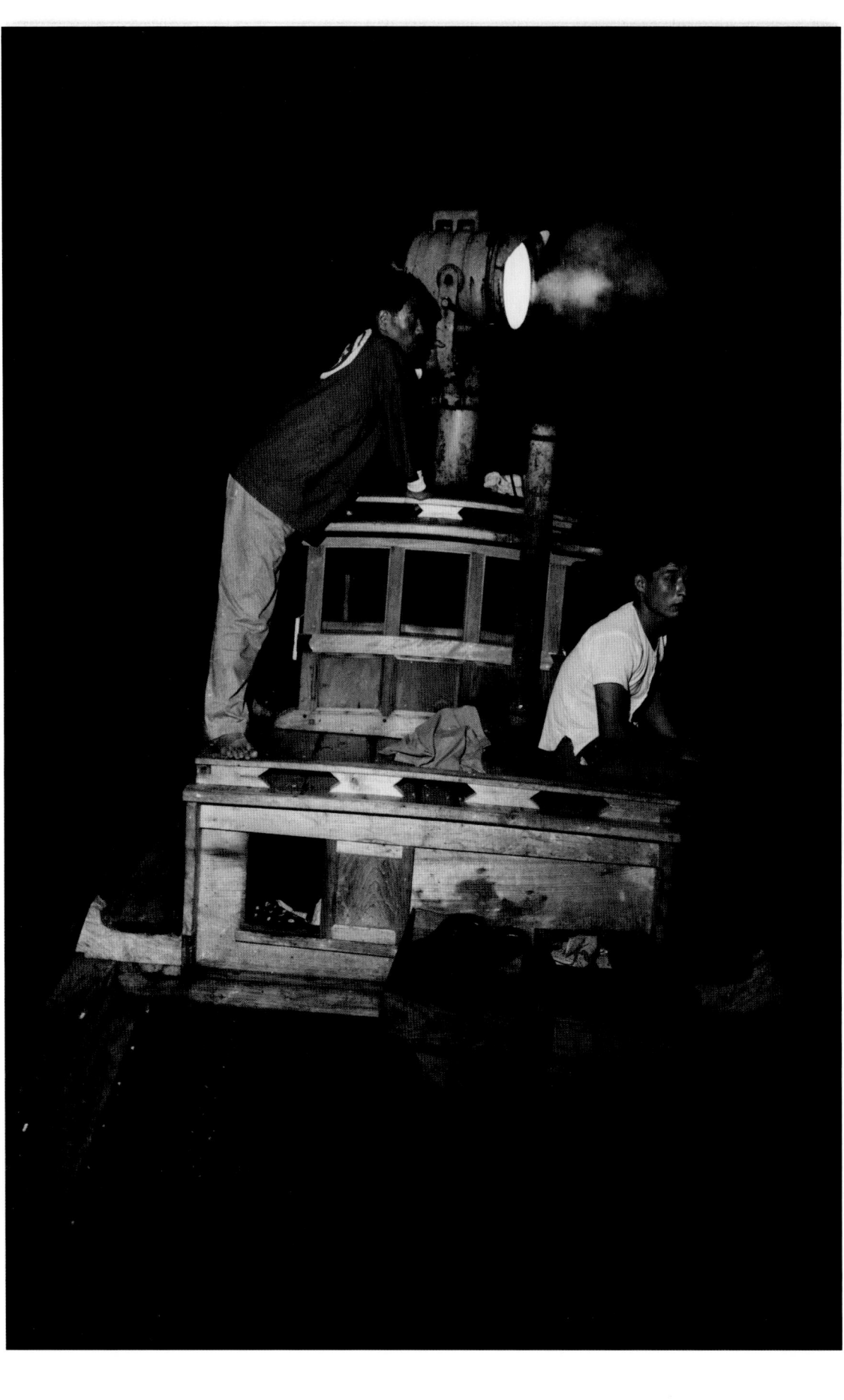

"密漁"を防げ。湾内は操業自主規制、漁協は自らの船で夜も監視した　一九六二年八月

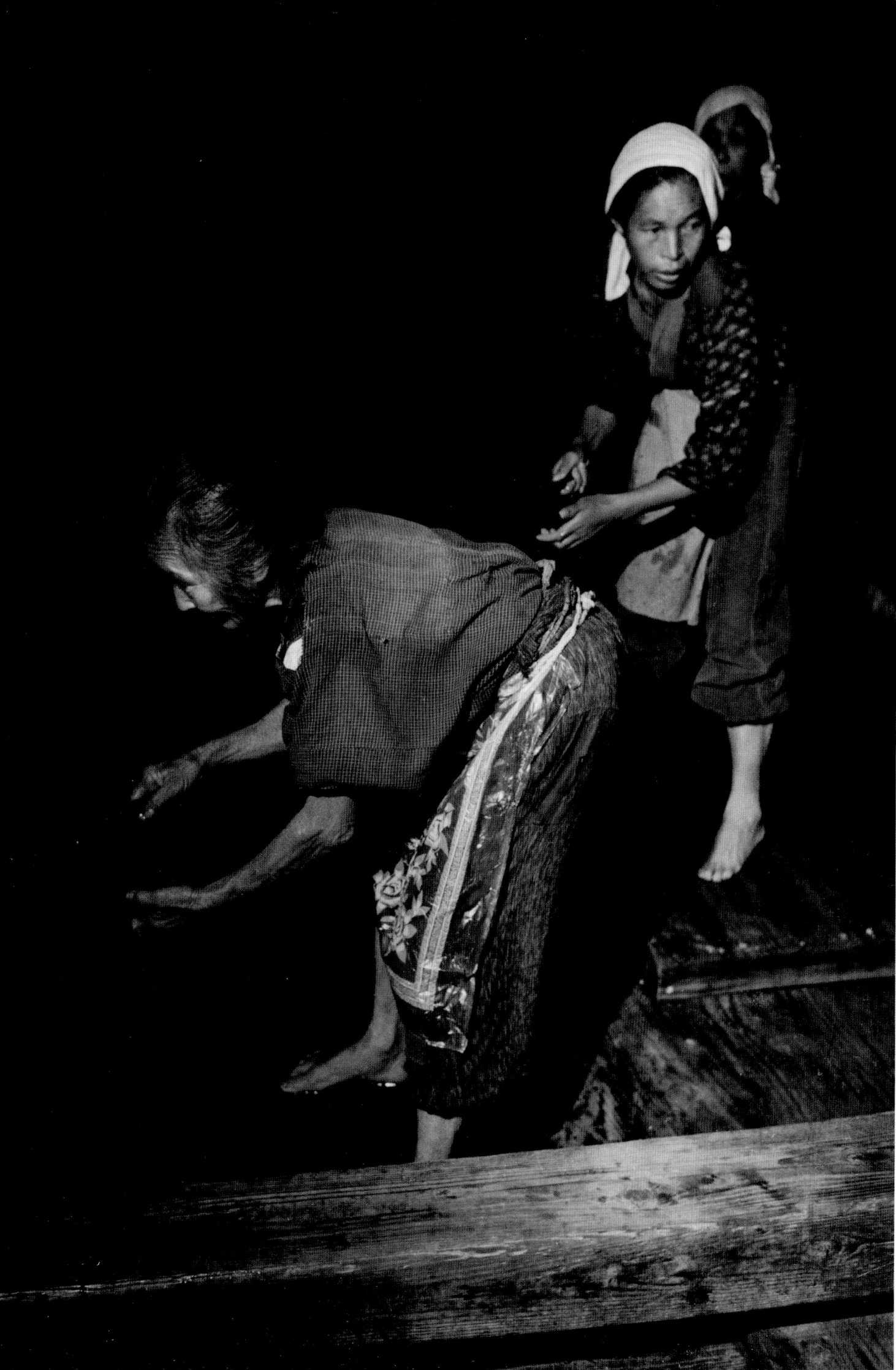

自主規制のない湾外へ、暗いうちから仕事の網子　一九六〇年八月

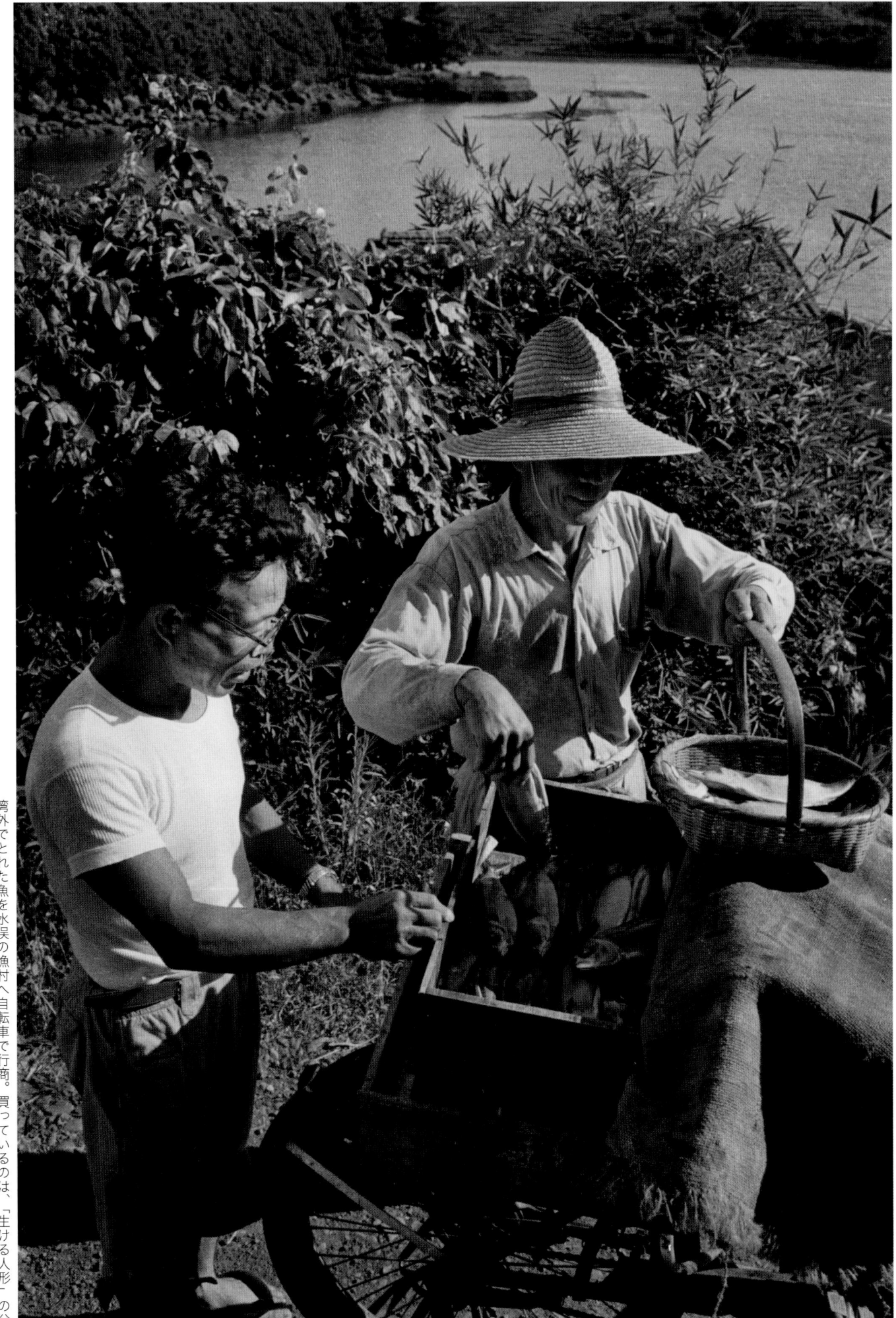

湾外でとれた魚を水俣の漁村へ自転車で行商。買っているのは、「生ける人形」の父、松永善一44歳　一九六〇年七月

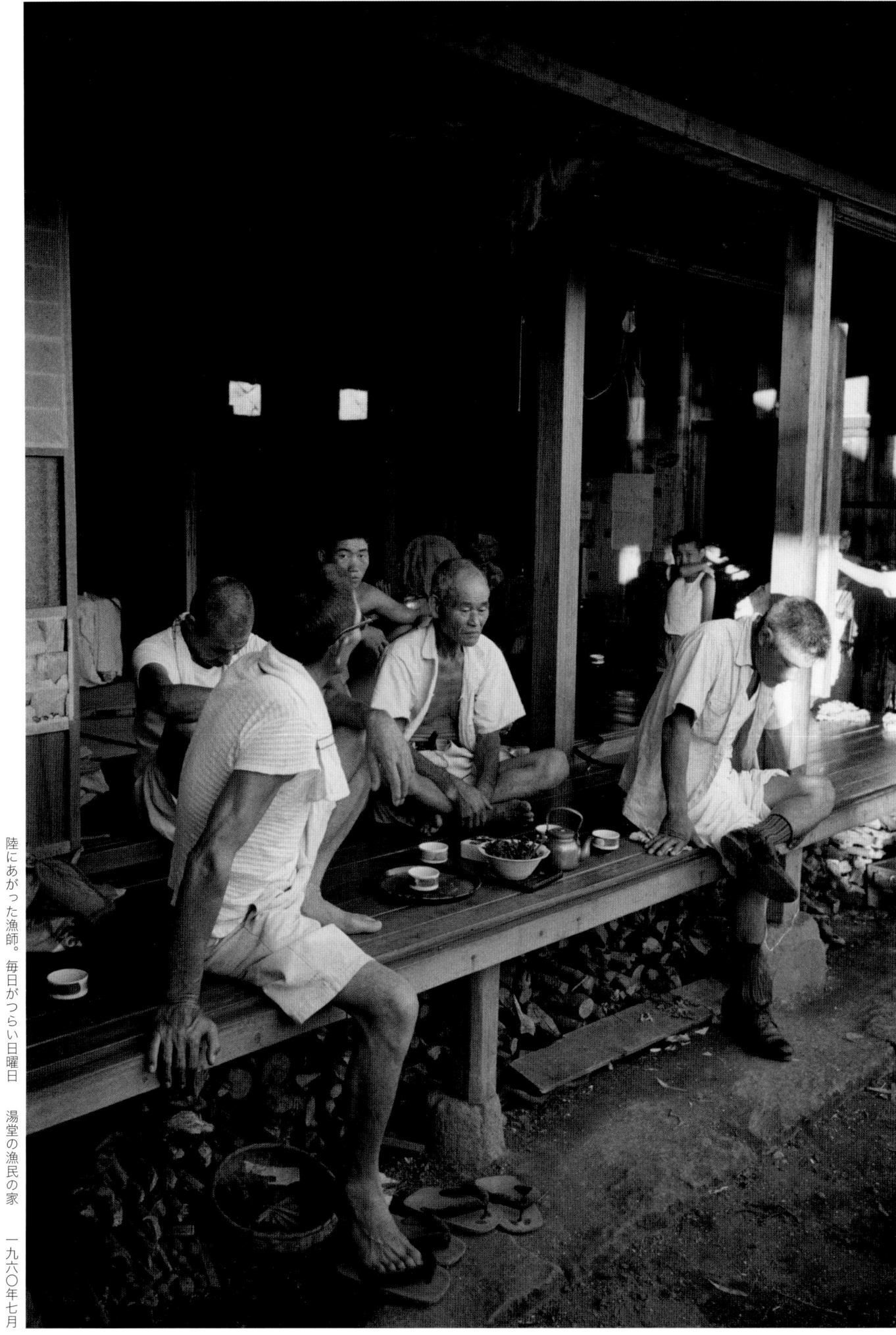

陸にあがった漁師。毎日がつらい日曜日　湯堂の漁民の家　一九六〇年七月

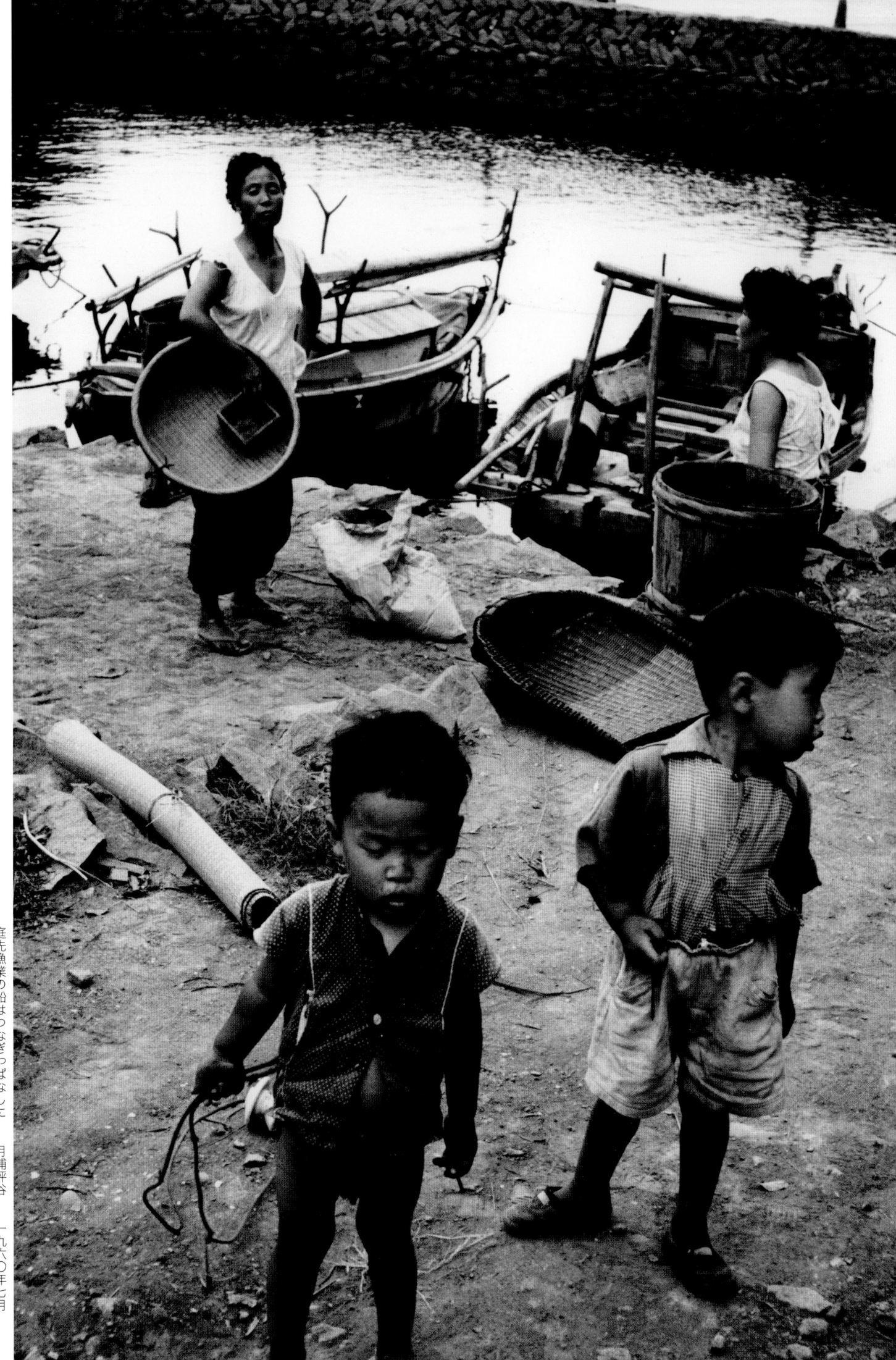

庭先漁業の船はつなぎっぱなしに　月浦坪谷　一九六〇年七月

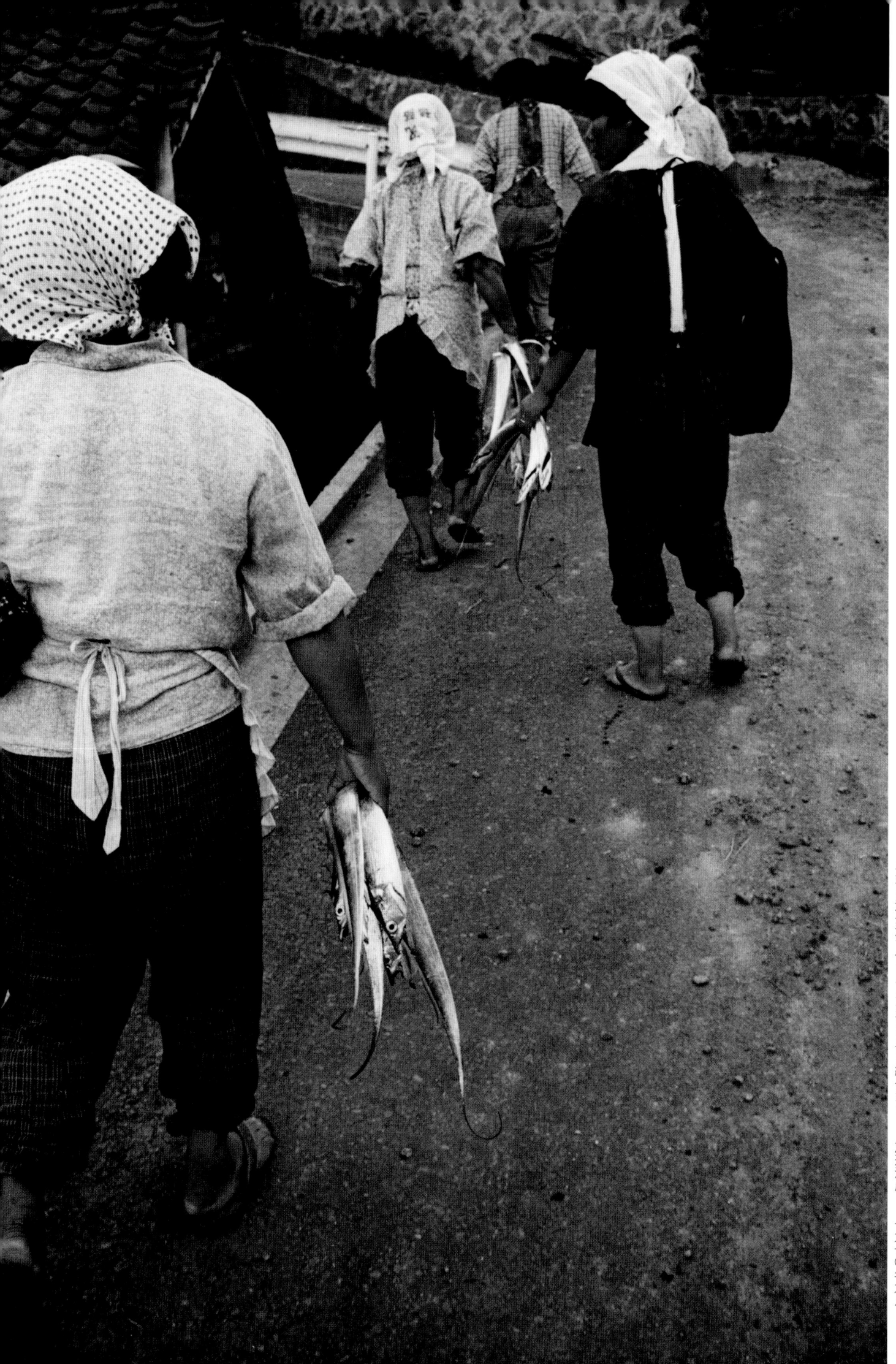

早朝の湾外漁で今日のおかずを手に網子たち　茂道海岸　一九七〇年九月

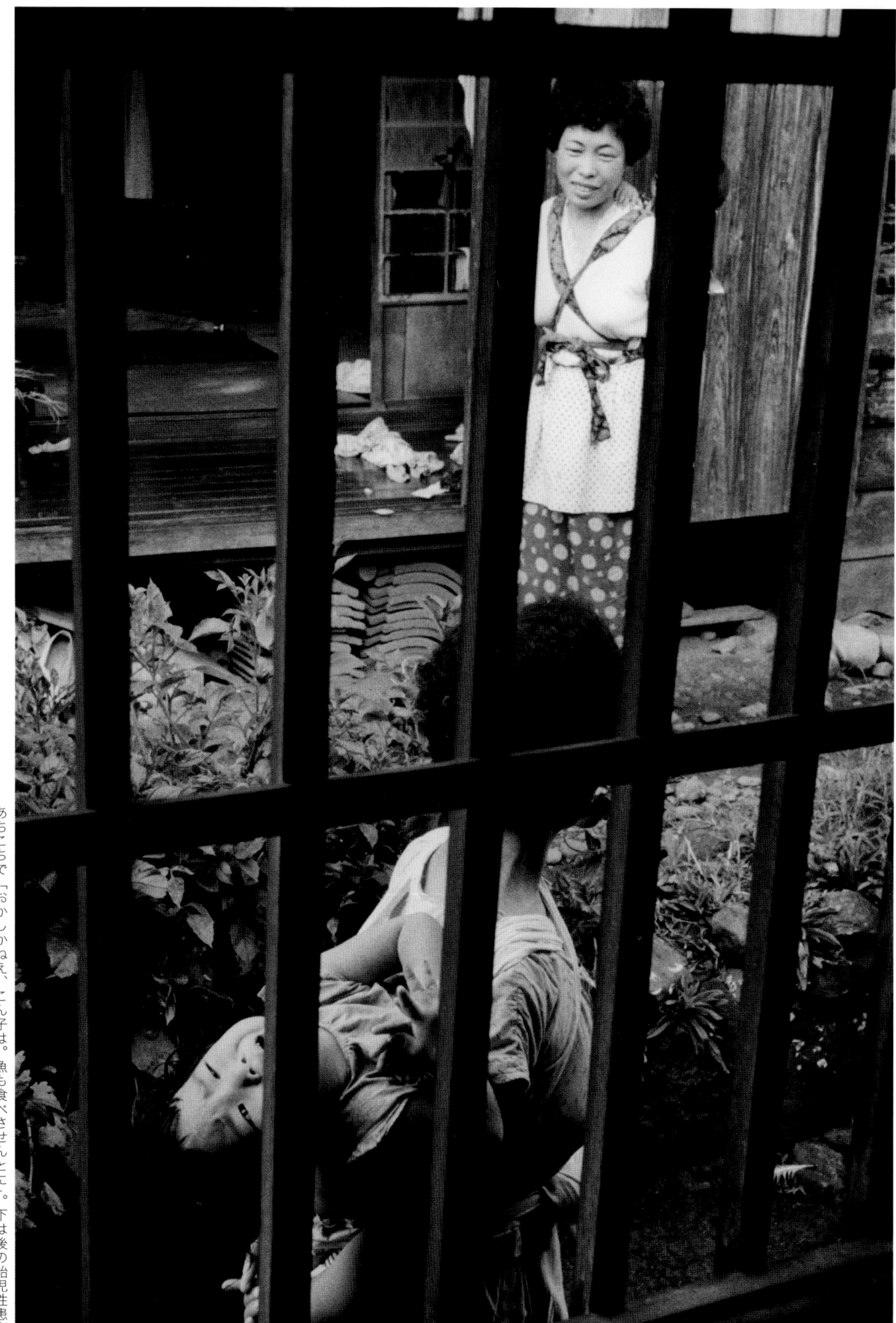

あちこちで「おかしかねえ、こん子は。魚も食べさせんとに」。下は後の胎児性患者、森本久枝3歳　茂道　一九六〇年八月

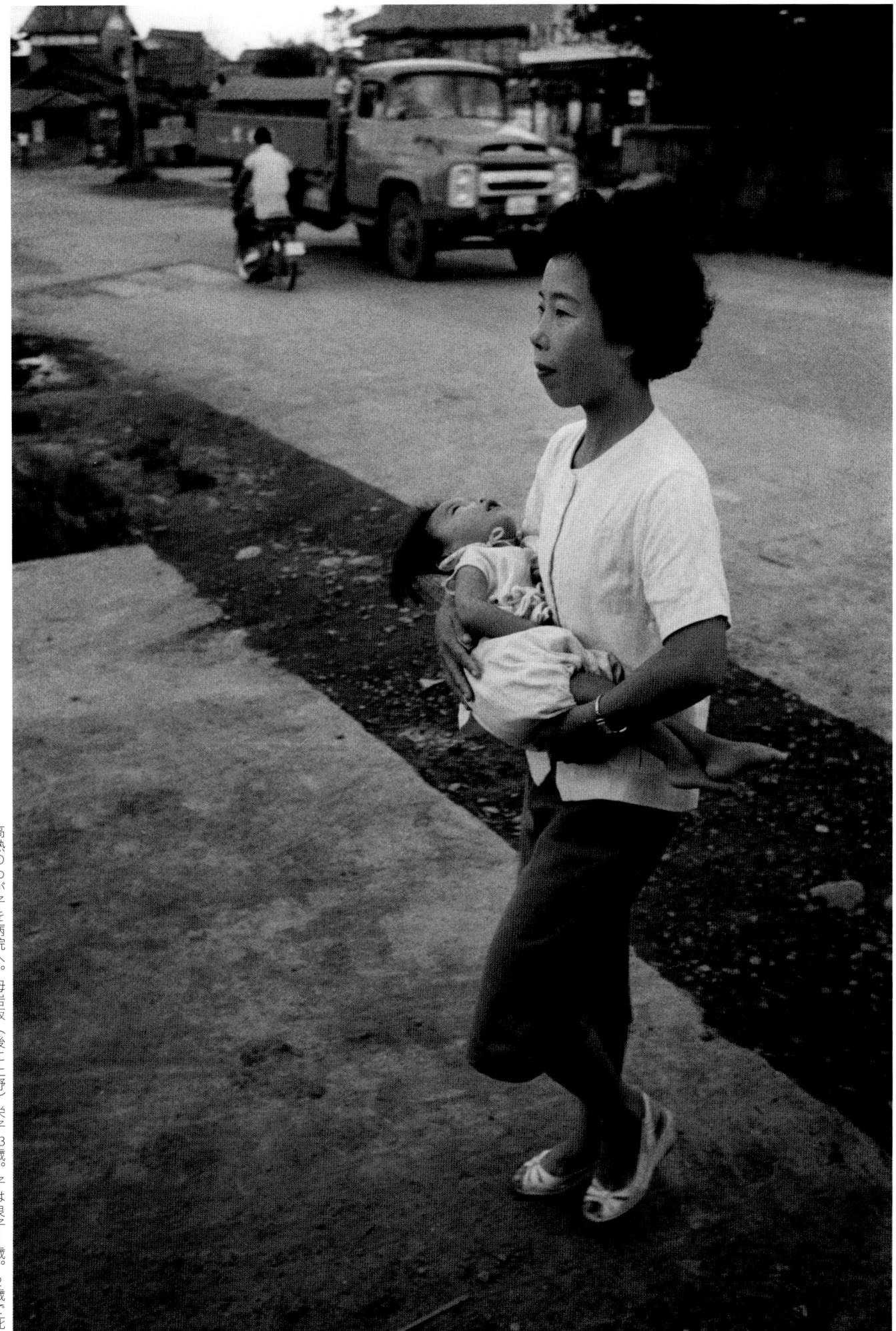

高熱のわが子を病院へ。母岩坂（後に上野）栄子33歳。子は良子1歳。2歳で死亡。死んだ後で、胎児性患者と認定　一九六〇年七月

娘を浜であやす患者、坂本タカエ31歳。入籍を拒まれ未婚の母　湯堂　一九七〇年九月

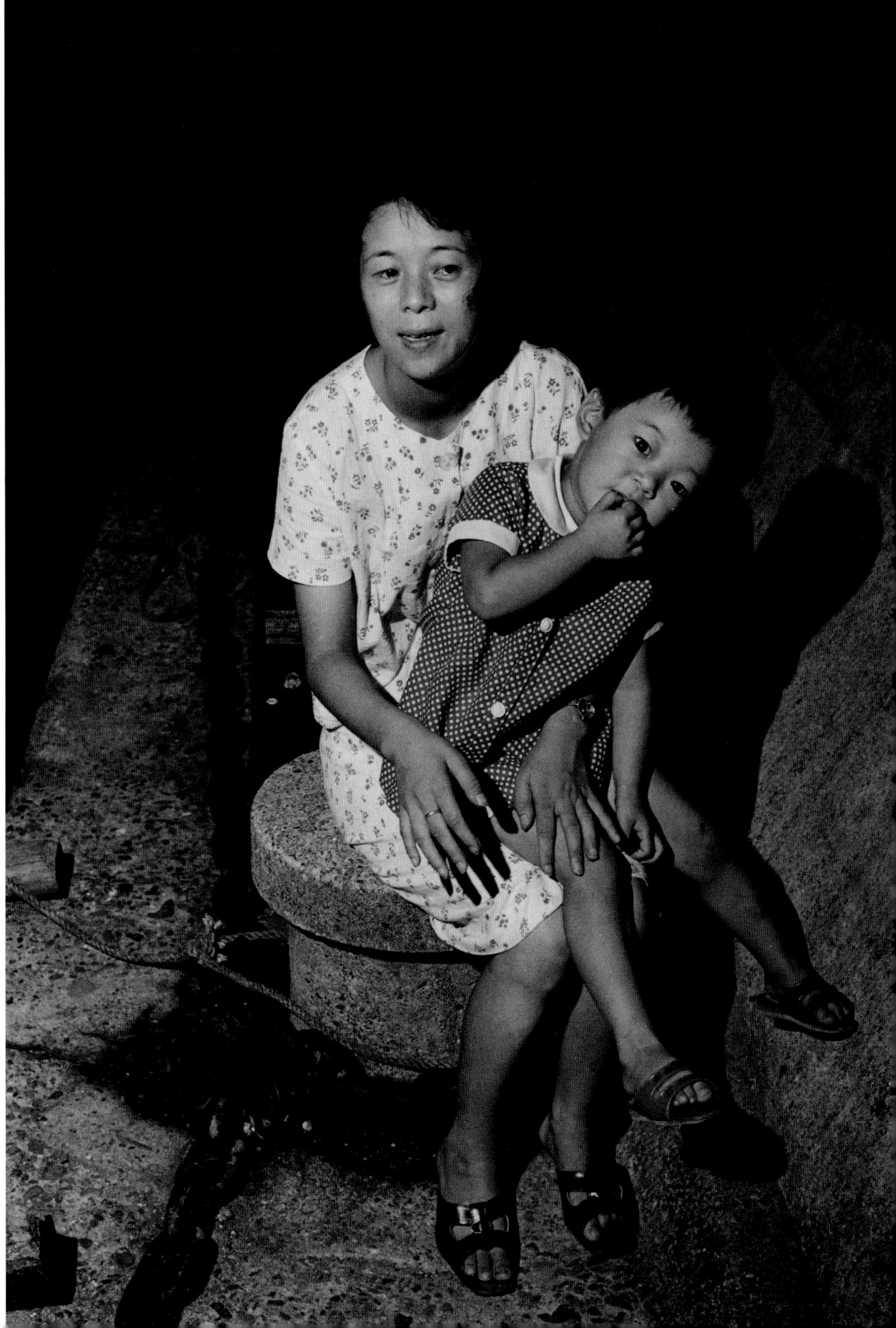

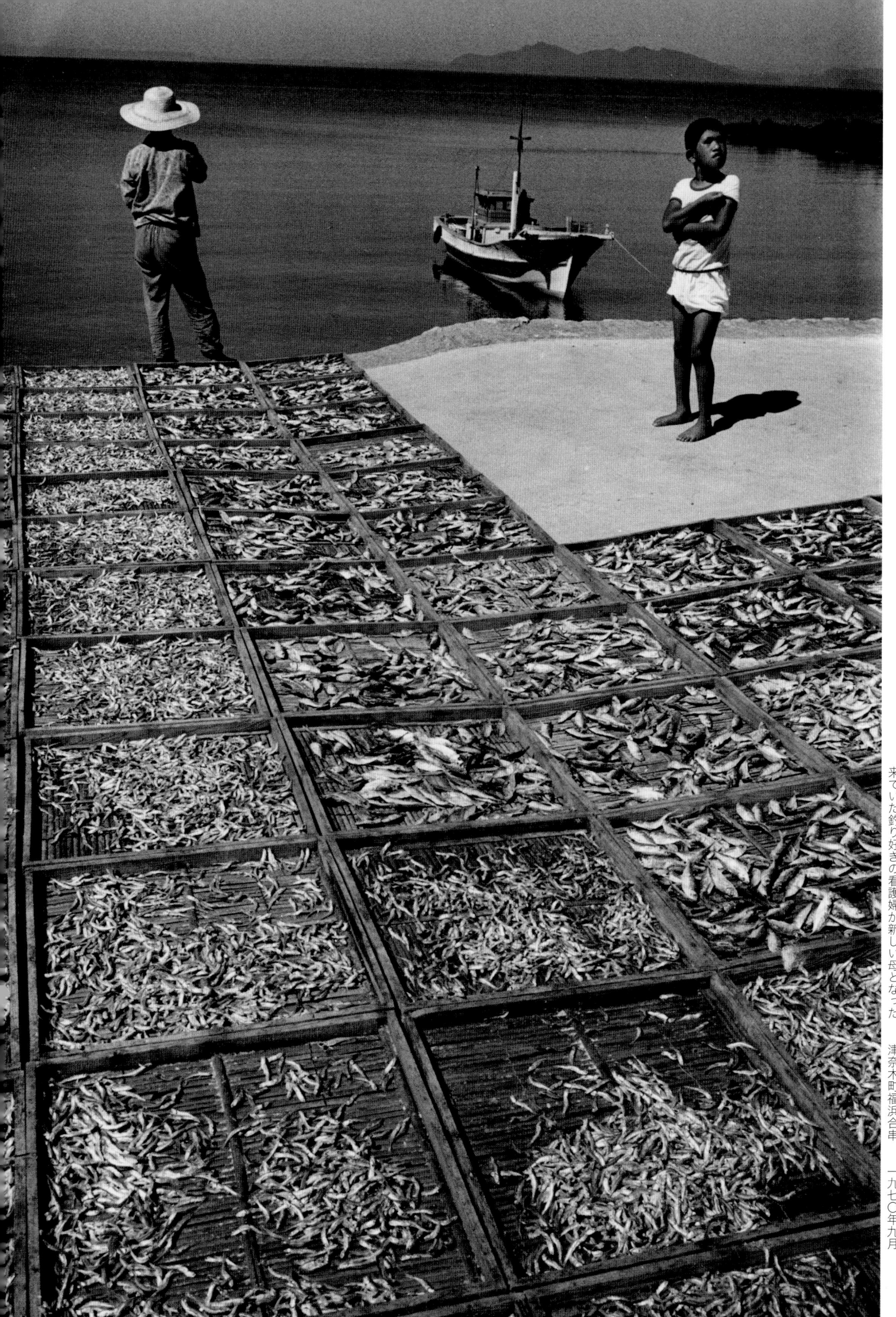

イリコ干しの浜で一人遊ぶ胎児性患者、浜田良次13歳。母シズエは64歳で後に死亡。浜によく来ていた釣り好きの看護婦が新しい母となった　津奈木町福浜合串　一九七〇年九月

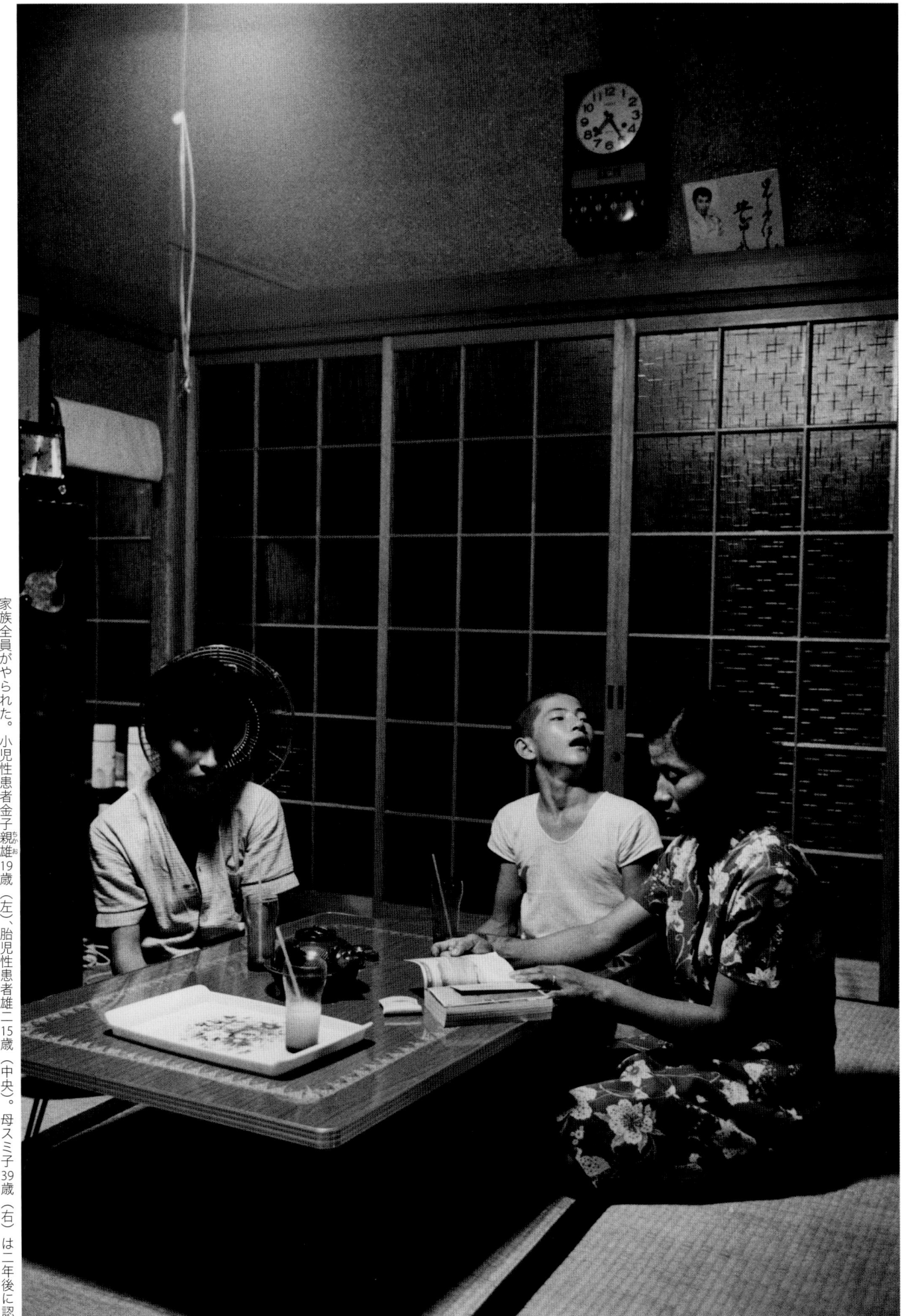

家族全員がやられた。小児性患者金子親雄19歳（左）、胎児性患者雄二15歳（中央）。母スミ子39歳（右）は二年後に認定。父の近は劇症で、奇病公式発見前の一九五五年に、34歳で死亡　明神町の自宅　一九七〇年九月

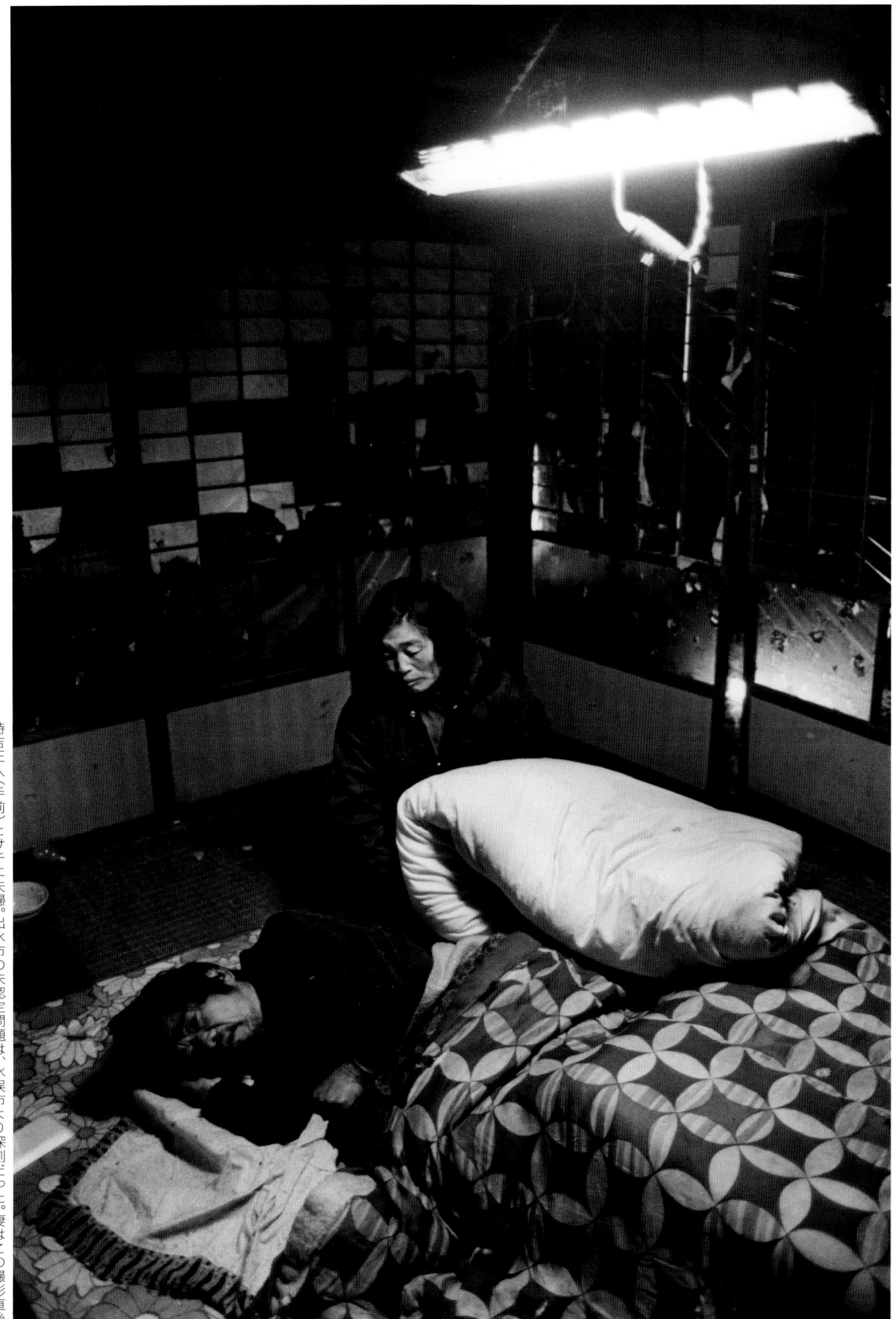

時吉正人（手前）とサチエ夫婦。出水市の未認定問題は、水俣市より深刻だった。妻はこの撮影直後に認定されたが、夫はアル中とされ、この一年半後に未認定で死亡　出水市荘の自宅　一九七七年一月

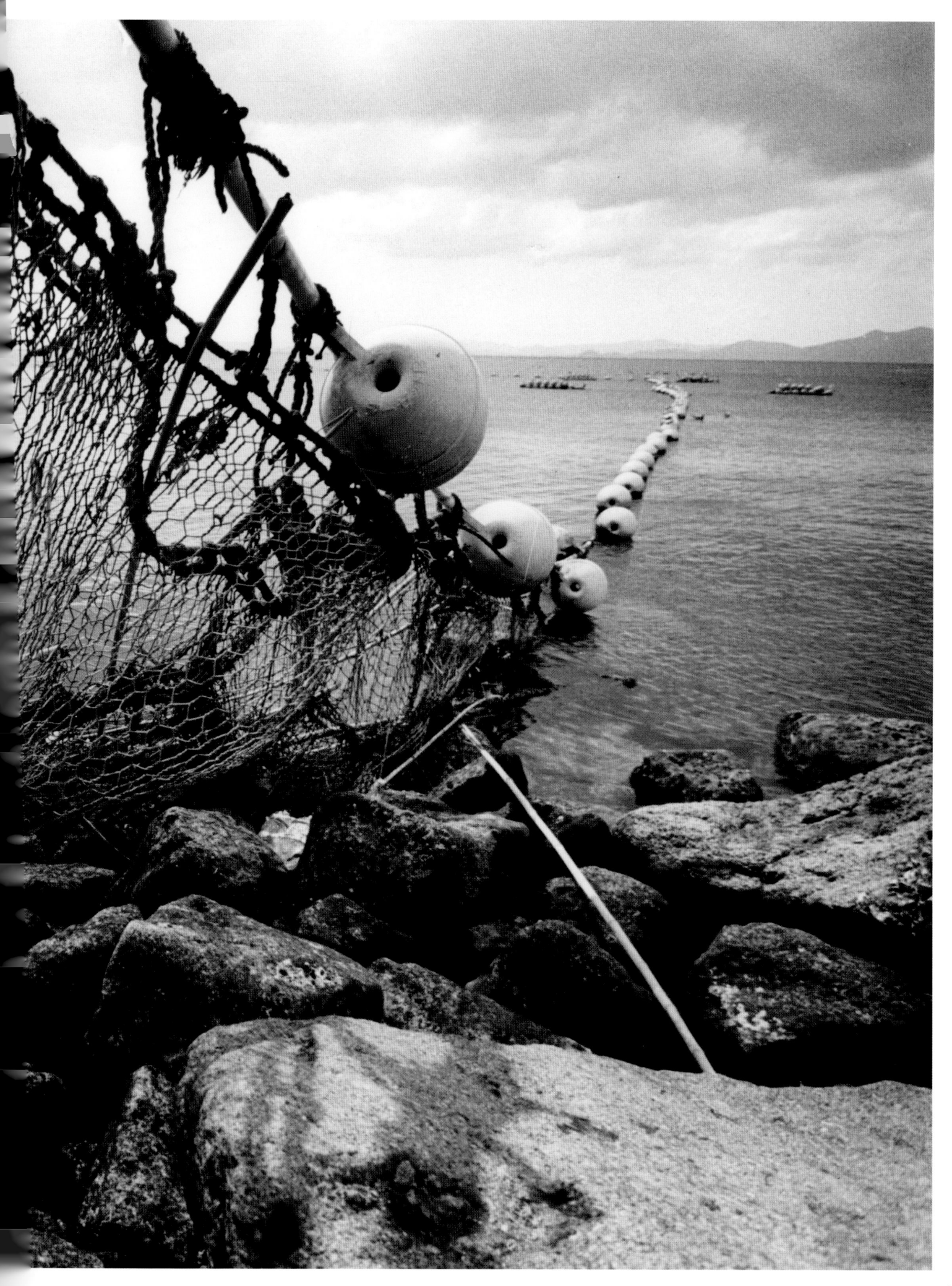

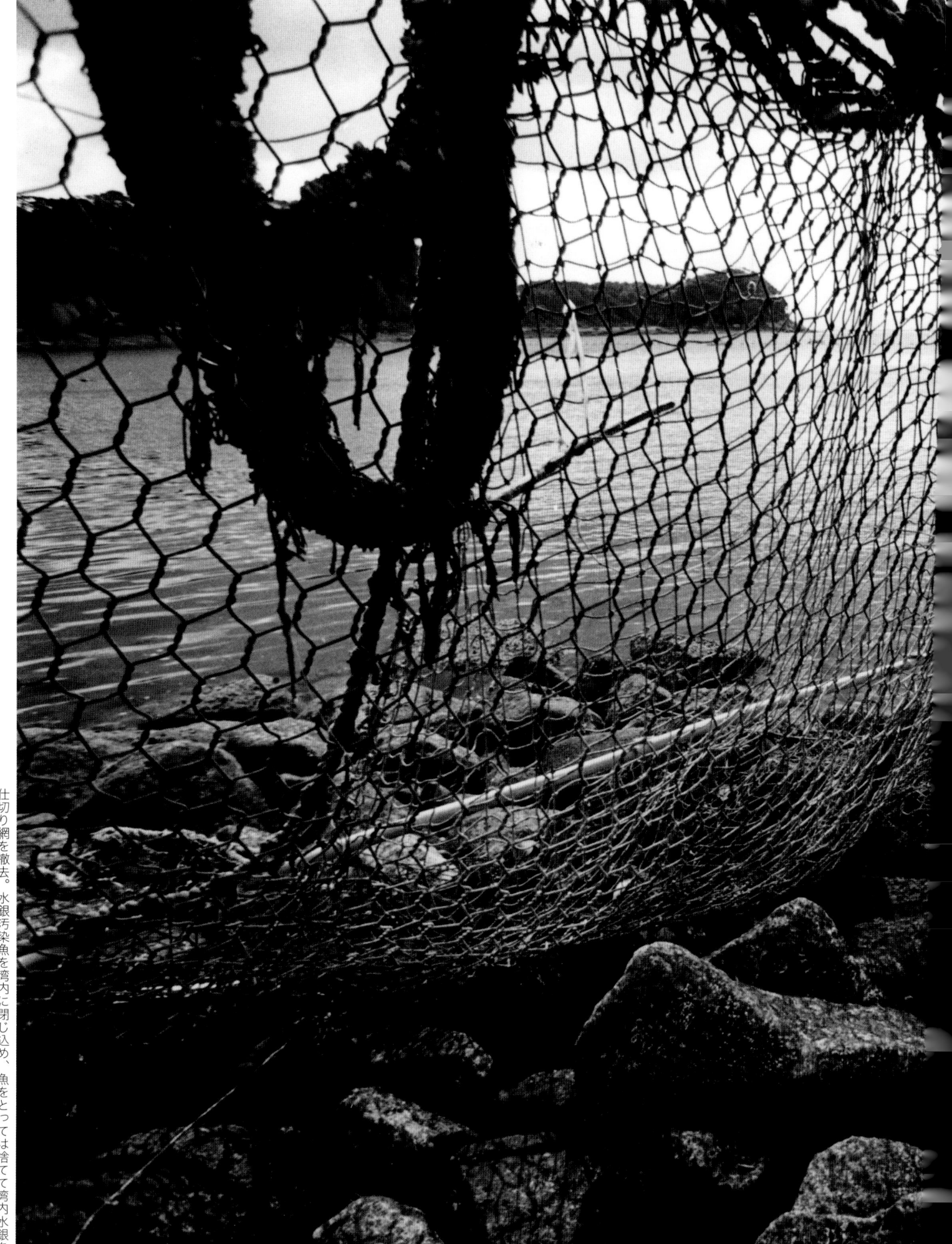

仕切り網を撤去。水銀汚染魚を湾内に閉じ込め、魚をとっては捨て湾内水銀をうすめる漁を二三年間もやった　一九九七年八月

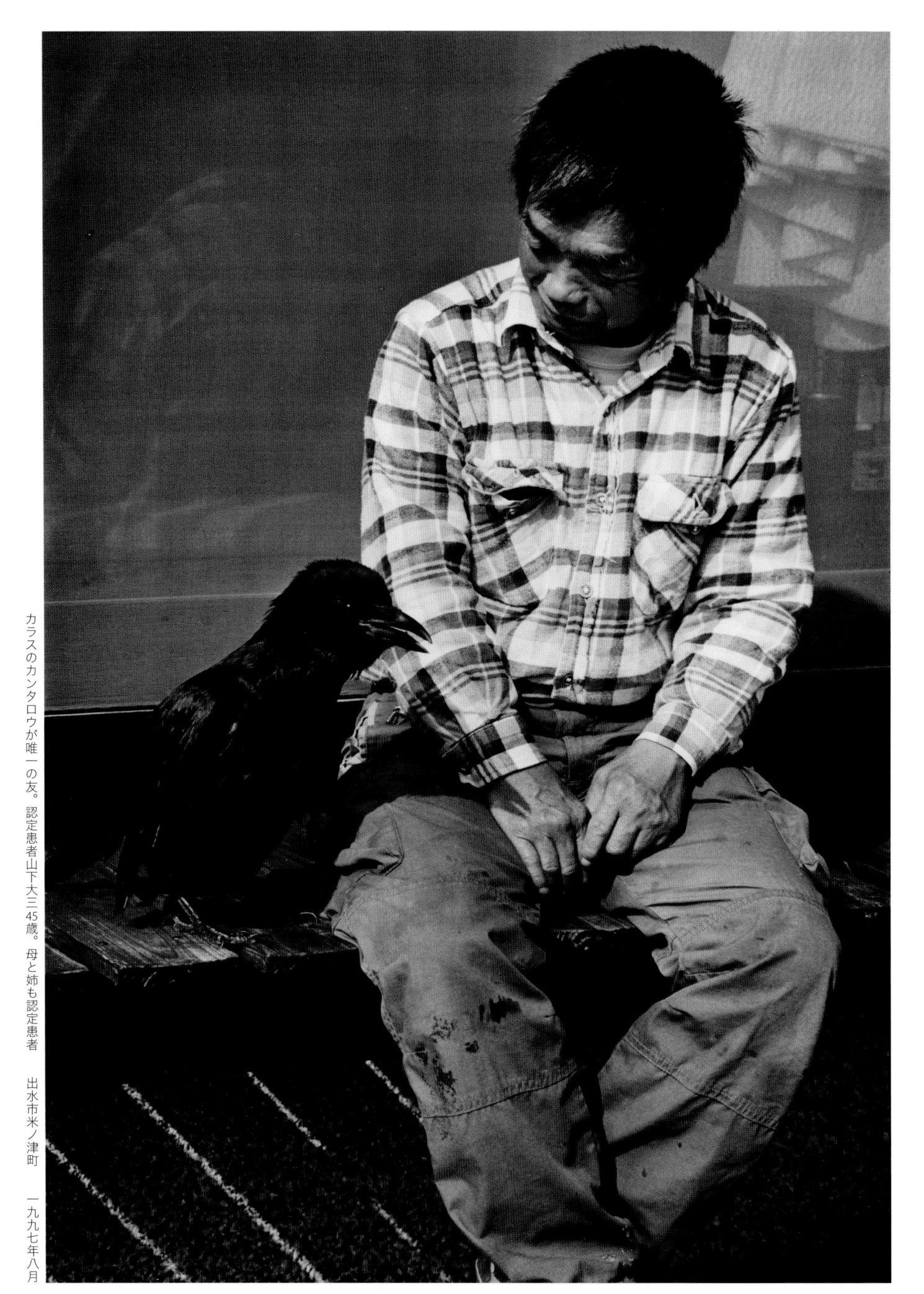

カラスのカンタロウが唯一の友。認定患者山下大三45歳。母と姉も認定患者　出水市米ノ津町　一九九七年八月

←〈次頁〉患者家族たちの五〇年。私が撮った人々に、昔の写真を手に並んでもらって
記念撮影　水俣湾埋立地船溜まり　二〇一一年五月一日

胎児性世代による第二世代訴訟の原告。最高裁で認定義務づけ訴訟の〈患者勝訴に笑顔
最高裁前　二〇一三年四月一六日

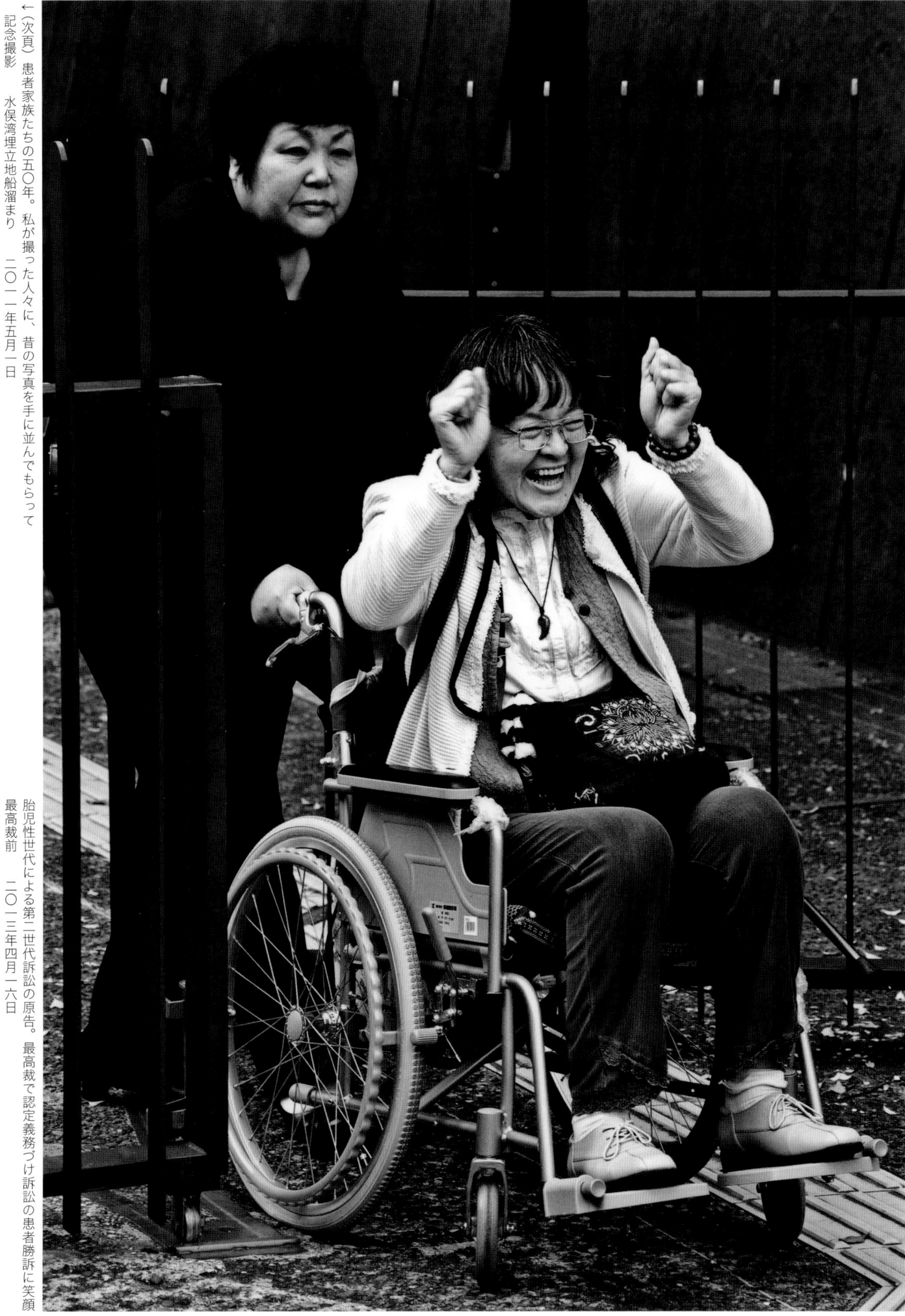

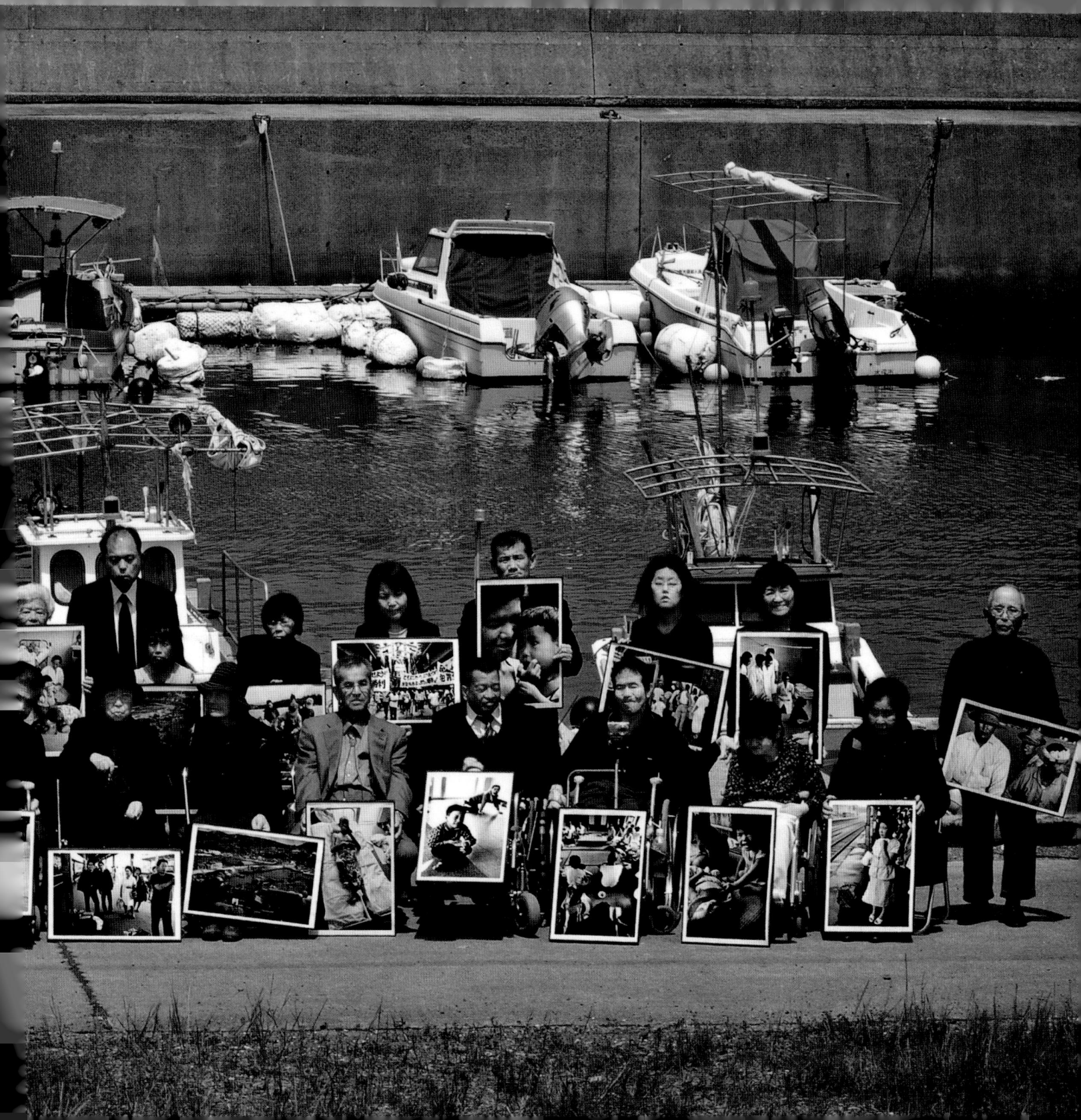

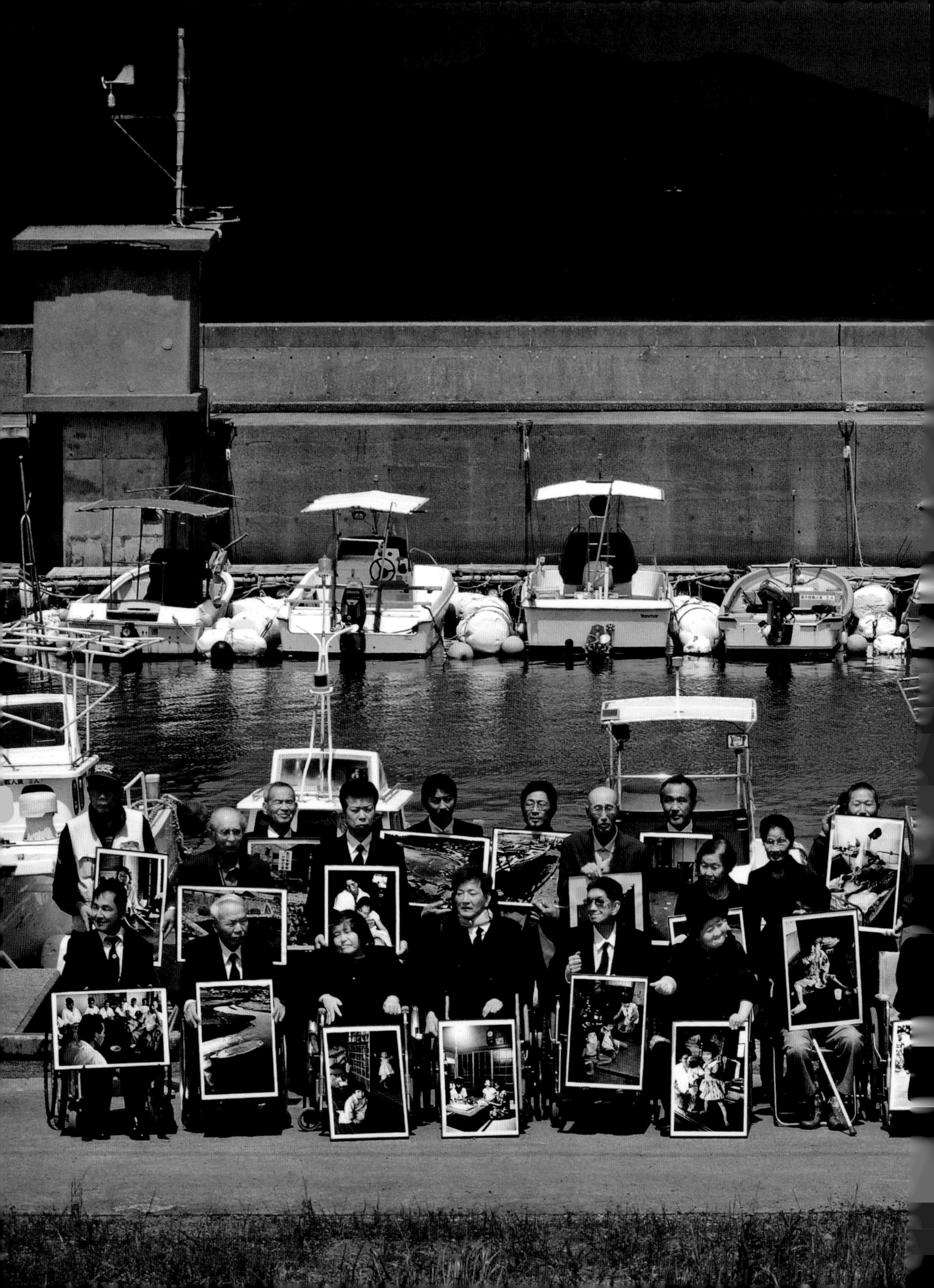

私の水俣病事件

「特措法」の暑い夏

西 貴晴

「議員の涙ですよ」記事の根拠を問うデスクに、携帯電話で怒鳴るように答えた。東京・永田町の参院議員会館前。いぶかるデスクに事情を説明し、電話を切った力が抜けた。

二〇〇九年夏、水俣病被害者救済特別措置法（特措法）成立に向けた自民・公明の与党（当時）と民主党の駆け引きが大詰めを迎えていた。「特措法、与野党合意へ」。この見出しがついた記事をいつ掲載するか、どの記者も虎視眈々とタイミングを見計らっていた。

「水俣病問題の最終解決」を掲げる特措法の骨格案を与党水俣病問題プロジェクトチームが示したのは、その二年前の二〇〇七年一〇月だ。「公害の原点」といわれる水俣病は、一九九五年の村山富市内閣当時に実現した政治決着でいったん「終わった」とされた。

しかし、患者勝訴となった二〇〇四年の関西訴訟最高裁判決をきっかけに、「厳格すぎる」といわれる国の認定基準見直しと新たな認定を期待する被害者が急増し、水俣病は改めて政治問題となっていた。国や与党が選んだ収拾策が特措法だ。「認定基準を満たさないものの救済を必要とする方々」を対象に、批判の声が強かった認定基準は維持したまま、新たな救済策をつくる。水俣病の代表的な症状とされる手足のしびれなどが確認されれば二一〇万円の一時金などを支給する。最終的な申請者は熊本、鹿児島、新潟の三県で六万五一五一人に上った。

これに対し「認定基準そのものを見直し、根本的な解決を図れ」という意見も当然出た。国や熊本県、原因企業チッソを相手取った裁判を続けていた水俣病不知火患者会や、胎児性水俣病患者の生活支援施設「ほっとはうす」のメンバーらが相次いで上京し、国会前で

二〇〇七年から六年間、毎日新聞水俣通信部で勤務した私を含め、当時水俣で勤務した記者たちは法案の行方を巡る取材に忙殺された。昼は東京都内の自民党本部や衆参議員会館を訪ね、夜は赤坂の議員宿舎前で関係議員の帰宅を待ち、あるいはチッソ役員の自宅を回る。記者たちが「スジ」と呼ぶ重大なニュースをめぐる会合の開催が前日に急きょ判明することも多く、私自身、熊本空港から最終便の飛行機に慌てて飛び乗ることもしばしばだった。

政権交代を見据え決着へ

与野党間の協議が一挙に動いたのが二〇〇九年の夏前だ。当時、迫りつつある衆院選で、民主党への政権交代が確実視されていた。民主党内では水俣病をめぐる対応を政権交代後に持ち越したくないと考える幹部らと、与党プロジェクトチーム案を批判して対案をつくった若手議員らに溝が生じていた。

やがて民主党の最終的な方向性を決める会議が党本部で開かれた。はたして幹部らが法案成立で押し切るのか、あるいは若手議員らが粘ってなお議論を続けるのか。固唾をのんで廊下で待つ記者たちの前を鳩山由紀夫代表（当時）が通り過ぎた。「鳩山さんっ」との問いかけにも無言のまま。他の幹部も次々と部屋を出て行く。最後に若手議員の一人が記者の前に現れた。しかし、どんなやり取りがあったのか、言葉を聞いた私だけではどうもはっきりしない。

私を含めて水俣から来た数人の記者が議員と一緒に建物から出た。ふと議員の顔をみると、うっすらと涙が浮かんでいる。法案成立で幹部らに押し切られた涙であることは私たちには明らかだった。議員と別れた私は「与野党合意へ」の記事を掲載するよう、その場でデスクに連絡した。この日の会議は事実上、特措法成立を決定づけた。記事は翌日の毎日新聞一面に掲載された。

認定制度はどこへいく

確かに一日も早い救済を求める患者は多かった。四〇年も続いてきた今の認定基準と認定後の補償制度を見直すのは社会全体でたいへんなエネルギーがいるのも分かる。ただ、認定制度をきちんと作り替えないと水俣病問題は終わらない――私を含め、水俣の記者の多くはこんな思いを持っていたのではないか。

しかし、そうした疑問は特措法による早期決着を優先する政治の動きの前で跳ね返され、認定基準は見直されないまま法案は与野党の多数で可決された。「僕たちは負けたってことさ」。その晩だったか、水俣の記者が冗談めかして言った言葉は、半分は本音だったろう。

その特措法成立から四年近くたった二〇一三年四月、水俣市の溝口秋生さんが母親（故人）の水俣病認定を求めて起こした裁判で、最高裁は原告勝訴を言い渡した。「水俣病、最高裁が初認定」「審査、運用見直し必至」――こんな見出しが翌日の新聞に躍った。判決を受けて認定制度はいったいどこへいくのか。水俣病問題の行方は今もなお見えていない。

（にし・たかはる／毎日新聞下関支局長）

16 行商人の魚は山間部でよく売れた

水俣事件は海の話だと、私は思っていた。行商ルートの水銀汚染の山へ行ったのは、初撮影から五二年後。湯浦、芦北、田浦、天草など、水俣漁民の先祖の地の漁民は、水俣の魚をとりに行っても拒まれなかった。奇病情報がない山では、ダシをとったイリコも捨てずに食べた。

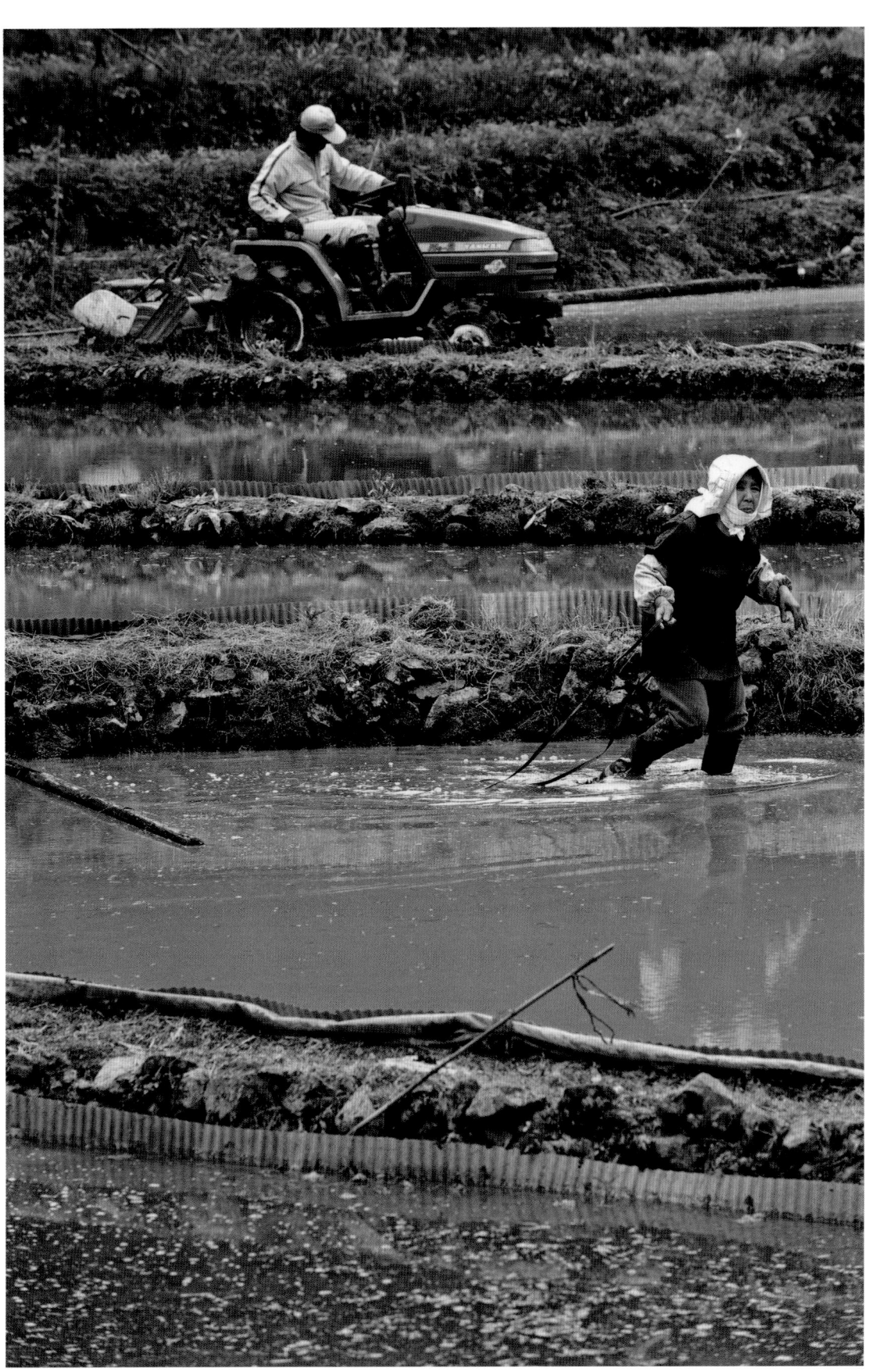

「からだは変なのだが、しびれる、かっとなる、カラス曲り（足の痙攣）など、起こったり起こらなかったり。『その他まあいろいろ。歳だから、みんながそうだから、水俣病だ、なんて思うとらんしなあ」　芦北町大岩　二〇一二年五月

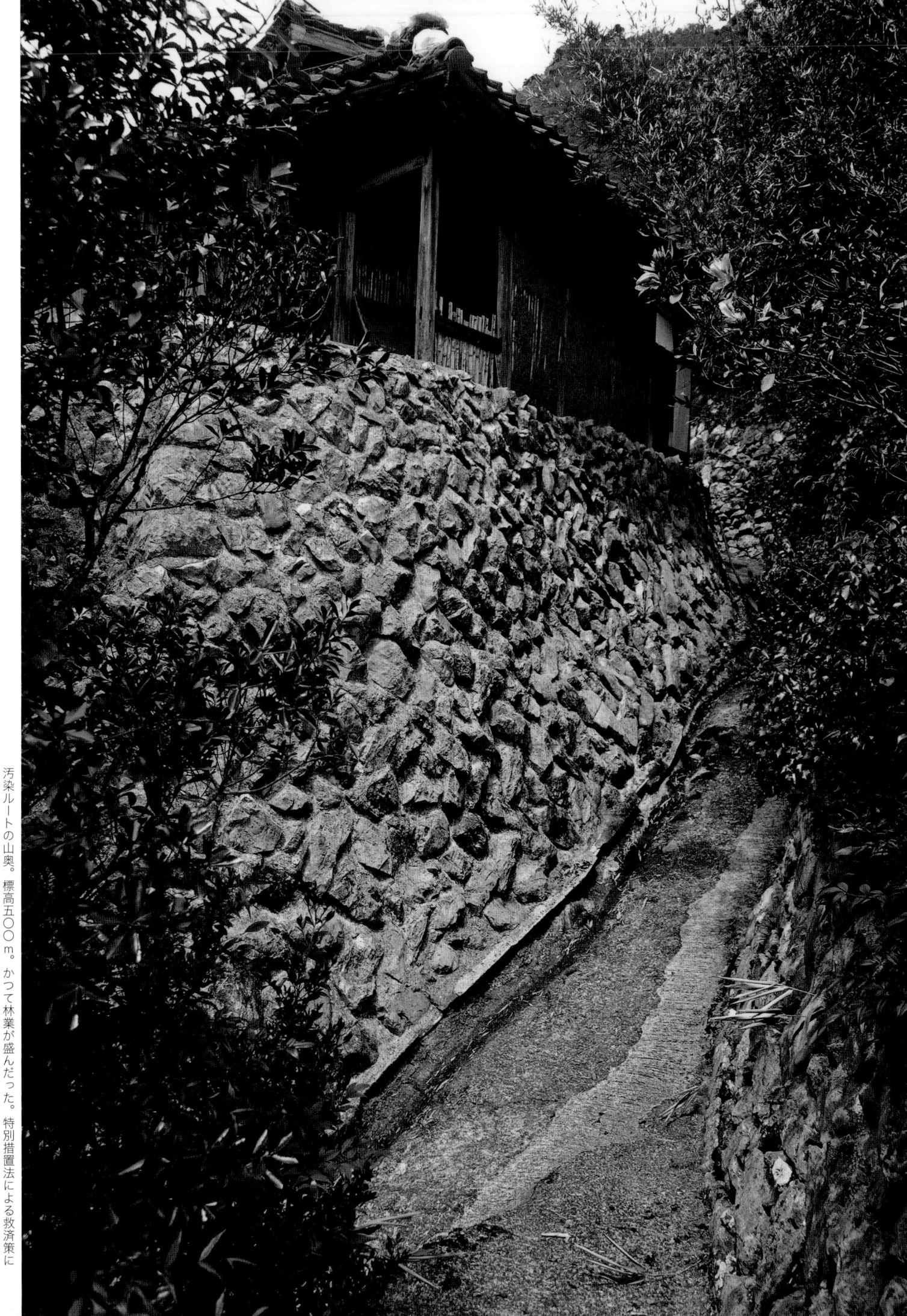

汚染ルートの山奥。標高五〇〇m。かつて林業が盛んだった。特別措置法による救済策に申請者が多数出た　芦北町黒岩　二〇一二年五月

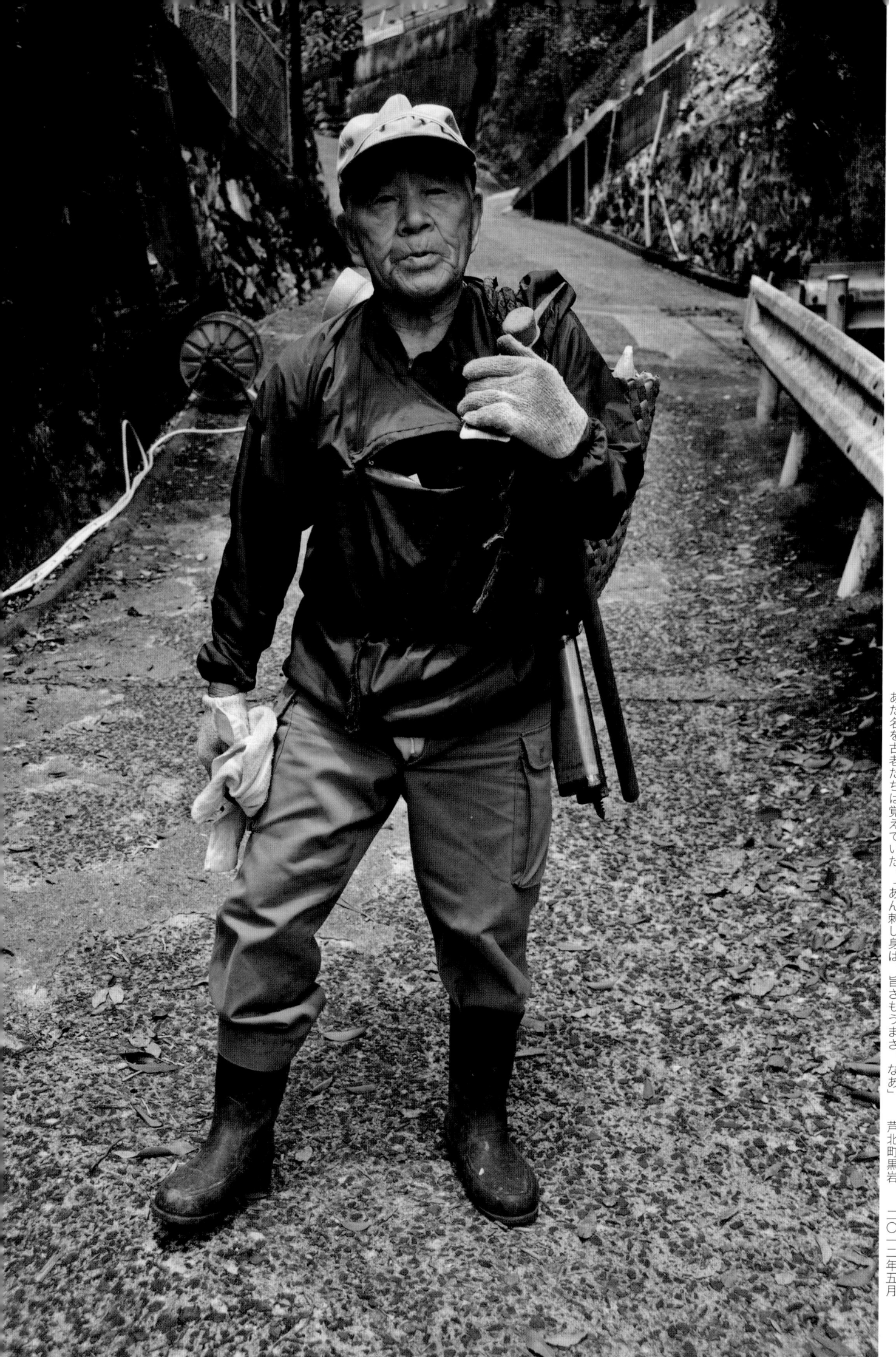

エーと、林田、門宮、藤井……。焼酎をひっかけて天秤棒負うて海からきた「一気どん」。行商人の名前やあだ名を古老たちは覚えていた。「あん刺し身は、旨さもうまさ、なあ」 芦北町黒岩 二〇一二年五月

17 隠れ患者の島

獅子島は水俣の目前一四キロ。隣県の島民は、チッソの都・水俣と生活も縁戚も近い。水俣病のことは長年、島のタブーだった。一九七三年に島から認定者が出ると、石を投げられた。別の認定漁民は直ちに漁協を除名された。今は、ほぼ島民全員が救済策の申請者となった。

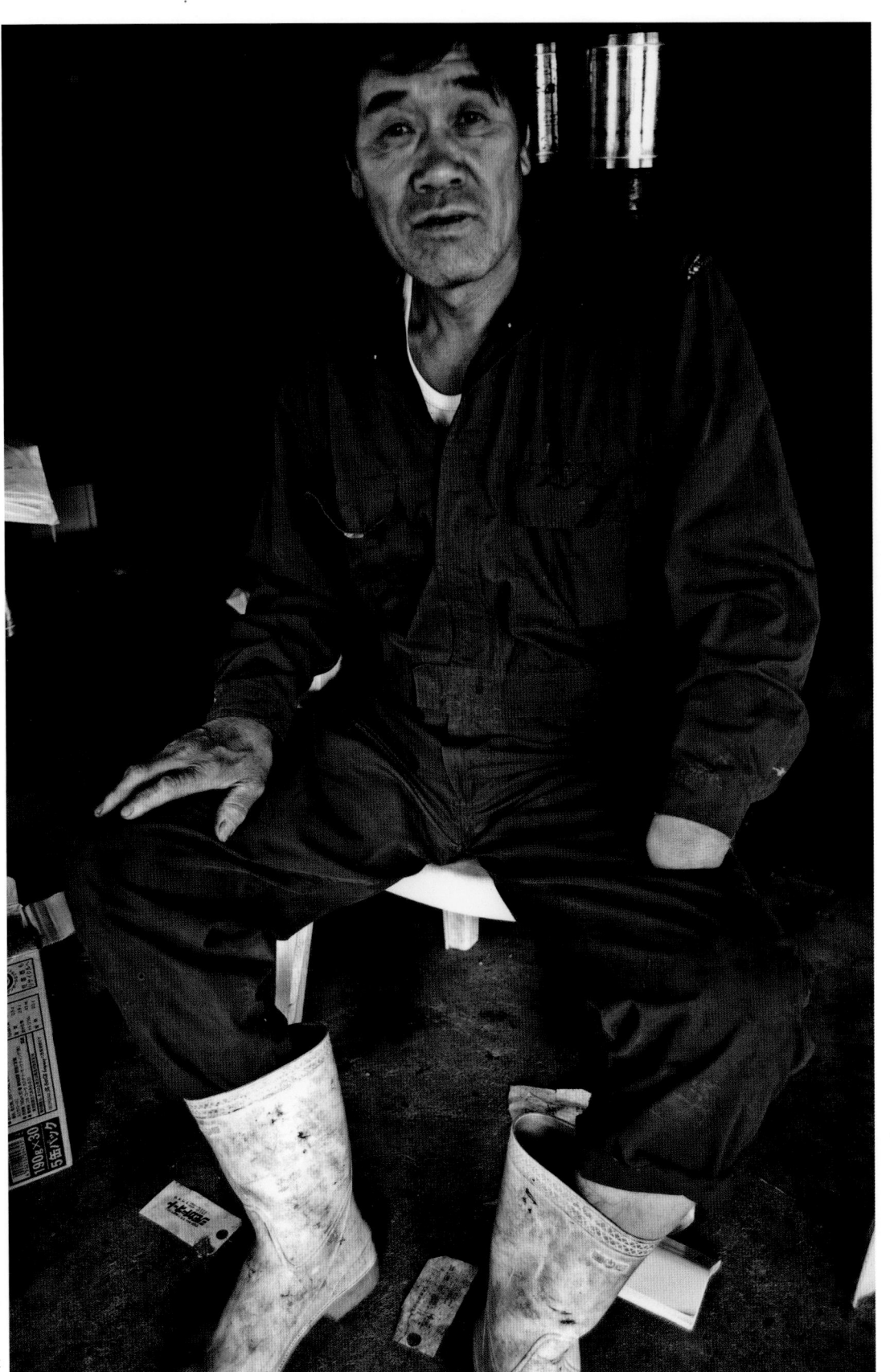

未認定の坂口澄夫58歳。働きに出た大阪の鉄工所で左手を四度もプレス機につぶされた。「お前の体、おかしいのんと、ちゃいますか」といわれ、島に帰った　獅子島御所浦　二〇一二年五月

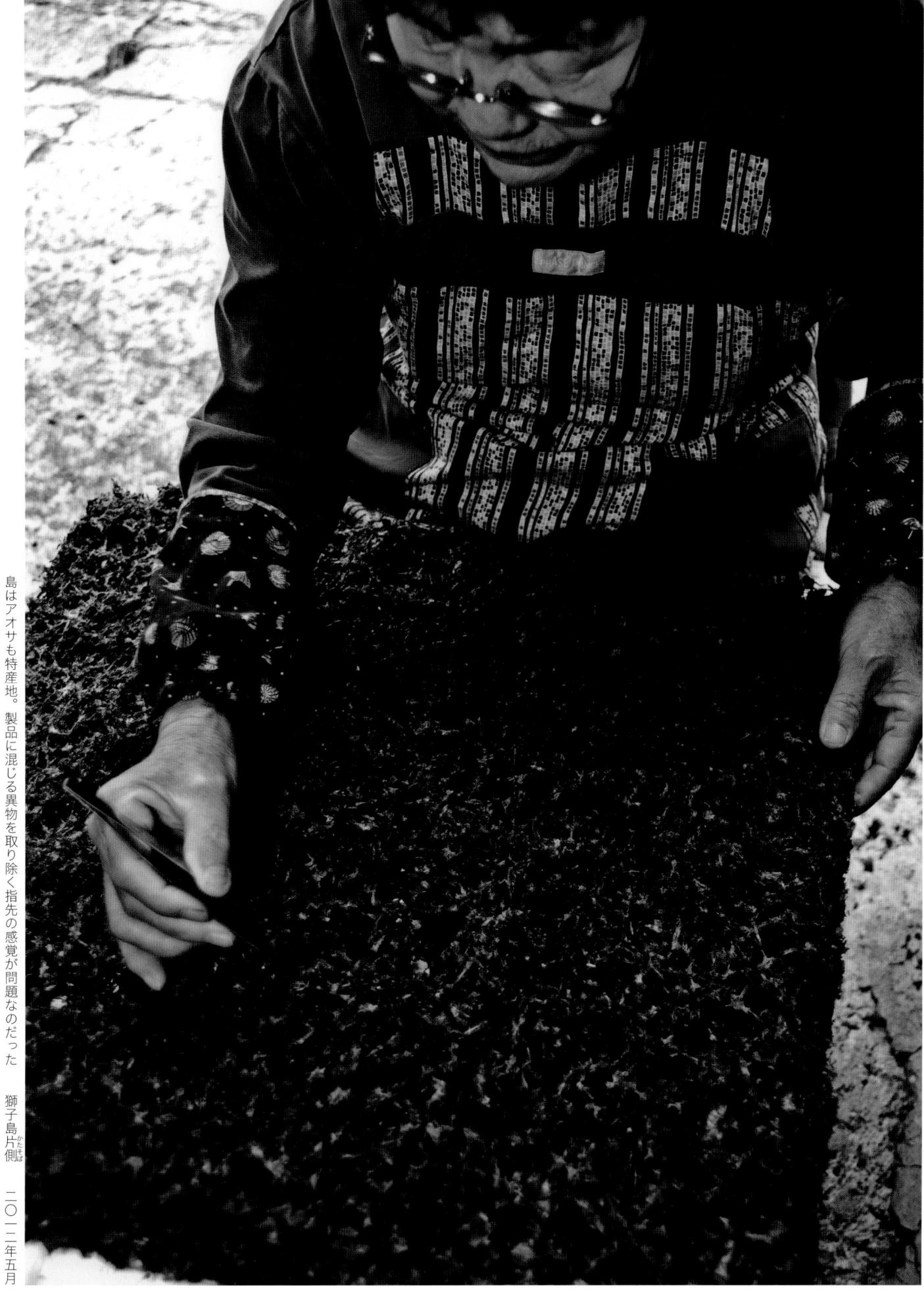

島はアオサも特産地。製品に混じる異物を取り除く指先の感覚が問題なのだった　獅子島片側(かたぼ)　二〇一二年五月

18 支援者たち

宇井純と私が東京から水俣へ行った八年後に、水俣事件の受難者への支援が、全国へと広がっていった。政府が水俣病を公害病に認定し、加害企業の名前を世間に表明した。それ以前の一二年間、受難者はひっそりと世に隠れていた。

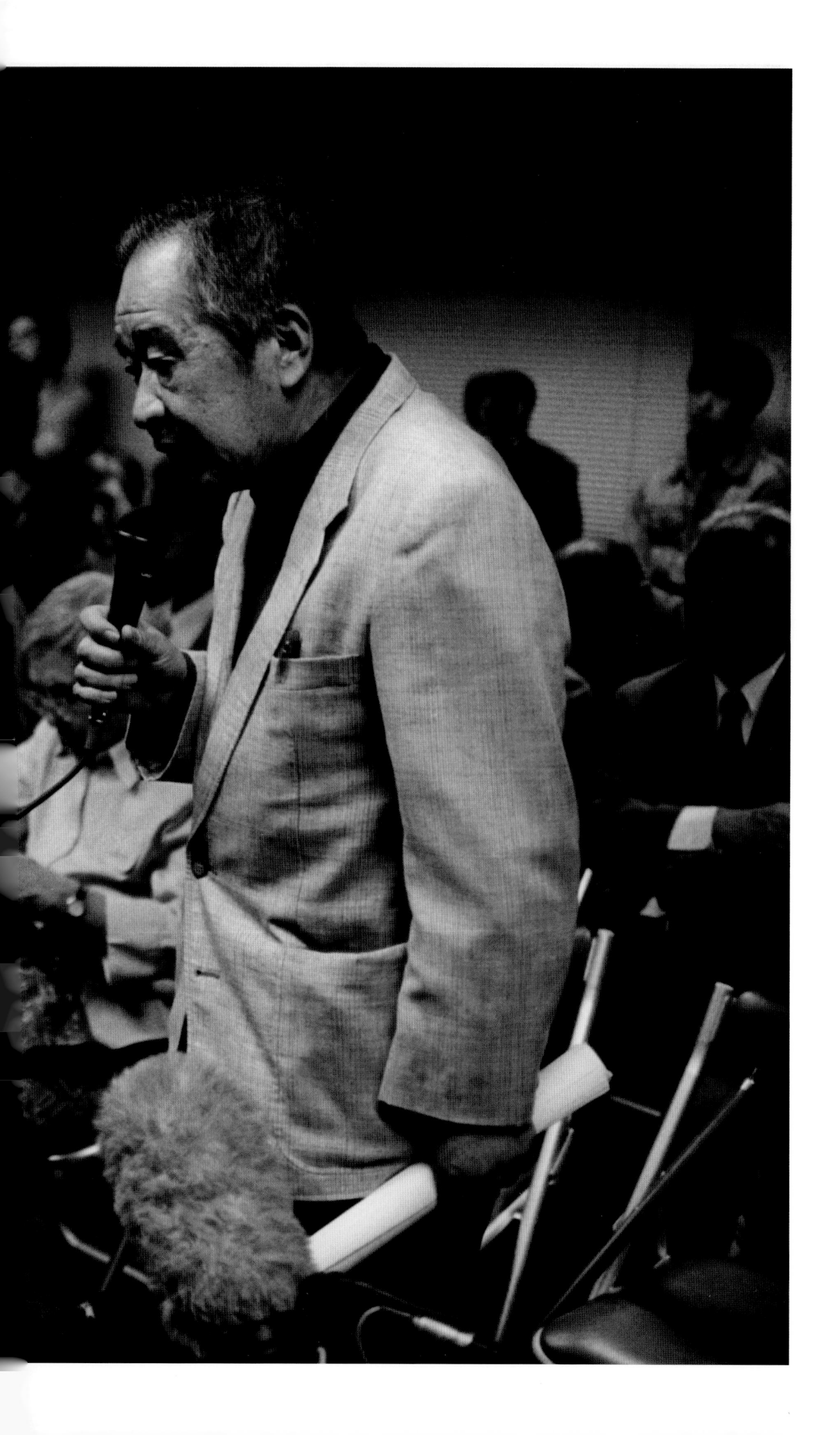

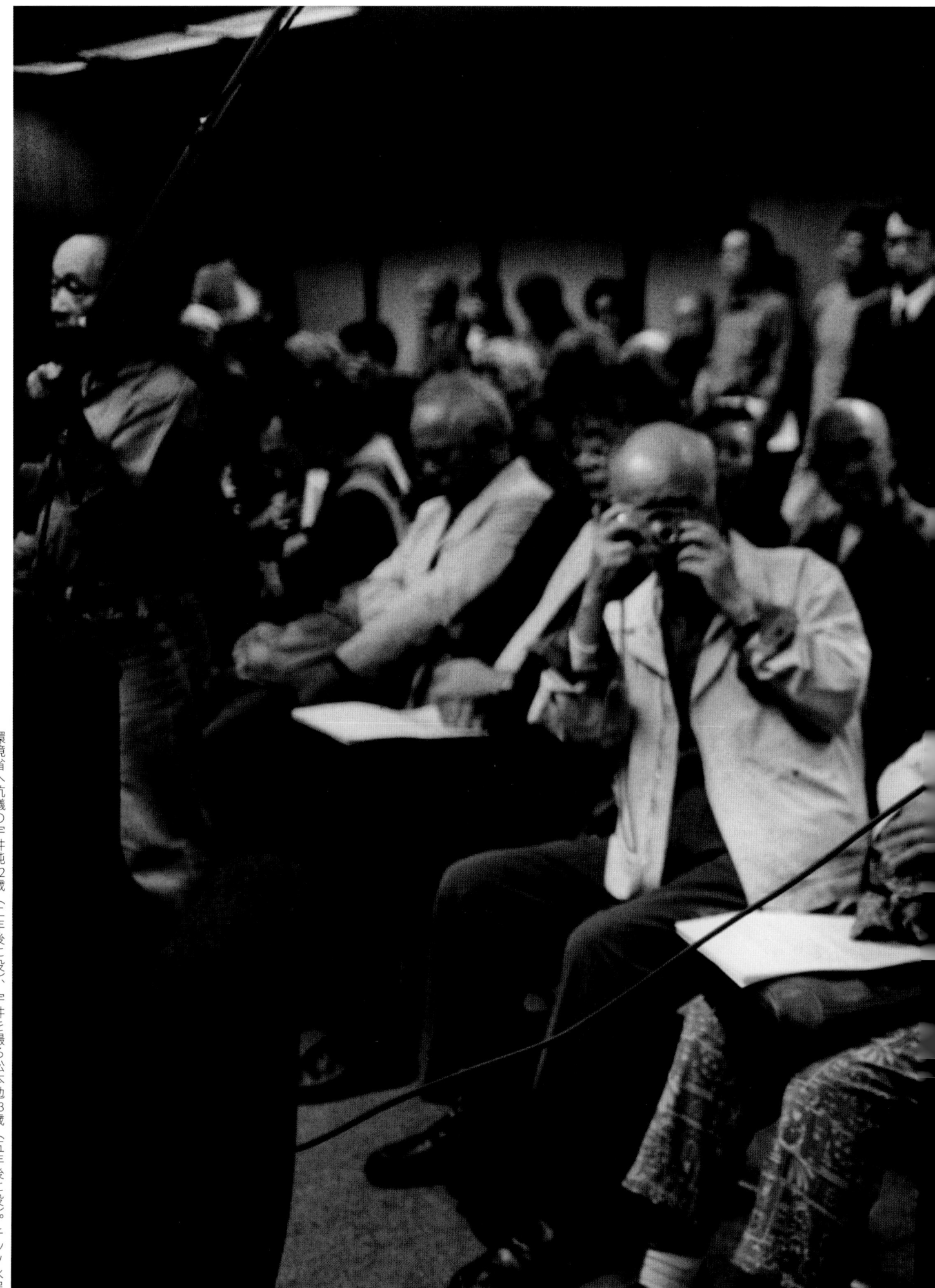

環境省へ抗議の宇井純72歳（二年後に没）、宇井を撮る松本勉73歳（五年後に没）。チッソ水俣病関西訴訟の最高裁判決で熊本県と国の上告を棄却、患者勝訴確定で　二〇〇四年一〇月一五日

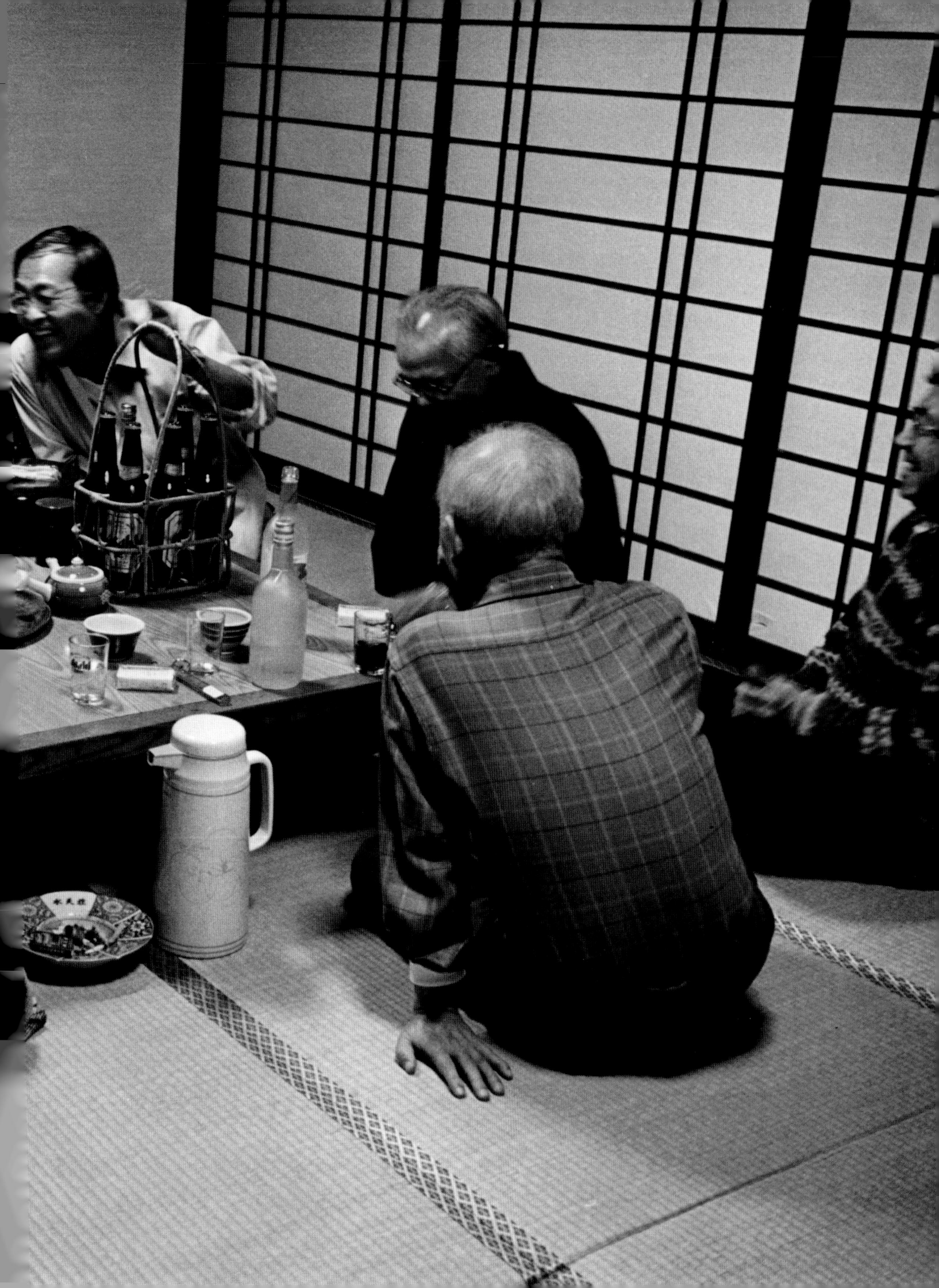

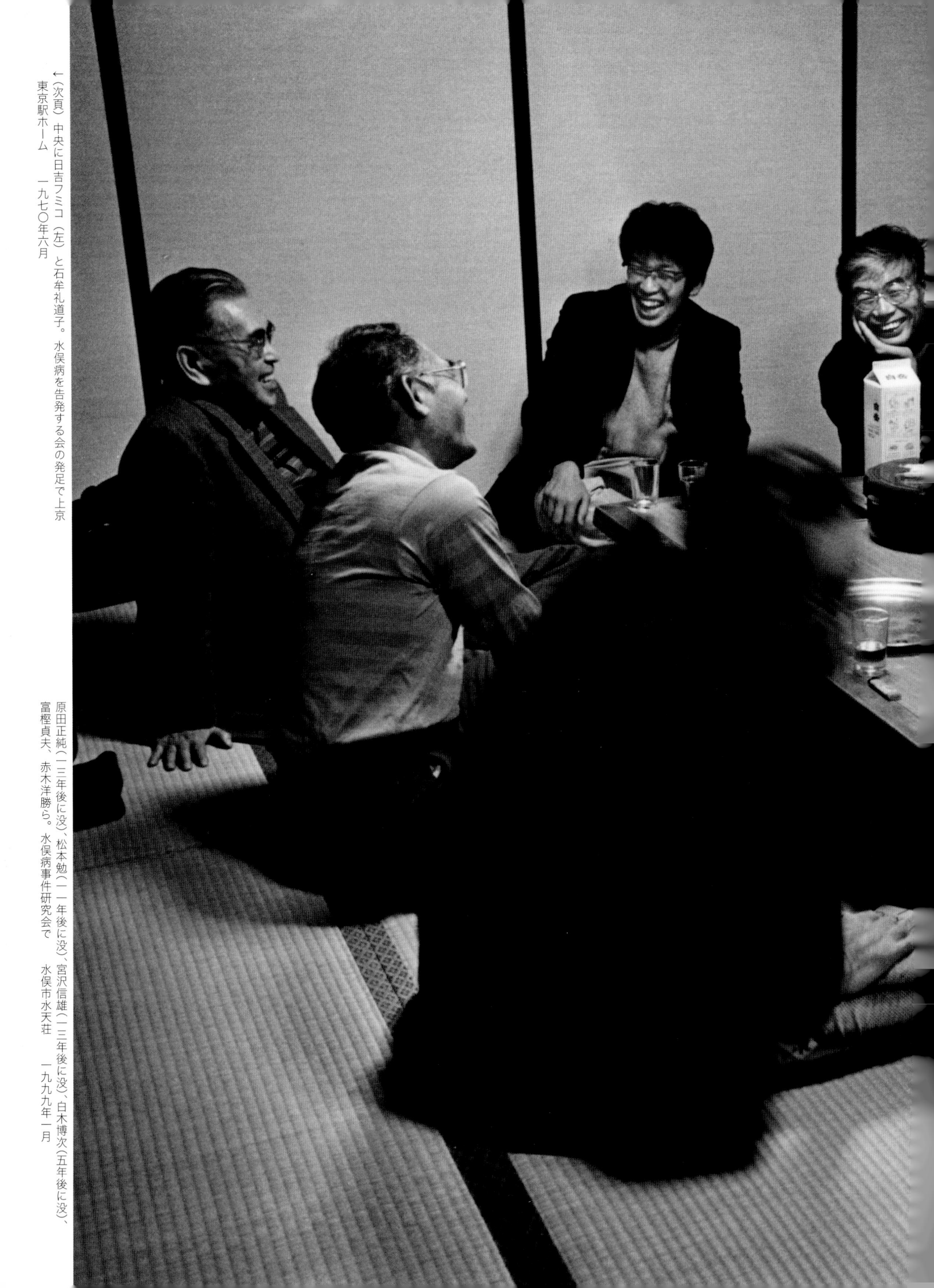

←〈次頁〉中央に日吉フミコ（左）と石牟礼道子。水俣病を告発する会の発足で上京　東京駅ホーム　一九七〇年六月

原田正純（一三年後に没）、松本勉（一一年後に没）、宮沢信雄（一三年後に没）、白木博次（五年後に没）、富樫貞夫、赤木洋勝ら。水俣病事件研究会で　水俣市水天荘　一九九九年一月

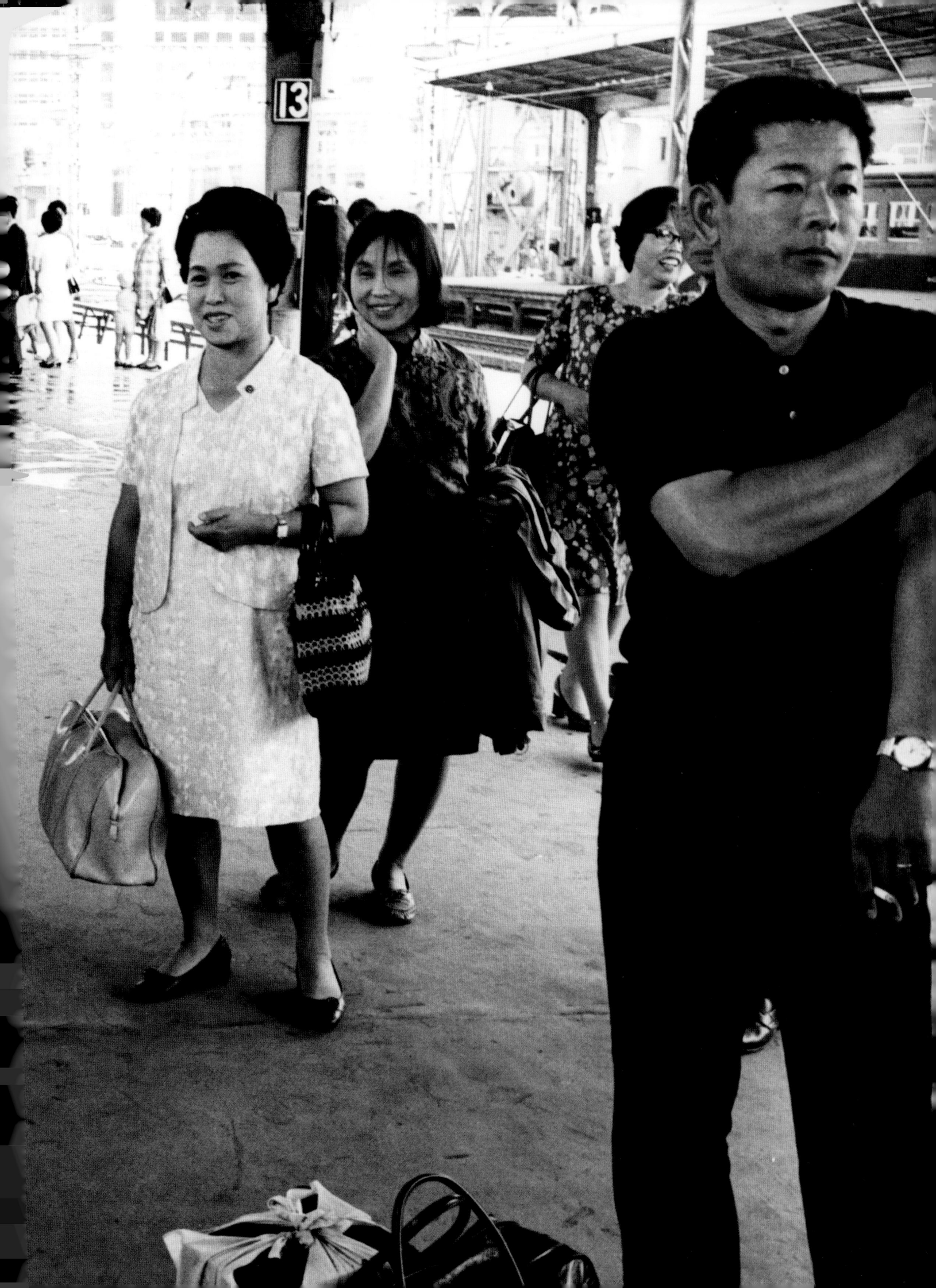

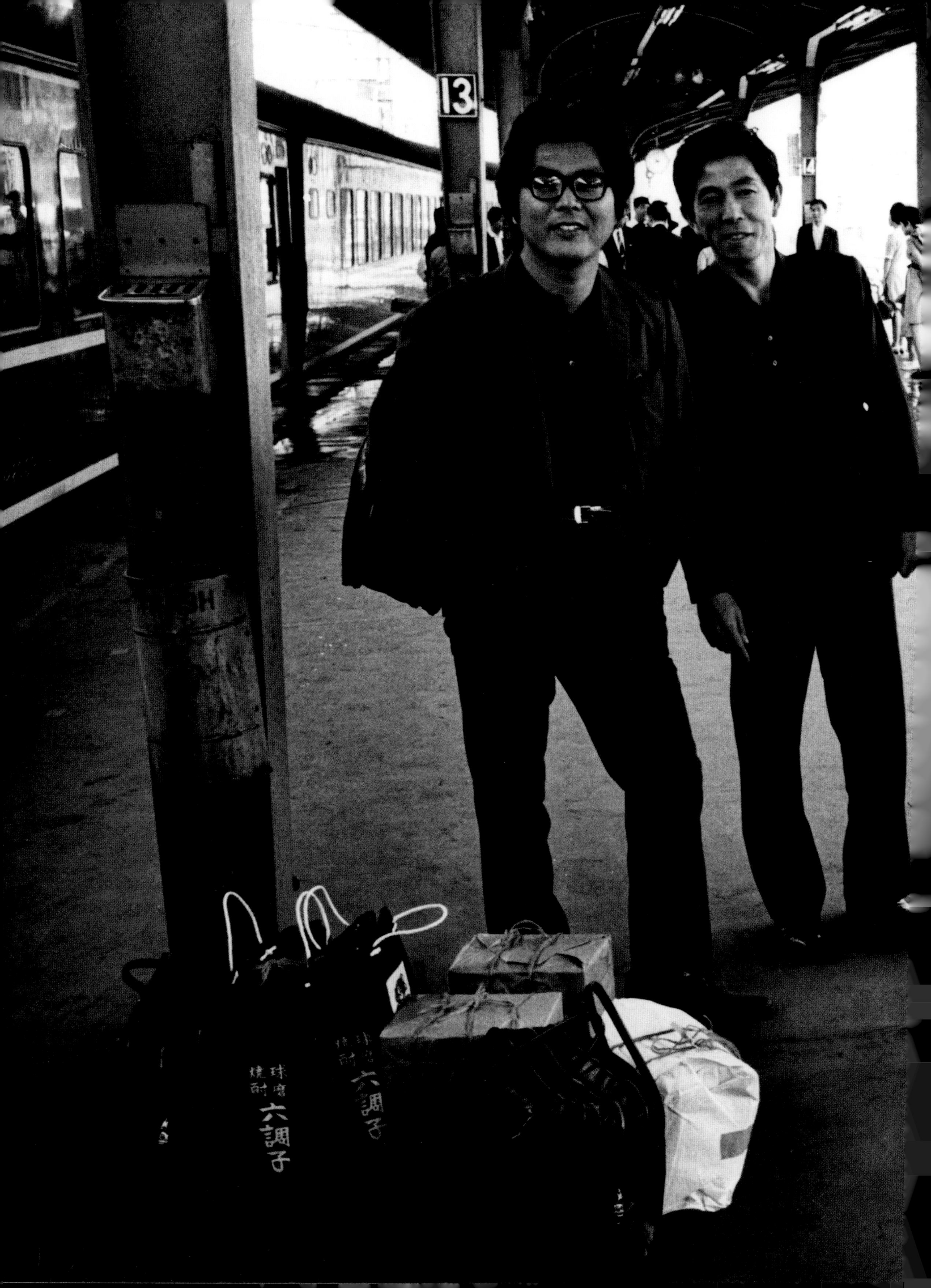
13
14
球磨焼酎 六調子
球磨焼酎 六調子

私の水俣病事件

ネコ四〇〇号実験記録の発見

宇井紀子

夫・宇井純の回想

娘が小学校に入学した時、ポプラ社から子供向けの本を書いてと言われ「自分の子供達への伝言」として夫の宇井純が書き始めたのが『キミよ歩いて考えろ』です。以下、桑原史成氏との出会い、ネコ四〇〇号実験との出合いについて書かれた箇所を抜粋します。

一九六二（昭和三十七）年八月十一日、桑原氏に同伴を願って新日窒付属病院を訪れて細川一博士に会おうとすると、もう博士は会社をやめて、郷里へ引退したと言われた。それでは博士と協力して研究していた人からちょっとでも話をきいて帰りたいとたのみ込むと、若い真面目そうな医師が出て来て、会社には秘密にしろと言われているのでと言いながら、結構親切にいろいろ教えてくれた。先生がデータを説明している最中に看護士が先生を呼びに来て先生はそそくさと出ていった。

私と桑原さんはそっと目くばせしてノートを覗いてみた。そこに一枚の紙が挟まっていて酢酸工場の廃水の中に水銀がどの位含まれているかのデータがあるではないか。はっとして、続きを読んでみると、その廃水をネコに飲ませて完全な水俣病の症状が出た事、廃水を濃縮していくと、有機水銀の結晶が出た事、それをネコに食べさせるとやはり水俣病がおこる事、つまり工場の中で、水俣病の原因は工場廃水の有機水銀だったことを、疑う余地なく証明した報告書の写真をとった。その間五分とはかからなかっただろう。写しり終わってしばらくすると先生が戻って来て、静かに一言いった。

『もう私達の申し上げられる事は全部お話しました。私達は先生に心から感謝の言葉を述べて宿へ帰って来た。さあ、これからどうしたものだろう。会社側が水俣病の真相を知っていて、しかもそれを隠していた証拠が手に入ったのだ。

桑原さんと一夜眠らずに相談して私はやはり細川先生を訪ねてみることに決めた。

引退した老医師夫婦二人きりの静かな生活を送って居た細川博士にとって、確に私は不意の客だったろうが、暖かく迎えてくれた。

その細川先生に向って私は自分の調べて来た事を説明してから頼んだ。『最近私はこんな報告書を手に入れました。書いてある事が本当なら、これは大変な事です。先生には会社に対する先生のお立場も有るでしょう。この報告書が本当なら、何も仰らなくて結構です。もしこの報告書が間違っていて、その結果私が考えている、会社が水俣病の犯人だという考えが間違っているなら、それだけを仰って下さい。』私は付属病院でみかけた報告書を読み上げた、そして是迄の私の調査でも酢酸工場の廃水に含まれていた水銀化合物が水俣病の原因だという結果が出ていることを話した。

細川博士の声は落ちついて冷静だった。『キミの持っている報告書は本物だし、キミの結論は正しい。実はもっと早くから水俣病の原因は解っていたのだ。熊本大学が有機水銀説を発表する少し前まで、つき止めたのだ。そこで沢山ある工場廃水を順ぐりに与える動物実験を始めた。すると酢酸工場の廃水を飲ませたネコだけに水俣病の症状がでた。そのネコを殺して工場の廃水を飲ませた動物実験もさまざまが環境問題の先進国だと胸をはって言っているのを夢のような思いで見ております。

桑原さんは得意のカメラでその報告書の写真を写した。私は自分のノートに必死になってその内容を書き写した。それだけではまだ心配だったので、

五十年が過ぎて

九州大学で脳の検査をしてもらった。その結果間違いなく水俣病になっていた事が解った。私はその結果を工場の幹部に報告した。それはあの漁民乱入事件がおこる直前だった。驚いた工場長はこの結果を絶対に秘密にすること、私が相談なしに、実験をしない事を命令した』（中略）『それから一年ばかり私は工場長の言う通りの実験しか許されなかった。しかしどうしても本当の事をつき止めずにはいられなかった。水俣病の騒ぎも収まり工場長も交代したのを機に、けっして外部に結果を漏らさないようにするというのが実験を許可する条件で、もう一度工場廃水の実験を始める。キミが見つけたのはその二度目の実験の報告書だ』と。

高度成長期の時代、大きな会社の力は特に強大でした。それに反するには勇気がいりました。私たちの家の周りを右翼の黒い車がスピーカーでがなり立てて嫌がらせをされたり、「子供を外へ出すな」との脅迫状が舞い込んだりと怖い思いもいたしました。丁度その頃、富山県のイタイイタイ病の原因を発表された荻野昇先生は批判の渦に巻き込まれて、奥様は自害されました。

私も、何で私たち家族まで苦しまなければならないのだ、私だって死にたいと思ったものです。宇井は一九七〇年五月には旧厚生省で「一任派低額補償処理委員会」に抗議して座り込み、逮捕されました（のち不起訴）。警察官が家宅捜索に訪れましたが、私は家には入れませんでした。その時の親戚や周りの態度もさまざまでした。五十年の年月が過ぎ宇井の七回忌も済ませた今、日本

（うい・のりこ／書家）

19 水銀国際会議

「全地球的汚染物質としての水銀に関する国際会議」二〇〇一年一〇月水俣市で。各国研究者が基礎的な研究を報告、展示した。実質運営は環境省だったが、会議の組織外の民間企画で、サテライト会議も多彩に開かれ、外国人も参加した。

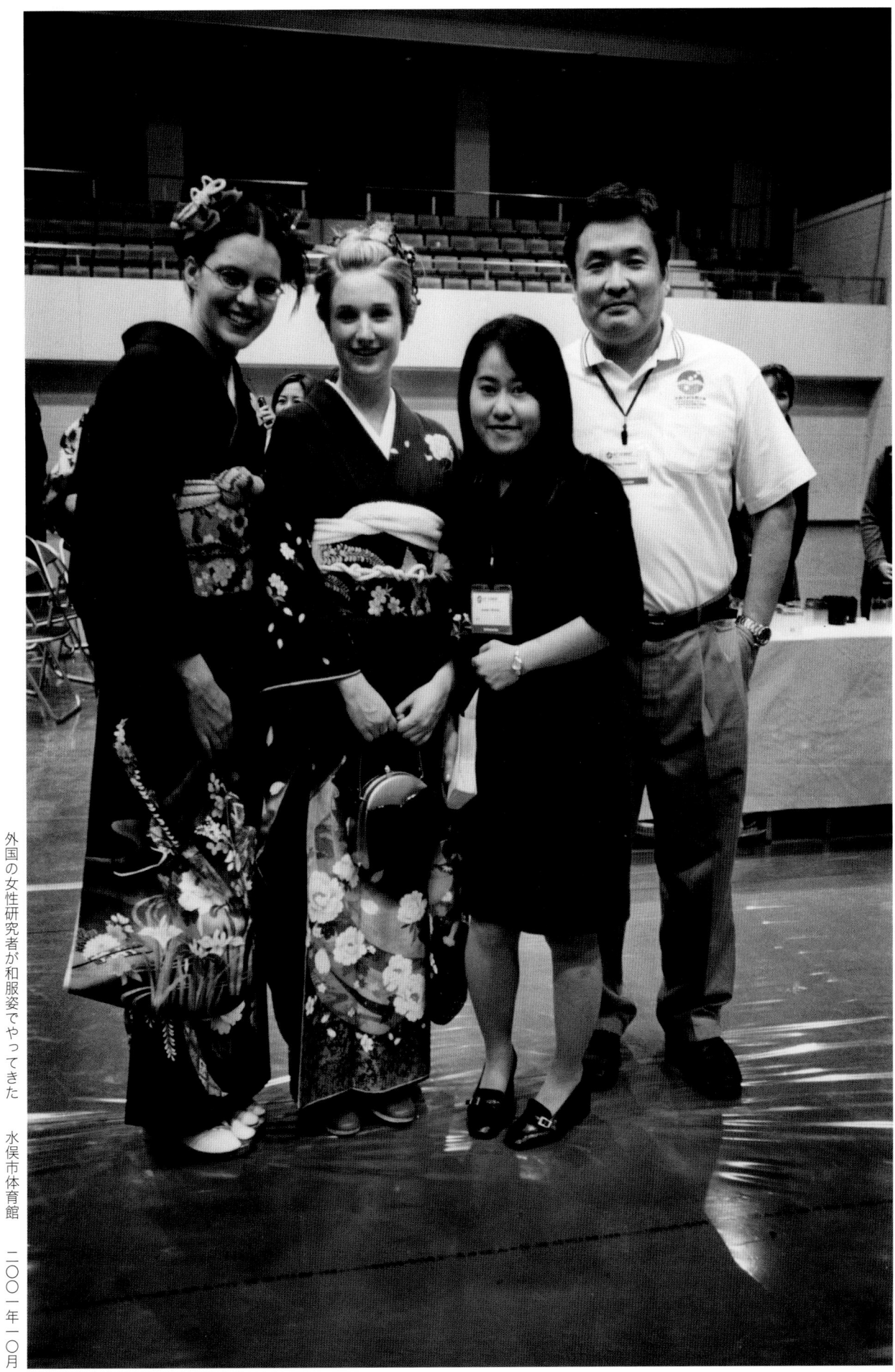

外国の女性研究者が和服姿でやってきた　水俣市体育館　二〇〇一年一〇月

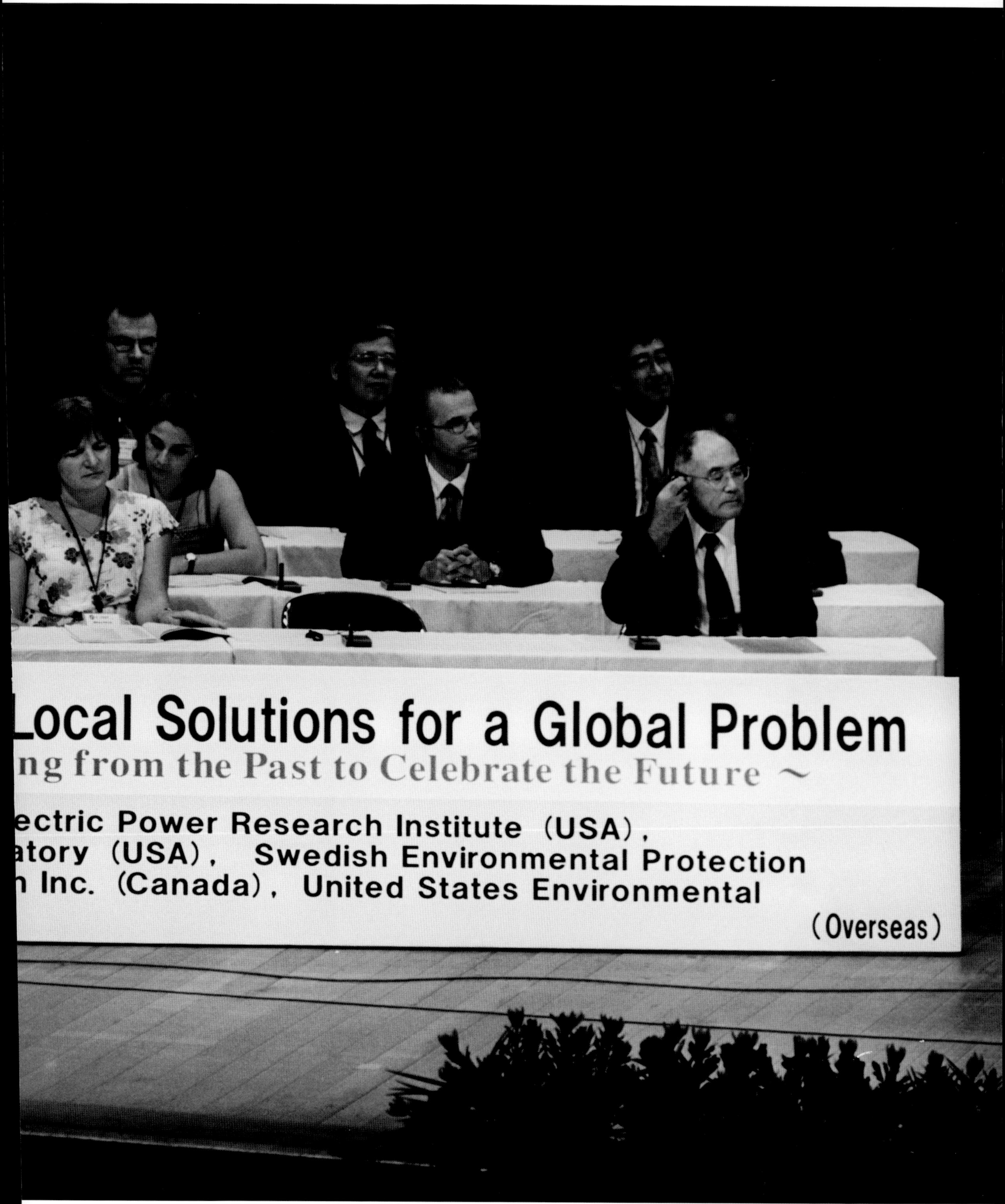
Local Solutions for a Global Problem
ng from the Past to Celebrate the Future ~
ectric Power Research Institute (USA),
atory (USA), Swedish Environmental Protection
n Inc. (Canada), United States Environmental
(Overseas)

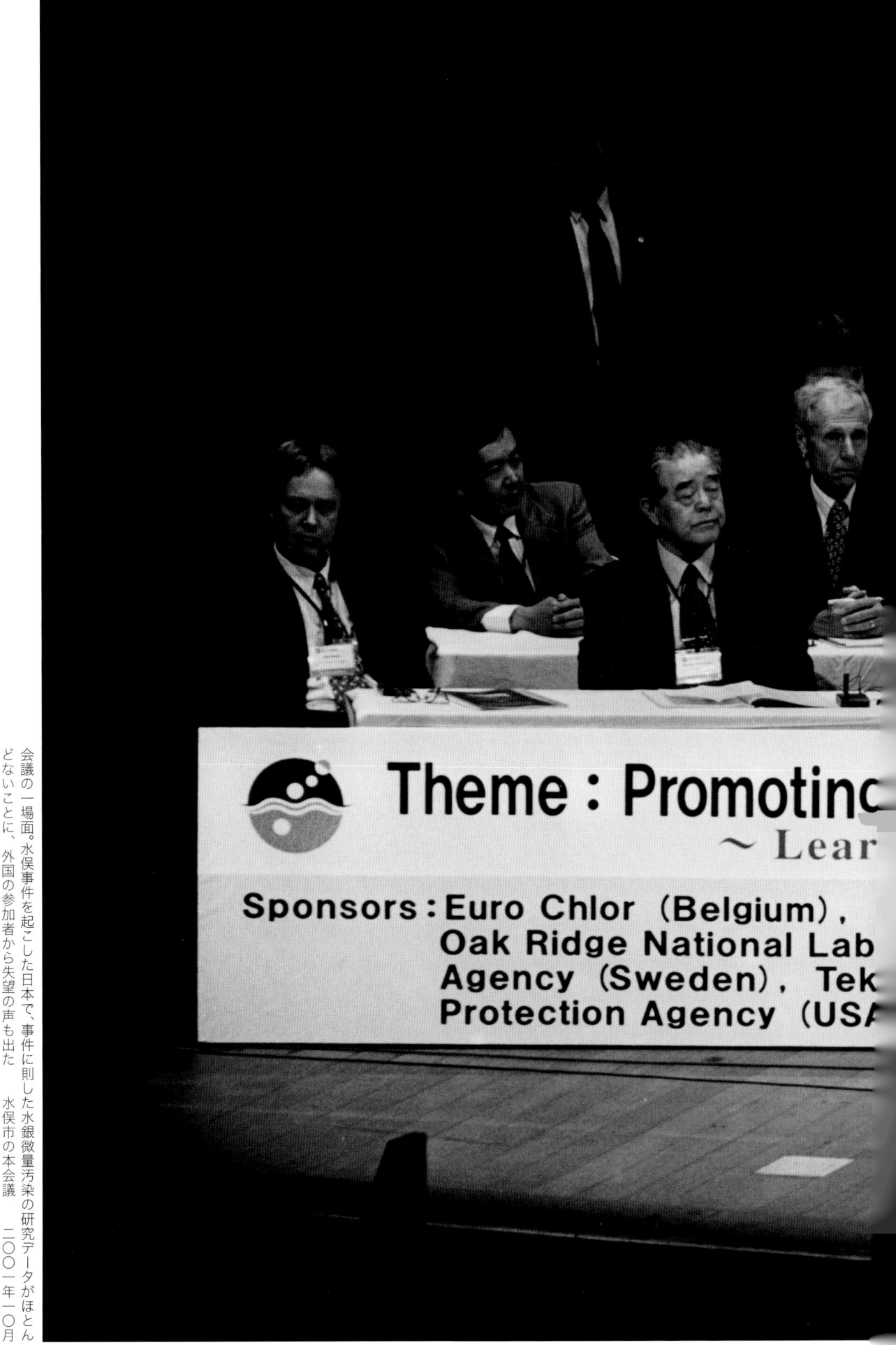

会議の一場面。水俣事件を起こした日本で、事件に則した水銀微量汚染の研究データがほとんどないことに、外国の参加者から失望の声も出た　水俣市の本会議　二〇〇一年一〇月

20 ある胎児性患者の一族

半永一光(はんながかずみつ)の写真を整理してみると、受難五〇年の歩みの断片がみえる。ヤウチ（親類）一族には、認定患者十数人。すでに死亡した人も少なくはない。一光は、成人後もずっと一人で患者の施設明水園で暮らしている。訳あって別の男性と結婚した母とは時々会う。

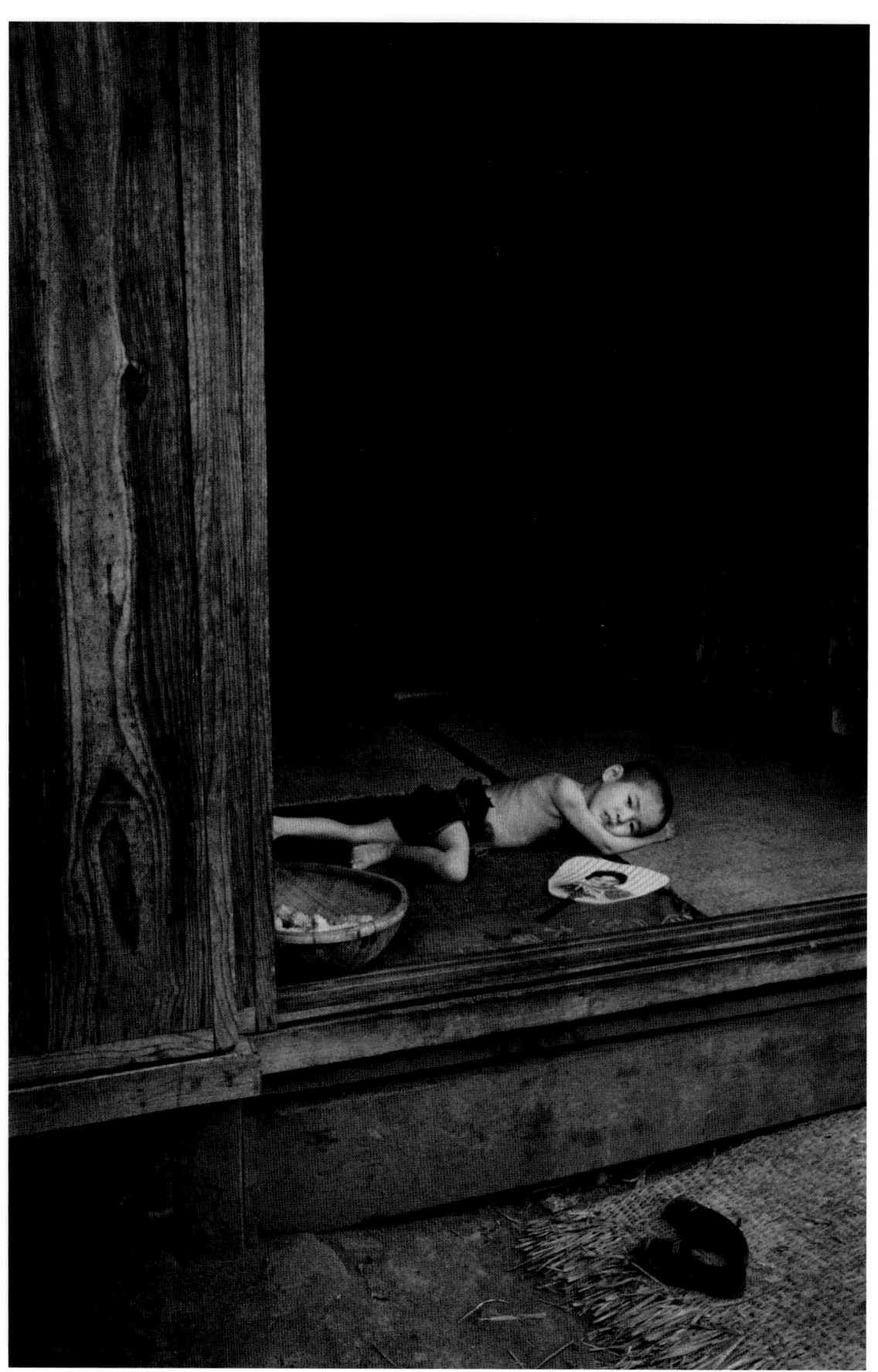

いつもひとり。実母はわけあって家にはいなかった　自宅　一九六〇年八月

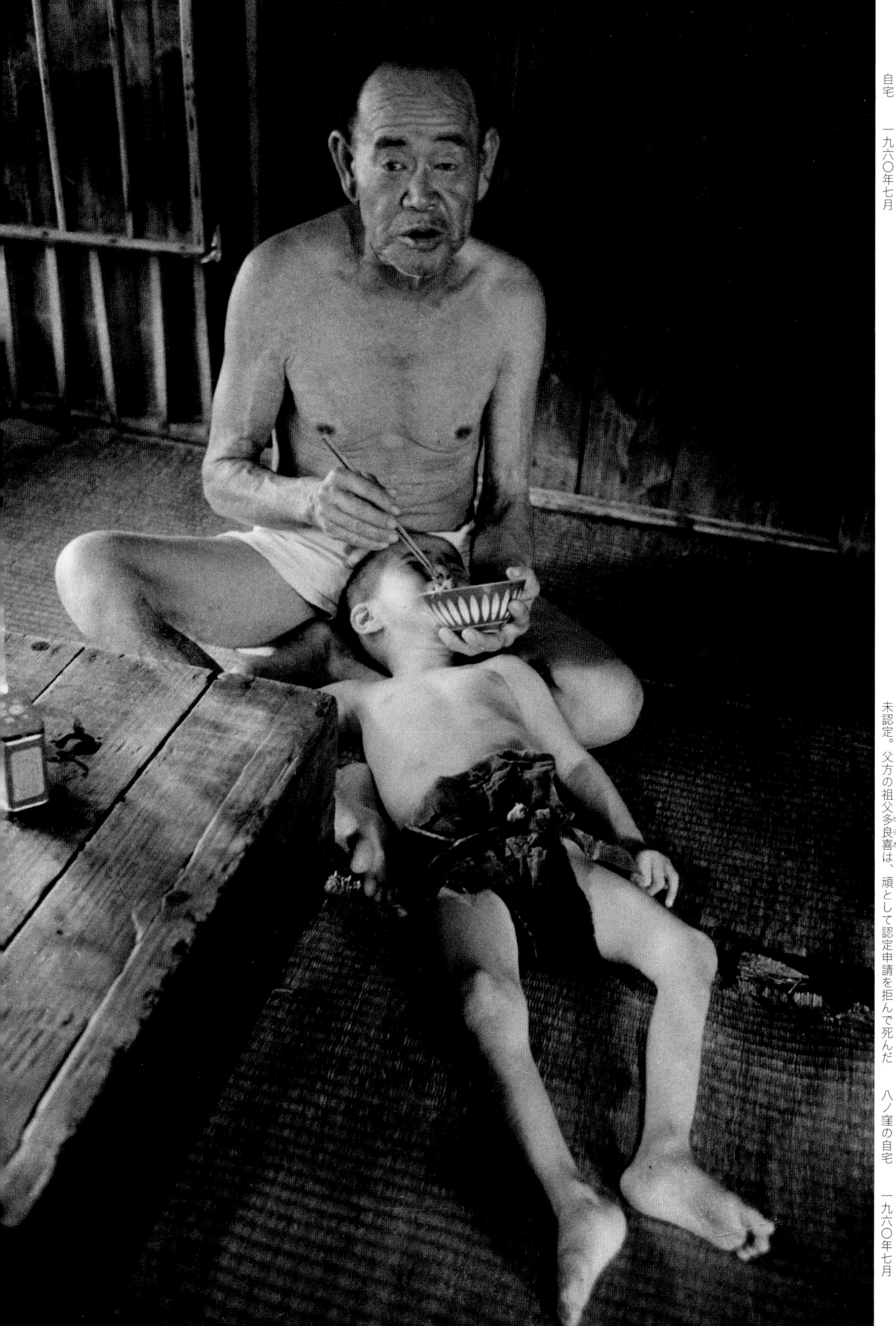

『←（次頁）どうやって寝るの、と私が聞く。居間に全員が寝た。夏にはゴザが布団
自宅　一九六〇年七月

一光4歳。石牟礼道子『苦海浄土』の杢太郎少年のモデル。奇病の公式発見の前年に生まれ、撮影時は未認定。父方の祖父多良喜は、頑として認定申請を拒んで死んだ　八ノ窪の自宅　一九六〇年七月

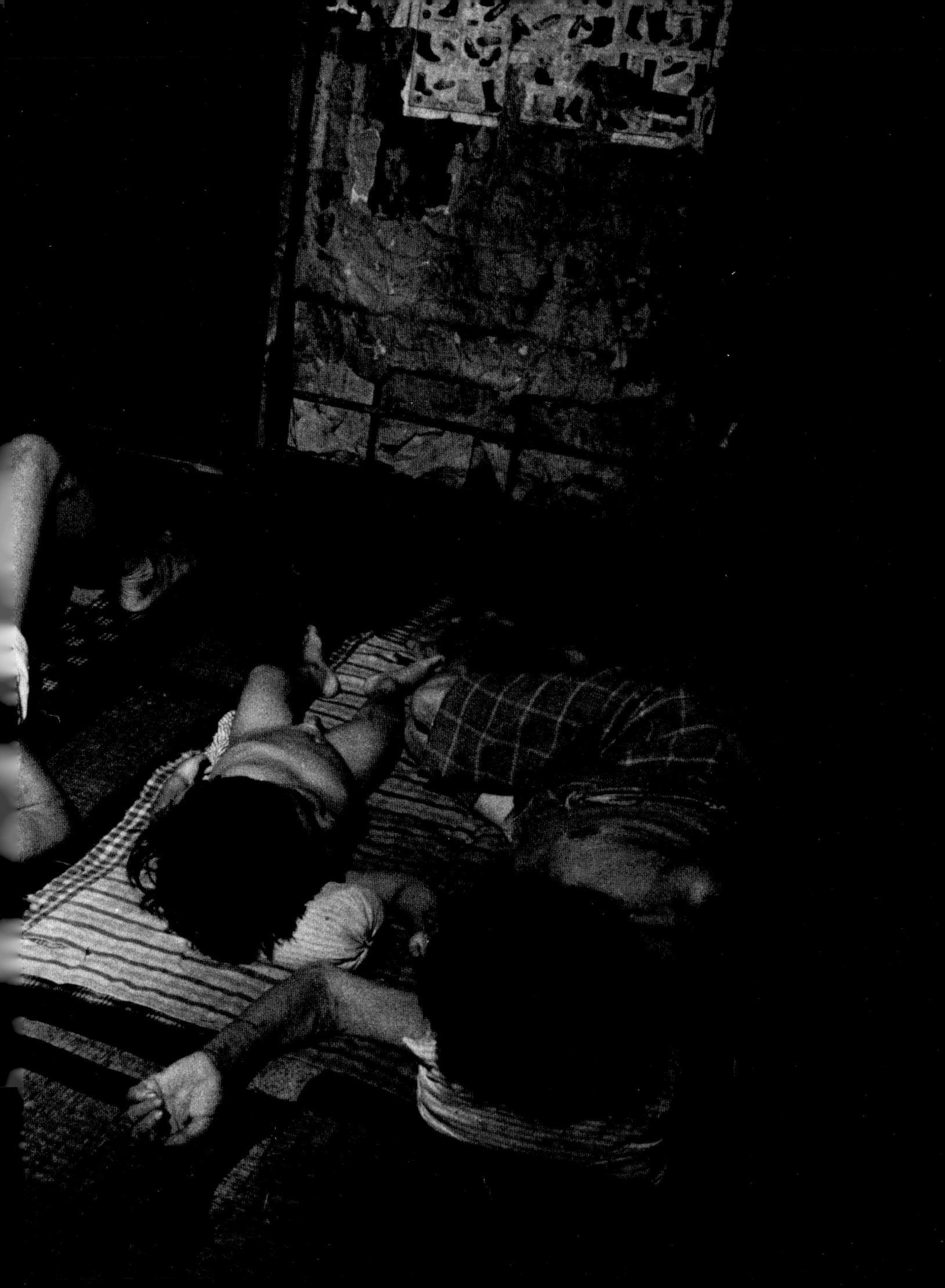

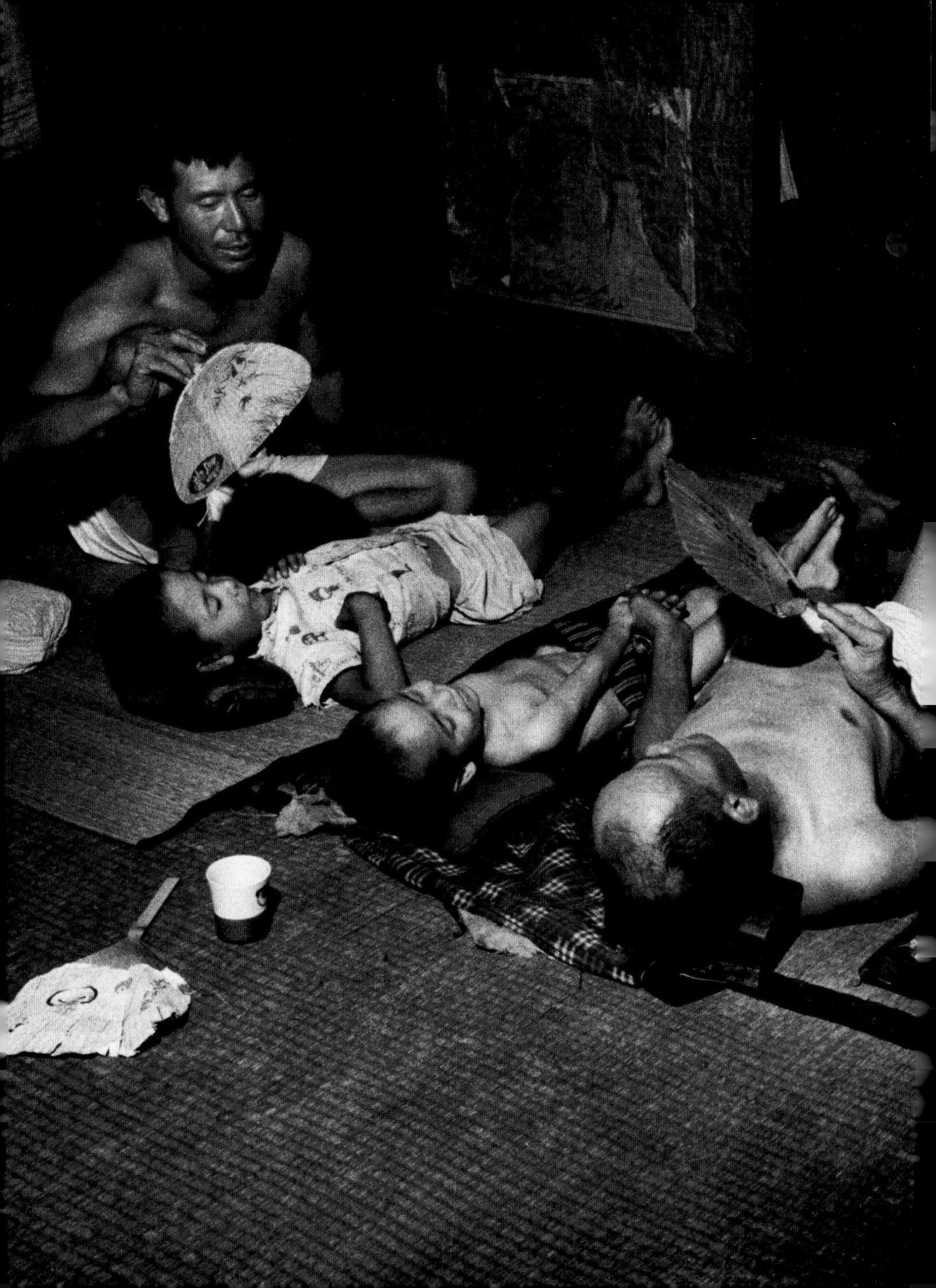

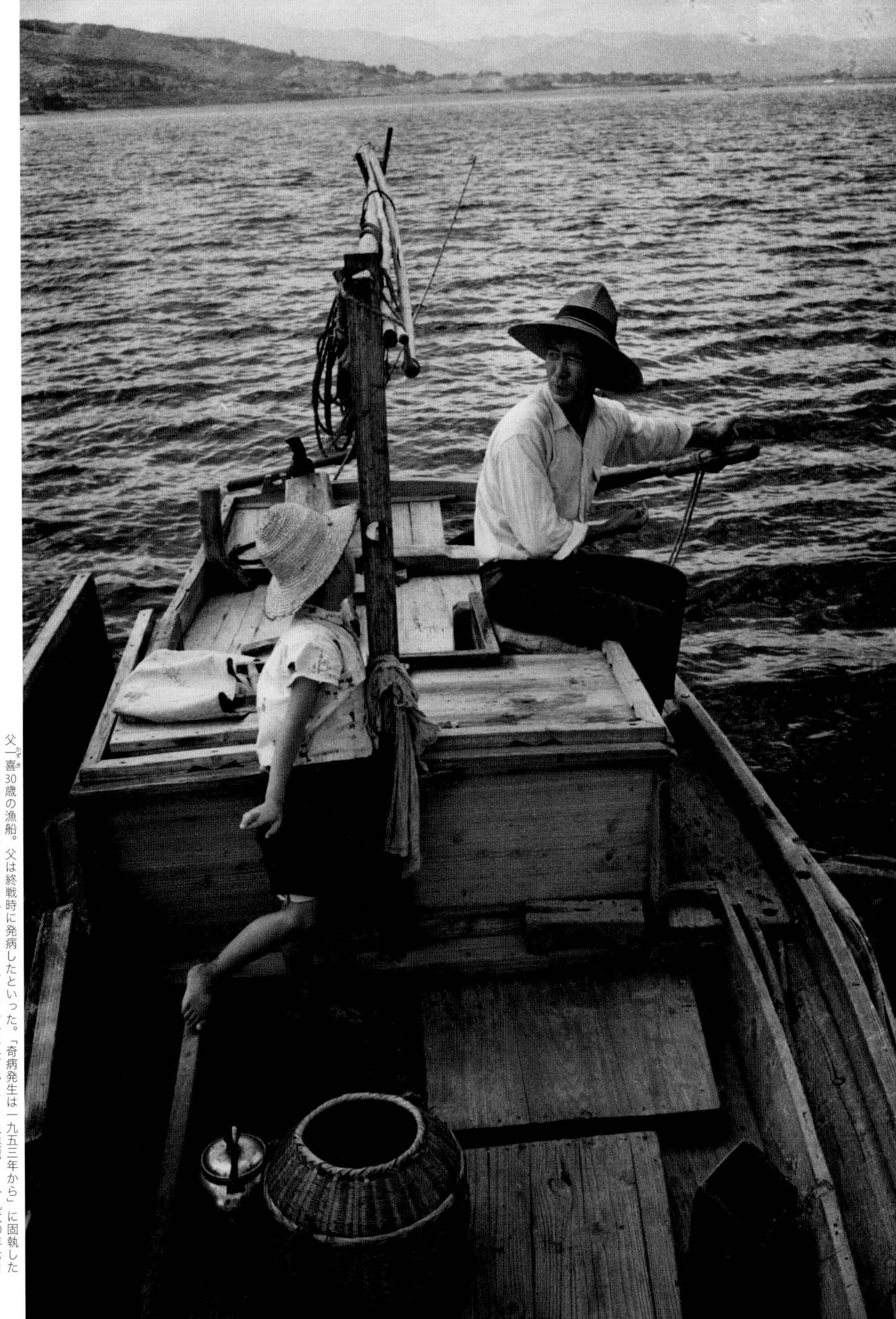

父一喜30歳の漁船。父は終戦時に発病したといった。「奇病発生は一九五三年から」に固執した審査会が発病時期不明として認定したのは、この二一年後だった　水俣湾　一九六〇年七月

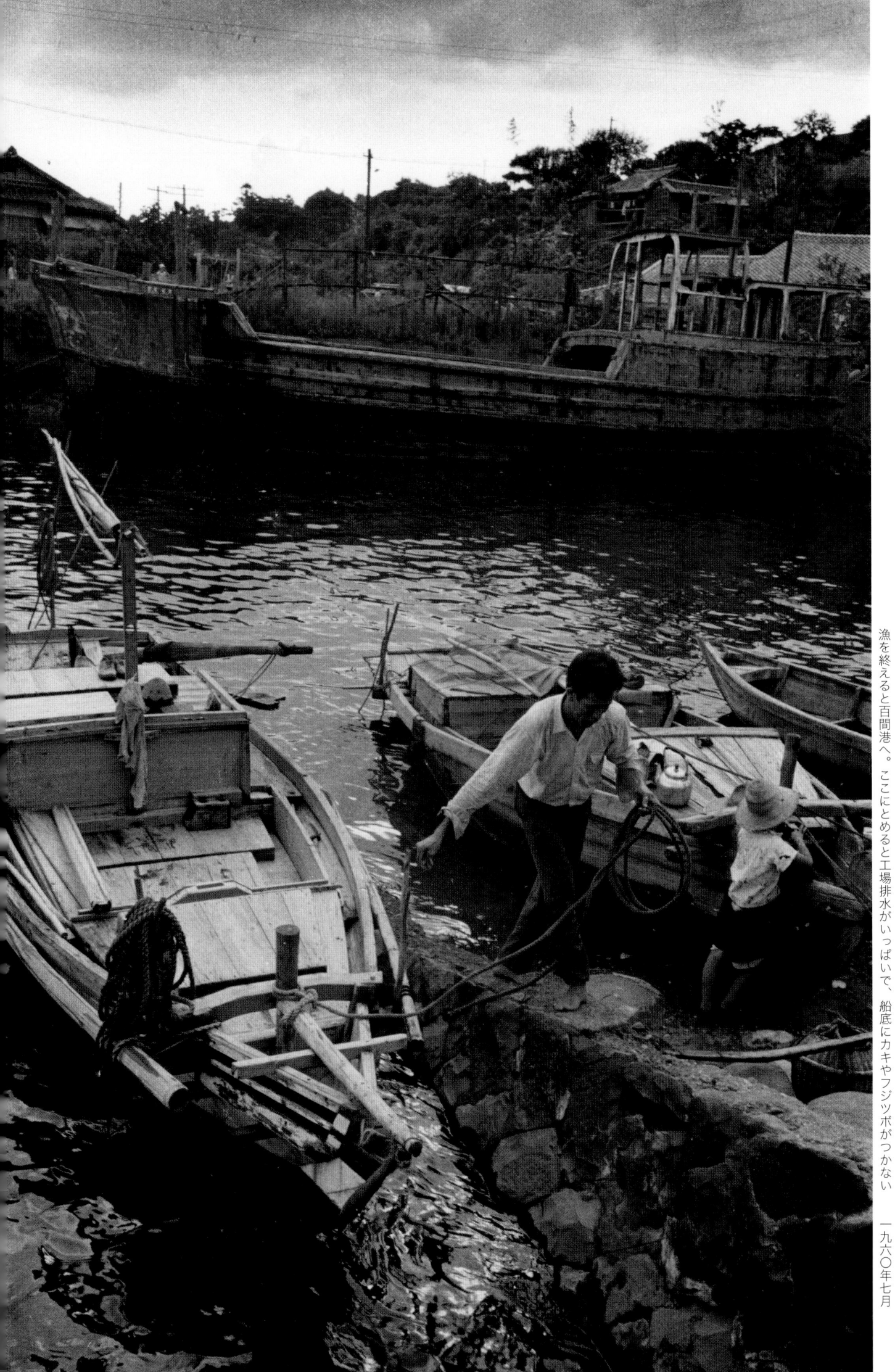

漁を終えると百間港へ。ここにとめると工場排水がいっぱいで、船底にカキやフジツボがつかない　一九六〇年七月

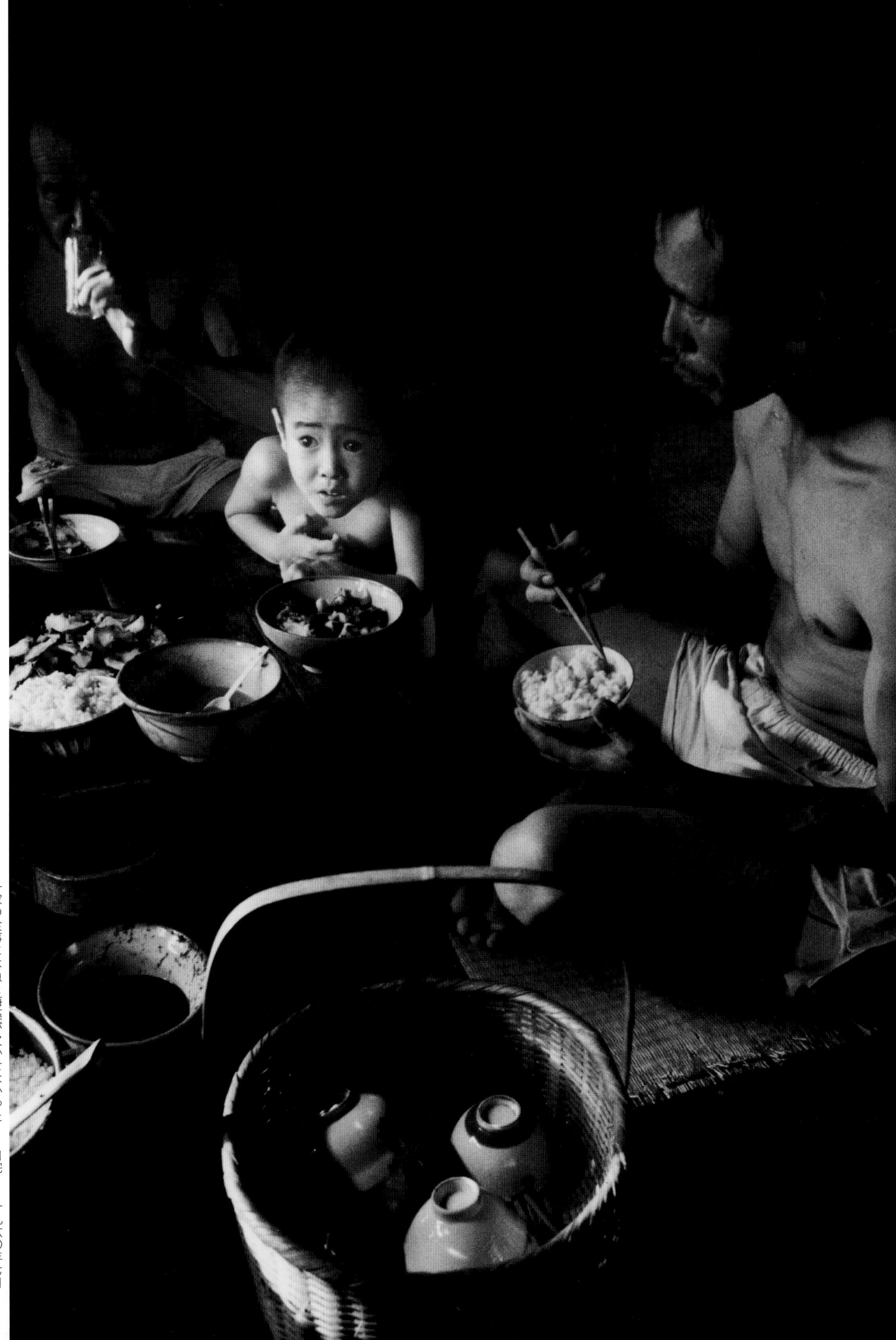

一家の食事には魚と海藻が欠かせなかった　自宅　一九六〇年七月

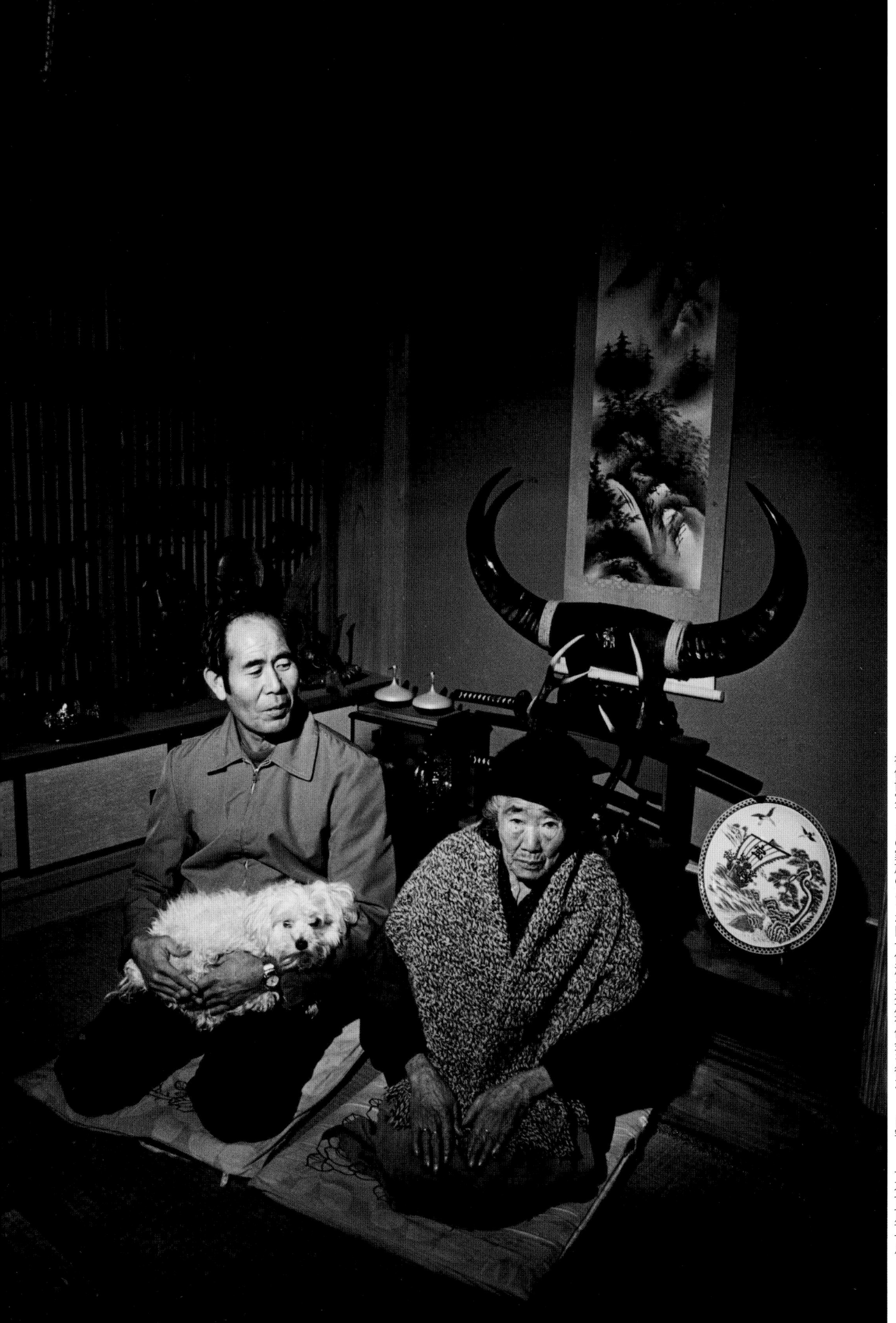

父一喜47歳と祖母スギヨ81歳。床の間も立派に。熊本訴訟判決後に東京交渉団がチッソと結んだ補償協定で、この家族のような旧一任派も追加補償金を得た　自宅　一九七七年一月

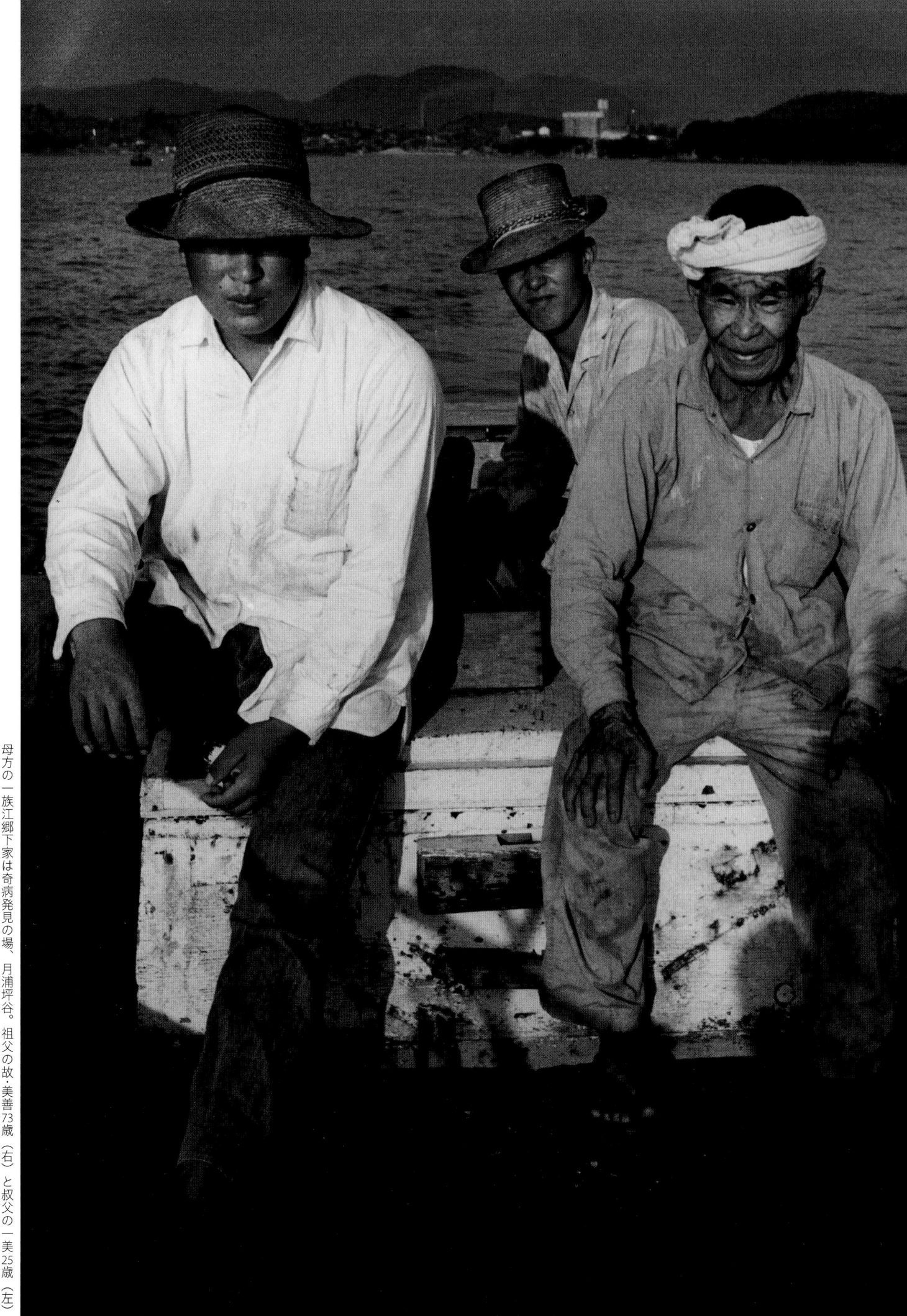

母方の一族江郷下家は奇病発見の場、月浦坪谷。祖父の故・美善73歳（右）と叔父の一美25歳（左）
水俣湾　一九七〇年九月

母のエミ子26歳（左）は、実家に戻っていた。下の叔父、故・美一13歳（中）、と祖母のマス48歳　月浦坪谷　一九六〇年七月

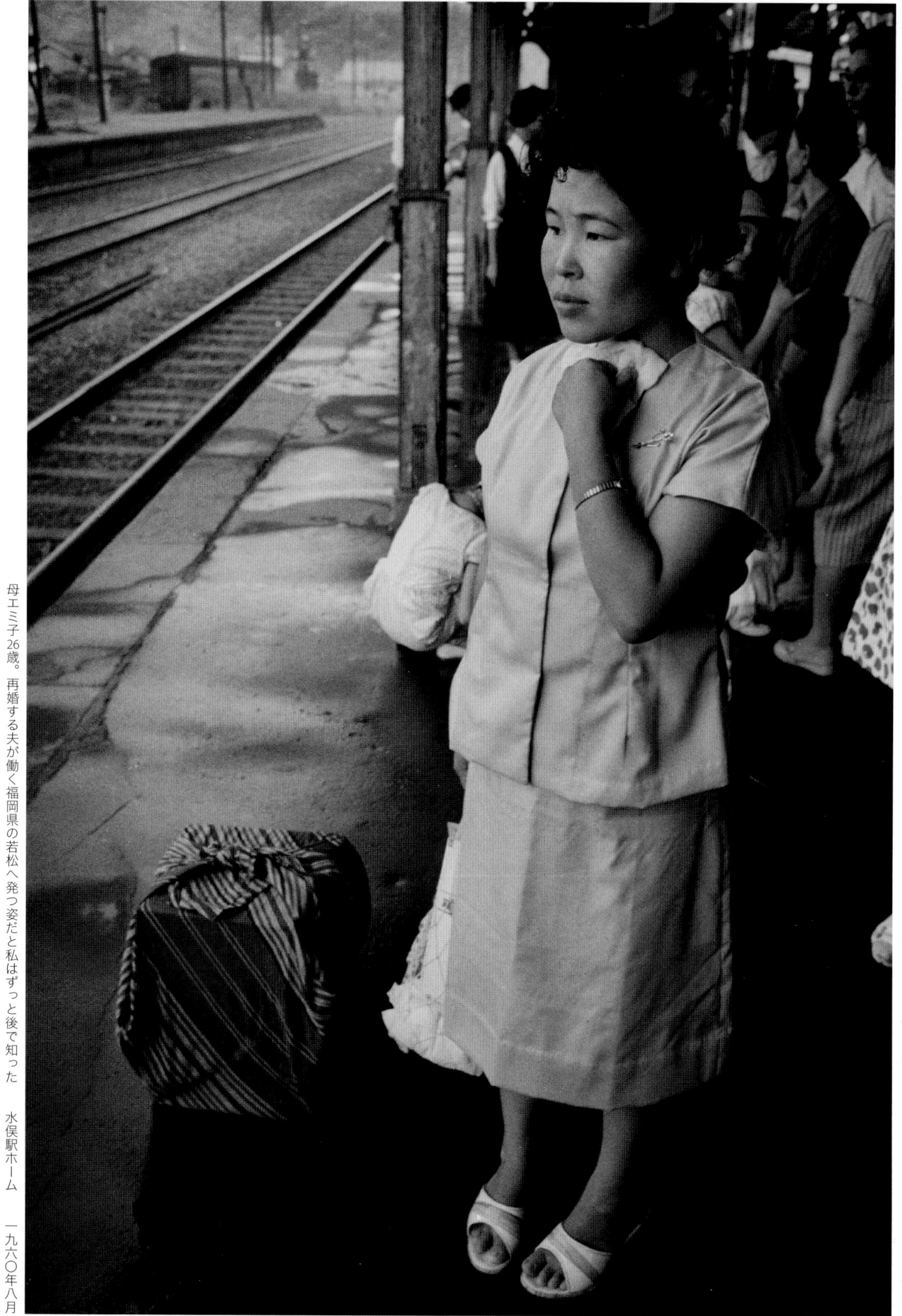

母エミ子26歳。再婚する夫が働く福岡県の若松へ発つ姿だと私はずっと後で知った　水俣駅ホーム　一九六〇年八月

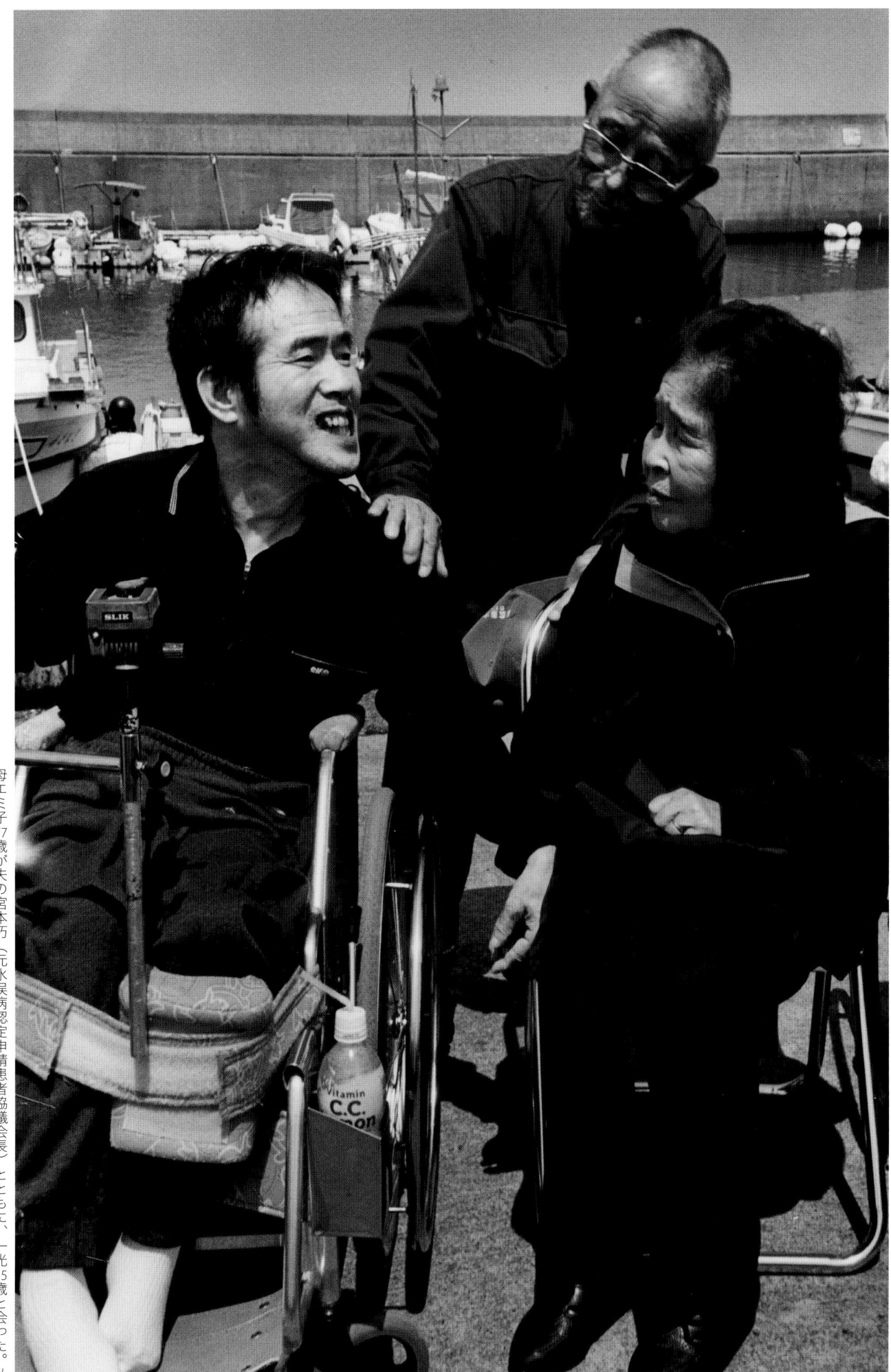

母エミ子77歳が夫の宮本巧(元水俣病認定申請患者協議会長)とともに、一光55歳と会った。私の被写体となってくれた人たちの記念集合写真を撮った日に　水俣湾埋立地　二〇一一年五月

全生類への鎮魂

不知火海の
水銀汚染を悼む

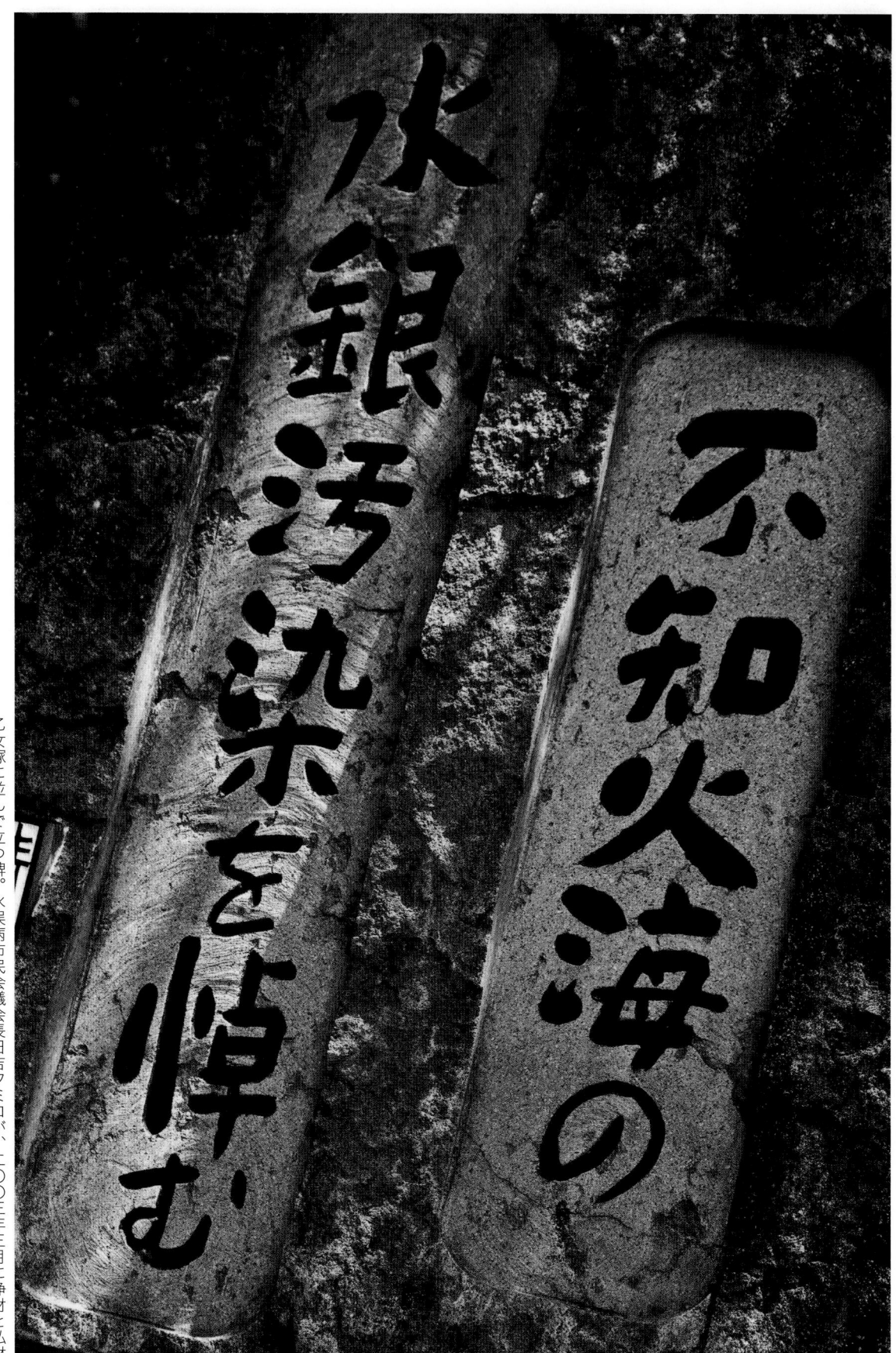

乙女塚に並んで立つ碑。水俣病市民会議会長日吉フミコが、二〇〇三年三月に浄財と私財で建立。「不知火海の水銀汚染を悼む」「忘れまじ人類の負の遺産」の字は淵上清園。趣意書はアイリーン・スミスが英訳して刻んだ　水俣市神ノ川　二〇一三年五月

[附]

あとがき ……………………………………… 桑原史成 162

Kuwabara Shisei's photo-documentary
The Minamata Disaster …………………… Kuwabara Shisei 163

偉大なノーテンキということについて ……… 西村幹夫 165

水俣事件と桑原史成の略年表（一九〇六—二〇一三年）…… 169

不知火海の地図／Minamata and the Shiranui Sea Area …… 173

An Abridged Chronology of the Human-made
Minamata Disease Disaster ……………………………… 176

Photograph Explanation ……………………………………… 180

The Minamata Disaster Abridged translation of
the expository essay on photographer Kuwabara Shisei
………………………………………………… Nishimura Mikio 182

あとがき

桑原史成

この写真集の書名『水俣事件』は、いくつかの候補の中から、出版を引き受けた藤原良雄さんが選んだものである。事件を知らない今後の若い世代が、水俣病という言葉を耳にして「病気の話か」としてしまいかねないという危惧は、私にもある。しかし、水俣病という言葉には半世紀を超える事件の重い経過と事実の積み重ねがあって、事件をよく知っているとはいえない私の体にも染みついている。ここに収録した作品は、いうまでもなく、水俣病の写真である。

水俣病の解明は、医学の今後の知見の蓄積をなおも待つ、ということのみならず、私が生きた同時代の経済活動や政治、行政、司法を含む社会の様相の中では、まともな取り組みや解決を期待できるような域を超えていた。そのような人類初の事件だった、とあらためて思う。事件の断片の羅列に過ぎないのだし、万というこの事件の受難者の中で撮った人は二〇〇人程度でしかない。しかし、何とかこの半世紀の記録をつなげる手がかりにはなろうとかとは思っている。

水俣病にはじまり、結局は水俣病に戻った貧しい写真家人生で、この本はおそらく最後の仕事となろう。写真展を今やるとしたら、どのような展示となるのか。そんな思いで約三万コマの中から並べてみたのが、この写真集である。報道写真家なのだから、最新のニュースとなった最高裁判決が冒頭になった。ついに勝訴確定となったその原告側死亡患者本人の生前の姿が、何と五三年前に撮影した私のフィルムの中にあると教えてもらったときの驚きを、読者は想像していただけるだろうか。それに続く二つの慰霊は、長い事件の末に至った今の風景である。この冒頭部を見て、若い読者がその意味するところをつかむのは、多分、容易ではなかろう。そこに至るまでの半世紀を超える事件の流れを研究したり、記述したりの作業はこれからの若い人にも期待したい。今の私ができることは、写真を残すことだけなのである。

写真集の配置レイアウトの作業をしてみると、二〇のセクションになった。それぞれのセクションは、どれをとっても、かなり大きな著作が要るテーマでもあろう。それを各一五〇字足らずの冒頭説明だけで読者への案内にできるとは思っていない。各セクションで選んだ写真の数にも制約がある。並べた順序は、大まかにいって、現在から過去へとたどった。うまくいったかどうかには自信がないが、次のページへとめくるごとに、過去の重い事実の姿が出てくるようにしたつもりである。また、「宝子」や「生ける人形」など同一の受難者と家族でまとめることもした。短い写真説明の中に、撮影時点の被写体の年齢や場所などのデータをつけたのは、五〇年にわたる撮影でその人たちの受難の人生を読者に少しは想像してもらえるかも、と思ってのことである。こうしたところでは、文章表現も含め友人のジャーナリスト西村幹夫さんの協力を受けた。

今にして思えば、一九六〇年に「週刊朝日」の記事「水俣病を見よ」に触発されて、これぞわがテーマと直感し、水俣へ行った若い私は、わき目もふらずにインパクトのある患者の姿を、とカメラを向けた。東京での写真展開催と処女写真集『水俣病』の出版で有頂天になった。そして、韓国、ベトナム、ロシアへと仕事を広げた。それでも、なぜか、幾度も水俣へと足を引き戻された。そして、見る人が目

Kuwabara Shisei's photo-documentary
The Minamata Disaster

Fujiwara Yoshio, the underwriter of this publication, chose the title *The Minamata Disaster* for this photo-documentary from among several candidates. I am fearful that the younger generations hereafter who do not know about this disaster will easily think, "this is a story of an illness" when they hear the term Minamata disease. However, within the term Minamata disease is the weighty passage of its tragic, half-century long-happenings and the accumulation of facts. The term Minamata disease is also steeped within my body, me who hardly knows any details about it. Needless to say, complied within this book are photographs of Minamata disease.

Minamata disease's clarification, in spite of still waiting for the information that medical science will accumulate hereafter, has gone through times in my life when it seemed that proper initiatives and a solution could not be reached from amidst social aspects that combine economic activities, politics, and governmental and judicial administration. I think that such a calamity is humanity's first. When I gather up all of my photographic films, it is just a fragmented listing of the disaster because the people photographed by me among the tens of thousands of sufferers only amount to two hundred. However, I think my photos will become a clue, among other things,

Kuwabara Shisei

connecting to its half-century long record.

This book will perhaps be my last work during my life as an impoverished photographer who began with Minamata disease and returned to it in the end. If I were to do a photographic exhibition now, what kind of exhibition would it be? With this thought in mind, I attempted to select photographs from among approximately 30 thousand frames of film. The result is this photo-documentary. I opened with the latest news of the Supreme Court judicial decision because I am a news photographer. I hope to imagine the surprise of the readers when they are told that an image of the deceased patient who finally won her lawsuit is among the photographic film I took 53 years ago while she was alive. The continuing scene of the two memorials is the present culmination of this drawn-out disaster. It is probably not easy for young readers to grasp what this disaster is about when they see the opening sections. I hope to describe and investigate more than a half-century of Minamata disease's passage up to the present to today's youth. The only thing that I can do is to leave behind these photographs.

When I tried to work on the arrangement and layout of this album, it became 20 sections. Each section, whichever one you take, is a topic in need of considerably more work and research. I do not think initial explanations of barely 150 characters can explain each section's topic to readers. There are also limitations on the photographs chosen for each section. The sequential order is from present to past, broadly speaking. I do not have the confidence to say whether or not I did it well, but, as you look through the following pages, I intend to make sure that the past's weighty reality emerges. I also consolidated the similar sufferers, the 'precious child' and the 'living doll,' together with their families. I thought that I might have the reader imagine a little these people's life of agony through 50 years of photography, while I was adding information in the short explanations about the places and ages of my subjects at the time each photograph was taken. As far as this concerned, I received the cooperation of Nishimura Mikio, my journalist friend whose essay is also included in this book.

In hindsight, I was triggered by the 1960 *Weekly Asahi* article "Look at Minamata disease!" I had the instinct to take Minamata disease as my subject, and go there. As a young adult, I pointed my camera at patients who had a strong impact without glancing aside. My photographic exhibition in Tokyo and the publication of my debut photo-documentary *Minamata Disease* was my ecstasy. After this, I diversified with jobs in Korea, Vietnam, and Russia. And yet, somehow, there were many times I returned, limping back to Minamata. I devoted all my finesse as a professional photographer to 'good photographs' of patients. I was so fearful that anyone viewing my photographs would avert their eyes, having seen disgusting and awful scenes.

Once my deceased friend, Kondo Kan'iti, who was a secretary of the Chemical Industries Labor Union and who assisted Ui Jun in his Minamata disease research, said this to me: "Really, your initial works are better than your later photos that have your skillful, professional tone!" Is that so? The appreciator's heart is something that does not necessarily coincide with the photographer's imagination. I can still hear Kondo's words: "a photograph implies a record." In the current photo-documentary, I did not necessarily choose photographs that have good composition and lighting based on these personal experiences. This is because my current thought considers photographs primarily as a record. Thus, several unpublished photos from my old work on Minamata disease were selected for this book.

Despite photographing the populace of Korea, Vietnam, and Russia amidst the heavy realities of revolutions, riots, and wars, I was always able to sincerely say, "Okay, my work has finished well. That was hard work!" feeling satisfied. However, I did not feel like this while photographing Minamata disease. Heavy-hearted and without a feeling of relief, I head towards Minamata. I cannot explain why I feel like this even to myself. But, I also think the reason for that is because I am Japanese.

If I could change my life, I would not want to be a professional photographer. I told my friends that I would like to be an Enka (a type of Japanese popular ballad) singer. I was destitute, and continually caused my family anxiety.

First, I have to express my gratitude to the sufferers and people who became the subjects of this photo-documentary. I am also grateful to friends and acquaintances from which I collected essays on my requested theme "Me and the Minamata Disaster." I also want to deeply thank Michelle D. J. Daigle who did the English translation, Tsunehiko Kanō who processed photos, and the people at Fujiwara-shoten publishing company to whom I am indebted for publishing this work.

偉大なノーテンキということについて

ジャーナリスト　西村幹夫

報道写真家の桑原史成が水俣事件を撮りはじめてから半世紀を超えた。この事件は「もはや戦後ではない」というころに表面化し、二〇世紀に初めて人類が体験した惨禍であり、二一世紀のいまにも及んでいる。新鮮な魚が、気がつけば全部毒魚、人も生物も破局という異様さに、自分の生活とは遠く離れた水俣へ東京から単身で別個に突っ込んだ青年が一九六〇年に二人いた。東大工学部大学院生の宇井純とまだ写真家でもなかった桑原史成である。筆者が作成中の「水俣病事件の年表」から、今回この写真集のために桑原と宇井の項目を重視して取り込んだ略年表（本書一六九―一七二頁）を作ってみた。二人が結果的には事件を世界へ警告したということを読み取ってもらえるだろうか。

水俣湾や不知火海の魚に安全宣言が出されて久しい。しかし、長年「水俣」を名乗るのもはばからざるを得なかったという風評被害は、すべてが消え去ったわけではない。「俺っどもはな、生涯『水俣』を負うて、いかんばんとじゃもん」という網元の妻の言葉を筆者が聞いたのはこの六月だった。東京電力福島第一原発の爆発事件でも、多くの人々が今後「福島」を負うていかねばならないことだろう。

この写真集は、「写真の第一の特質は記録である」という桑原が、現在に至るまでの三万コマを超えるフィルムの中から、水俣事件の作品をあらためて選び直し、集大成したものである。

桑原史成とは、一体何者だろうか。残念ながらそれを研究した記録はほとんどなく、文献もない。桑原の写真を長年、掲載してきた小さなメディア「月刊社会運動」誌（市民セクター政策機

構）に、筆者が書いた一文（二〇一一年五月一五日号）があるので、それを書き変えて、あまり知られてはいない彼の特質に触れてみよう。

大きな敬意を払いつつも冷やかし半分の老友として筆者がいわせてもらうと、桑原の行動を支配していた特質の一つは「ノーテンキ」ということであろうか。ノーテンキとは、江戸時代からあった俗語で「呑気で軽薄なこと。または、そのような人」（ウェッブ辞書サイト日本語俗語辞書）。桑原は今七六歳で、七三歳の筆者が年上の彼を「ノーテンキ」というのは、かなり失礼ではある。だが、そのノーテンキも彼のようなケタ外れのものとなると、話は別である。時と場合によっては大変な美点でもあり、本人も気づかぬ才能となり、まさに天才的な特質となる。水俣事件が世界に関心をもたれるようになったのも、彼の存在、ノーテンキのおかげだと筆者は思っている。

桑原は一九三六年、島根県の寒村、木部村（現在津和野町）に生まれた。終戦間もなくの子どものとき、村で見かけた木炭車に近寄ってのぞき込み、高温ガスの突沸にあって、右目を失う。役場勤めの父は後に、独眼の息子に、本物のカメラを買い与えた。カメラならできる、残りの目を大事に生きろとの思いからだったのだろう。カメラは当時とびきりの高価、田舎の中学生が手にするなど、及びもつかない。村の知人を撮っては、喜ばせて得意だった。大人になってからも、たとえば凄絶な水俣病患者の写真でも、その家族に〝プレゼント〟して得意気でいる風に見えるのもその名残かと筆者は思っている。

少年時代に、反戦水兵として知られた木村荘重が木部村に乗り込んで無投票で村長となった。保守的な村に、突如、共産党村長が生まれ

赤い村と有名になる。それで、オルグだの細胞だのという左翼前衛用語は子どものころから目にする。だが、左翼に心を動かすようなおませでもなし、政治向きのことにはむしろ鈍感だった。村長を追放しに連合国総司令部（GHQ）の米憲兵がジープで村へ乗り込むと、チョコレートはないかと近寄った。「左翼用語には免疫ができていた」という。一九六〇年の安保騒動でも、感激することはなかった。彼は、田舎の赤い村騒動からの影響もいくぶんかはあったのであろう。その後生涯、戦争や動乱、事件の中の民衆の姿を追う写真家となっていった。水俣作品がその登竜門となった。

「大学出となれば、村の役場勤めなどで安穏にできる」という父の言葉により東京農大へ入ったが、学業もそこそこに、東京綜合写真専門学校へ通いつめる。

一九六〇年五月、都会での就職を求めず写真家としてのテーマを求めて帰郷する列車に、写真仲間が届けてくれたお茶や弁当の中に「週刊朝日」があった。同誌小松恒夫記者が水俣の現地をルポした「水俣病を見よ」が目にとびこんでくる。記事に「公害」の文字がある。彼が子どものころから知っていた文字は「鉱害」だった。郷里木部村は、近くに天領の銅鉱山があり、そこから出る砒素で水田はしばしば赤いカナヤケ田となり、自分も砒素汚染の水を飲まざるを得ないという体験があった。この水俣では何十人もの死者まで出ているし、写真では手つかずのテーマである。そうだ、コウガイだ、と思った彼は、郷里で父母に会った翌日東京へ引き返し、小松記者を訪ねて準備に入る。壮絶な患者の写真など新聞や雑誌には載せにくいだろうな、と思うでもなく、まずはテーマに出会って心高まるのだった。さらに彼は後に「わが身を震撼させる出会い」をこう書いている。

「驚くべき事実が記載されていた。水俣の魚を直接に食べたこともない乳児までが胎児性の水俣病にかかり一五人も倒れているというのである。急に、誰かに話しかけたくなるような、身体を思いきり動かしたくなるような衝動にかられた」（桑原史成『報道写真家』岩波新書、一九八九年、二八頁）

この記述には、実は困る部分がある。水俣への衝動はその通りだが「胎児性の水俣病にかかり」はちょっと違うのである。この時期、医学者たちはそれを胎児性水俣病だとは、まだ認めていない。後で知る事実であるにすぎないことまでも、既に学問的に認知されていたように読者に思い込ませかねないことまでに書いてしまう。これも彼のノートンキに、まっしぐらに悲劇の子どもたちにレンズを向け、漁民の母と同様に、この子らを本心奇病だと思い続ける。こうして、桑原は後に医師の原田正純がいう「ヒトの命の原初の場である子宮環境を侵した世界初の事件」を、真っ先に写真でとらえたジャーナリストとなった。

この半年ほど前に後の作家水上勉も奇病を見に水俣へ入ってはいる。
「NHK『日本の素顔』は、奇病の実態をうつした。骨と皮だけの人間が大写しにされ、コップの水さえ呑めぬほどにふるえている老人。地獄草紙をみるような光景に、すぐ熊本ゆきを思いついて……。奇病などというものではなく、これは白昼下に起きている企業殺人だった」（推理小説『海の牙』あとがき、中央公論社、一九七七年、六三九頁）。そして後にこう話した。

「私は洋服の行商をしながら小説を書いていた。……実際（私は）頭が混乱していたんです。もっと追及していかなきゃならない問題なのを人殺し小説にまぶせてしまわなきゃなんないこの当時の小説商売の悲しさでございました」（水俣病三十年記念講演で「水俣」紙、一九八六年六月五日）。小説商売はもとより、技術者、行政官、医者、文化人、学者、経済人、芸術家、宗教家、政治家、マスコミ、ジャーナリズムの商売も、それぞれに自分の高度成長に忙しく、事実上この事件を黙殺するという状況にあった。

このしばらく前、不知火海沿岸漁民が新日窒（チッソの旧社名）水

六頁）。目前の海にいる魚は怖くて手が出せないが、「魚食べずに何の人生か」という庭先漁民のつぶやきが聞こえるような風景である。普通にみえるが実はすごいこんな写真がほとんど未公表なのだ。若い桑原の目からは、こうした写真は、写真集に載せるに値する図柄とは思わなかったのかもしれない。そうした点まで見直して「写真の特質である記録」に徹したのが今回の写真集なのだろう。

桑原はマスコミに水俣病作品を売り込めると思っていた。これもノーテンキの一つであろう。病院での患者の姿など紙面に出せるものではない。悲惨な姿を載せないのは、戦争報道で死体を載せたがらないのと同様である。こうして、売り込めなかった桑原作品が現存の唯一の偉大な記録となる。桑原は貧乏だった。

アルバイトで資金を得て水俣病の真相を追った宇井が桑原の旅費を出して、二人が決定的な証拠を握ったのが一九六二年八月である。新日窒水俣工場付属病院を訪問した二人の目前に、会社の極秘資料を置いたまま、医師小嶋照和が電話に呼ばれ部屋を出た（多分、見てもいいよという小嶋の暗示だったのだろう。無名の青年と大学院生なのだから）。宇井が記録をめくり、桑原が次々に接写した。水俣病の原因が工場排水の有機水銀であることを最終的に実験で確認したデータとフィルムから解読した宇井は、後に膨大な記録で患者運動の原典となった『水俣病』の執筆をはじめる。だが、それを大手のジャーナリズムで載せてくれるようなところはなかった。

このフィルム記録「精溜塔廃液について」の原文は、一三年後に熊本県警による会社への強制捜査で押収されるまで、内容を知っていた部外者は宇井純だけであろう。文字を接写した写真など絵にならない。桑原はフィルムごと宇井に渡してしまい、現在は行方不明である。

極め付きの偉大なノーテンキについて書こう。

土門拳の弟子で写真家の心があった富士写真フイルム勤務石井彰の好意で「水俣病――工場廃液と沿岸漁民」（一九六二年九月、東京銀座の

俣工場へ乱入し、漁業補償、患者見舞金契約を経て、乱入事件の漁民たちが大量逮捕され、事件が終わった。水俣病問題本体の追及もついでに終わってしまう。東京では「国会は『安保』と『ベトナム問題』に焦点を合わせてしまって"水俣病"はケシ飛んでしまった感」（月刊「水」一九六〇年一月号）となり、その後の九州では、三池争議、炭鉱爆発、新日窒の安定賃金闘争、蜂の巣砦騒動などでケシ飛んだ。

事件がケシ飛びつつある中で、彼は水俣市立病院長大橋登に会い「水俣病専用病棟で患者の写真を撮らせてきるとぅ？」と院長に一喝された。桑原はご託を並べず「患者を撮って写真家になりたい」と答えた。まさに本心だった。これほどノーテンキな答えはあろうか。それが院長の心を動かした。

この青年に撮らせてもトラブルになるまいと院長は思ったのだろう。小児性患者田中実子に付き添う母アサヲらの手引きで、漁村を歩き回る。この時期、魚の水銀汚染はまだかなりのものだったのだが、彼は漁家のあばら家に泊めてもらい、その魚も食べた。変な青年がいると漁村は好奇と好意との目で彼を受け入れた。

初めて撮った熊大第一内科による"集団検診"で、漁民が公民館に詰めかけた。筆者がそのコマを全部見ると、検診とは違う。漁民の体を診ているコマがない。下を向き問診表に住民の答えを書いているだけである。それでもわが子を頑としても水俣病とは認めなかった。

漁獲自主規制で食うや食わずの漁民が、工場からもらった見舞金で新調したらしい夏着を子どもにきせている（本書五、六三三頁）。医者がじっと子へ目を向けるコマもあろうかと探したが、ほとんどなかった。なぜか。医学は普通の脳性マヒと区別できないこの子たちを頑として水俣病とは認めなかった。毒物が胎盤を通過するはずがないという医学だったからである。

別のコマには、このとき水俣湾以外でとった魚（これも多分水銀汚染魚）を自転車で水俣の漁村へ売りに来る風景までもある（本書一一

富士フイルムフォトサロン）をやれた。「私のデビューは順風満帆」と桑原は得意だった。早くも写真家の登竜門突破である。

そこで、彼はその写真パネルを全部、水俣市役所に送り"寄付"した。水俣病では食えないから、韓国やベトナムの仕事にも一〇年ほど出た。その間も、終始寄付したと思い込んでいた。

しかし、市役所は桑原作品を公民館の床下に放りこんで、ほこりまみれにしたのである。実はこれが、すごい結果を生んだ。

新潟水俣病事件を経て一九六八年に政府が水俣病を公害病に認定すると、ようやく、訴訟など患者支援運動が勃発する。水俣病市民会議にプリントされ水俣市立水俣病資料館に常設展示となっている。「それでいいんですよ」と桑原はいうのである。

桑原の写真に触発されて記録映画作家の土本典昭が水俣へ行った。桑原の写真集を見せられた米国の著名な写真家ユージン・スミスも水俣を撮って世界へ広げた。その他多数の青年写真家が桑原の後を追うように撮った。桑原はだれに対しても親切だった。しかし、五〇年前に撮った患者がいまどうしているか、同じ人物や家族ごとに時代を追って記録できるのは、桑原だけである。そうした時代の流れが分かるように今度の写真集では注意深く配列されている。

桑原は写真家であって、水俣事件の研究者ではない。彼がノーテンキに書く文字には、とんでもない事実誤認や筆禍事件寸前といったものまであって、油断はならない。彼が書く著作物は日本ではあまり敬意を払われてこなかったようにも見える。未公表の作品を含め、桑原作品の評価が本当に高まるのは、これからであろう。

その一方で、韓国の心ある人たちは、韓国人が撮れなかった激動の現代韓国を残してくれた桑原を、とりわけ尊敬している。そして、水俣作品も含め、韓国での展示がどれほど行われ、韓国の「知性」がどのように「韓国現代史の目撃証人」として彼を遇してきたか。その一端も筆者が「社会運動」誌二〇〇九年八月一五日号に書いたので、暇があったら参照してほしい。

「桑原さんの写真集を隠してあるところは知っているんですよ。出し

（本書一二二頁）。

市立病院長は桑原の処女写真集『水俣病』（三一書房、一九六五年）一〇〇冊を、売れない写真家のために、おそらくは院長裁量で買った。院長は市役所のどこかにその一部を保管させたのだが、水俣病を封じ込める市の行政は多分備品扱いにはしなかったのだろう。桑原はその本がどう扱われるか気にもしなかった。

またも「無主物」となった写真集を目ざとく見つけたのは、水俣病市民会議会長で水俣市議の日吉フミコである。一九六九年熊本市であった日教組全国教研集会で、先生たちが大勢水俣病の勉強に来た。

「生ける人形」松永久美子の姿を無断で運動に使われた一任派の親は、かつて桑原を自宅に泊め、貧しい食事をともにした仲だった。親は桑原に絶交を告げた。写真を出したら訴えるという「人形」の遺族に「かなわんな、かんべんしてくださいよ」と桑原は菓子折りを差し出すのだった。

市役所の備品でもない「無主物」を松本は、市職労事務局の部屋に移す。そのパネルを見つけた熊本水俣病を告発する会など全国に広がった運動団体は、桑原に無断で、街頭デモの先頭に掲げたのである。

事務局長の松本勉が、ほこりまみれになっているのを見つけたのだった。市役所は桑原作品を公民館の床下に放りこんで、ほこりまみれにしたのである。実はこれが、すごい結果を生んだ。

「だれがみんな持って行ってしまった」とのことである。かつて、ほこりまみれにされたことにも意に介さず、市長からの謝罪の言葉も得ないまま、桑原作品の特大パネル約二〇点が、今は新たという桑原は、何と、自分の処女写真集を、いま一冊も持っていない。「へえー、そうだったんですか」金名簿や貯金通帳にもいくら見てとれる。「へえー、そうだったんですか」にどれほどの威力を全国の学校に回覧されて、患者支援日教組職場カンパなさいよ」と日吉は役場職員を一喝し、一冊一〇〇〇円で先生たちに売る。写真集が全国の学校に回覧されて、患者支援日教組職場カンパ

（敬称略・二〇一三年七月）

水俣事件と桑原史成の略年表（一九〇六—二〇一三年）

年	事　項
一九〇六（明39）	1月12日　**曽木電気創立**　社長野口遵（したがう）〈一八七三年生、〇六年帝国大学工科大学（後の東京大学工学部）電気工学科卒、資本金二〇万円、本店は鹿児島県伊佐郡大口村〉
一九〇八（明41）	8月20日　**水俣村に日本初の電気化学工業**　曽木電気が日本カーバイド商会を合併、水俣村の水俣川川尻に日本最大のカーバイド工場、日産能力一〇トン 11月10日　**日本窒素肥料発足**　曽木電気が「日本窒素肥料株式会社」と商号改名、本店大阪市、公称資本金一〇〇万円（一九二七年五月朝鮮窒素肥料設立で興南工場に電気化学事業を拡大、四五年敗戦で水俣工場に引き揚げ、五〇年に新日本窒素肥料、六五年にチッソ、二〇一一年に事業部門を分社化しJNCへと社名変更）
一九三〇（昭5）	**有機水銀中毒の文献**　チューリッヒ大学法医学教授H・ツァンガーらが無機水銀中毒と有機水銀中毒とを区別し、アセトアルデヒド工程中の水銀触媒が有機水銀になる可能性とその中毒例を報告（慢性症状特に心臓障害、多発神経炎、多発性硬化症、詐病などとされた症例を有機水銀を含む要因による中毒と判断）
一九三二（昭7）	5月7日　**水銀汚染始まる**　水俣工場アセトアルデヒド設備稼働、廃液を無処理で百間港へ
一九三三（昭8）	3月24日　**物質的進歩への警告**　水俣出身の徳富蘇峰が水俣婦人会へ手紙「水俣ハ昔から風俗醇美人情敦厚肥沃に於ケル楽土デアッタ。最近物質上長足ノ進歩ヲ来シ工業地トシテ将（ま）タ商業地トシテ其ノ面目ヲ一新シタルコトハ寔（まこと）ニ祝著ノ至リテアリマス。ケレトモ此ノ物質的進歩ニハ必ラス精神的心霊的ノ進歩ヲ以テ調節スル必要カアリマス」
一九四一（昭16）	11月13日　**最も早期の胎児性患者が出生か**　水俣町袋湯堂に出生の女児が胎児性の疑い（七三年熊大医学部第二次水俣病研究班の報告書に記述）
一九五〇（昭25）	初夏　**海と生物に広範な異変**　水俣市袋茂道、袋湯堂などで魚が浮き、ネコが狂い、カラスや水鳥がおちる（以後毎年のように異変を目撃、と後の各種文献に記述される）
一九五三（昭28）	12月　**劇症奇病患者が続発**　漁民とその家族に精神症状、失明、運動マヒから廃人となり死者や重症者（アル中、精神病、神経炎などと誤診され、発病を隠し集落に潜む患者もかなりいた、と後の認定作業からも判明、奇病との認識もなくすでに死亡した者も）
一九五五（昭30）	1月　**乳児に脳性マヒ様の奇病続発**　漁民集落で相次ぎ出生（死産、流産、堕胎、乳児期に死亡」などの実態で総合的な調査研究資料はなし）
一九五六（昭31）	5月1日　**水俣奇病（後の水俣病）の公式発見**　新日窒水俣工場付属病院の医師が「脳症状を呈する奇病が発生、その四人（水俣市月浦坪谷の田中しず子、実子ら）が入院」と届け出 5月28日　**水俣市が奇病対策委を設置**　水俣市医師会が過去の誤診を見直す（7月27日奇病患者を隔離し患者の家や井戸水を消毒、8月24日熊大医学部に水俣奇病研究班を設置、11月3日同研究班が非公開で中間報告、同27日国立公衆衛生院が現地視察調査。奇病対策委が年末までに患者五二人を認定。ほかに隠れた患者も多数と後に判明
一九五七（昭32）	1月17日　**「汚悪水の放流、直ちに中止を」**　水俣市漁協が決議により水俣工場に要望書 3月4日　**自主的漁獲禁止の方針**　熊本県が水俣奇病対策連絡会で決定 3月22日　**ネコ飼育試験で発病**　熊大研究班員の依頼で水俣の漁家が熊本市のネコを飼育、全例が奇病を発病（4月4日に水俣保健所でも水俣の魚を食べさせたネコが高率に発病） 6月24日　**「水俣病」の用語を提唱**　熊大医学部水俣奇病研究班第三回報告会で病理学の武内忠男が「中毒性因子が確認されるまでは本症を水俣病と仮称することにしたい」。以後医学報告では「水俣病」の用語へ 8月1日　**水俣奇病罹災者互助会結成**　会長渡辺栄蔵、後に水俣病患者家庭互助会と改称 9月11日　**「食品衛生法を適用できない」**　熊本県の問い合わせに厚生省が文書で回答
一九五八（昭33）	6月　**行政文書に「水俣病」**　水俣奇病の厚生科学研究班主任松田心一が「いわゆる水俣病に関する医学的調査研究成績」を厚生省に提出（六〇年にかけ順次水俣病の用語が定着） 8月4日　**奇病の恐怖が再現**　袋湾のカニを食べ中学生が発病（この年新たな患者四人認定） 9月12日　**国家責任に触れた初の文書**　水俣病患者家庭互助会長渡辺栄蔵が熊本県知事桜井三郎に嘆願書「仮に工場の排水により原因があるとしても、何らの対策もなく排水を許可しているのは国でありその責任の一半は国にある。栄養費の支給を」 9月　**排水の出口を密かに変更**　新日窒水俣工場がアセトアルデヒド工程の水銀廃水の排出を百間港から水俣川河口へ（五九年春から河口や津奈木村方面の漁民に新たな劇症患者）
一九五九（昭34）	7月14日　**「水銀に注目」**　熊大水俣病研究班が魚介類の汚染毒物について厚生省に報告（病理教授武内忠男、第一内科助教授徳臣晴比古は有機水銀と主張、8〜10月水俣工場が数度にわたり反論） 7月21日　**細川実験**　新日窒付属病院の元院長細川一（はじめ）をネコに直接与える実験を独自に開始（10月6日ネコ四〇〇号発病、六〇年夏にネコに実験再開、工場内研究班で発病再現実験を経て六二年2月までに原因物質をメチル水銀基と確認と後に判明） 11月2日　**新日窒水俣工場へ突入**　不知火海三六漁協漁民が排水停止と補償を求め、事務機器を壊し投石

一九五九（昭34）	12月30日 見舞金契約 患者家族初の工場前座り込み（11月25日）、患者一人一律三〇万円の補償要求を工場が拒否、熊本県の調停で発病から死亡までの年数×一〇万円＋葬祭料三〇万円などで調印（将来水俣病が工場排水に起因と決定しても補償の要求は一切しないとの条項も）
一九六〇（昭35）	3月30日 単独で調査 東大化学工学大学院生の宇井純が新日窒水俣工場を訪問、事件解明を決意 5月 「週刊朝日」5月15日号で現地ルポ「水俣病を見よ」 記者小松恒夫の記事に触発された青年桑原史成が水俣事件の撮影を決意し水俣へ 7月14日 写真家を目指す青年桑原史成が水俣へ 水俣市立病院院長の大橋登の許可を得て水俣病専用病棟などで撮影開始、後に胎児性と診定される未認定の乳児と母など多数撮影 10月7日 「水俣病のために大きく報道していただくことを願う」 葦北郡津奈木村磐城の劇症患者船場藤吉（五九年9月発病、同月26日水俣病専用病棟入院、同年12月5日死亡、同じ時期に同じく入院した岩蔵の4男で網元の跡継ぎ）の妻恵美香が桑原史成に手紙
一九六二（昭37）	1月 宇井純と桑原史成が東京で出会う 「朝日ジャーナル」2月4日号ルポ「問題の地（4）水俣」で「水俣病事件は〝解決ずみ〟ということの中身があやしい」と書いた副編集長高津幸男が宇井と桑原をひきあわせる。以後宇井と桑原の協力で水俣事件の解明行動へ 4月27日 新日窒水俣工場で安定賃金闘争 九カ月の長期闘争へ。スト権放棄を求める会社側に労組が分裂（六八年以降、会社に差別された第一労組員有志が患者支援運動へ参加） 7月9日 桑原史成の写真個展 桑原史成「水俣病——工場廃液と沿岸漁民」東京有楽町の富士フォトサロンで一〇五点を展示（六三年日本写真批評家協会新人賞、富士写真フイルム宣伝課長石井彰が化学業界から個展中止の圧力を受けたが10日間開場 8月11日 桑原史成が極秘データを接写 宇井純と桑原史成が新日窒付属病院で医師小嶋照和に取材、社内研究班の水俣病原因物質追試実験報告書「精溜塔廃液について」のデータの一部などを接写（接写データを解読した宇井が真相をつかみ、後に膨大な調査記録をまとめる） 9月15日 水俣病事件で初の写真個展 桑原史成「水俣病」 11月1日 雑誌「世界」で桑原史成が写真報告 未認定患者半永一喜の家庭、タコ漁、食事風景など五枚を掲載。桑原が解説「暗い海——水俣漁民のその後」 11月29日 医学が胎児性水俣病を認める 水俣病患者診査会が七時間の議論の末一六人認定
一九六四（昭39）	3月1日 ネコ四〇〇号実験と経緯を記した細川ノートの存在を知る 宇井と桑原が愛媛県大洲市に元水俣工場付属病院院長の細川一を訪問、細川が告白。この後桑原が三度目の水俣取材 8月12日 初の患者支援活動 熊本短大社会事業研究会（顧問は同大教授内田守）の女子学生西北ユミ（後の永野ユミ）らが水俣病の子供を励ます会。熊本市で桑原作品の展示など
一九六四（昭39）	11月 記録映画作家土本典昭が水俣へ 桑原史成の作品に触発され日本テレビの番組「水俣の子は生きている」のロケハン開始（以後約三〇年間、水俣病事件の映画を連作）
一九六五（昭40）	3月10日 初の水俣病写真集 桑原史成が『水俣病』三一書房を出版。未認定患者の存在やマスコミ報道の欠落を批判する文章の巻末で宇井純が無署名で工場の秘密実験と記者発表 6月12日 第二の水俣病 新潟大学教授椿忠雄らが水俣病に似た有機水銀中毒と記者発表
一九六六（昭41）	5月1日 桑原史成が四回目の水俣取材 胎児性患者らのその後などを撮り、宇井純や石牟礼道子、松本勉（水俣市職労）らと交流 10月8日 桑原史成が五回目の水俣取材 水俣市湯ノ児のリハビリセンターで〝生きる人形〟松永久美子の瞳ほかを撮影、赤崎覚（元水俣市衛生係）らの協力で漁村風景など取材
一九六七（昭42）	6月21日 桑原史成が新潟水俣病事件を取材 「アサヒグラフ」記者と同行 昭電鹿瀬工場、住民検診風景など撮る
一九六八（昭43）	1月12日 水俣病（対策）市民会議発足 宇井純らの呼びかけで新潟水俣病訴訟原告患者らが水俣を訪問するに際し、同会議会長の日吉フミコ、事務局長の松本勉らが熊本勢に向けて広範な患者支援運動開始 4月5日 患者家庭互助会分裂 厚生省に多数の患者補償処理の白紙委任の時点で訴訟派（後に六四世帯）と自主交渉継続派（6月14日熊本訴訟提訴の時点で二九世帯）が以後別行動へ 4月20日 水俣病を告発する市民の会（熊本告発）発足 以後全国各地に告発する会が発足、水俣市役所に遺棄されていた桑原作品を無断で街頭デモに掲げるなどの支援運動も 8月21日 戯曲「告発・水俣病事件」作・演出は高橋治、上演は劇団泉座、東京・新宿の紀伊國屋ホールで初公演。以後東京・六本木の俳優座劇場ほかで公演、上演で桑原作品を映写 9月7日 水俣病研究会発足 水俣病対策市民会議の裁判研究班が、熊大若手学者、水俣病を告発する会と結成。岡本達明、花田俊雄、山下善寛、小坂谷義二塚信二（いずれもチッソ水俣工場第一労組）、原田正純（熊大神経精神学）、富樫貞夫（民事訴訟法）、丸山定巳（社会学）、本田啓吉（熊本県立第一高校教員）、宮沢信雄（NHK熊本放送局アナウンサー）、半田隆（同技術）、小山和夫（学習塾教員）、有馬澄雄、牟礼道子。東大助手宇井純、合化労連書記近藤完一、後の岡山大教授阿部徹（民法）らが外部から協力
一九六九（昭44）	1月28日 石牟礼道子『苦海浄土——わが水俣病』講談社から出版、桑原史成の作品二三点も収録。七〇年以降に多数の患者運動支援者が水俣訪問

一九六九(昭44)	10月5日 富田八郎(宇井純の筆名)『水俣病——水俣病研究会資料』 水俣病を告発する会が膨大な研究記録を非売品で出版
一九七〇(昭45)	5月25日 厚生省水俣病補償処理委が仲裁案 低額補償に抗議する宇井純、土本典昭ら一三人が厚生省に突入、逮捕(27日に仲裁確定、一任派へ死者一時金一七〇〜四〇〇万円、生存者同八〇〜二〇〇万円、患者年金一七〜三八万円など。当初の要求は死者一三〇〇万円、年金六〇万円) 8月18日 行政不服審査請求 川本輝夫ら認定棄却の患者が市民会議の協力で厚生相に申立て(七一年八月環境庁が県の認定棄却を取り消す。七三年三月の熊本判決を経て以降数千人規模の認定申請、認定棄却をめぐる患者運動と行政を批判する各種訴訟が相次ぐ) 9月3日 桑原史成が七回目の水俣取材 最新の認定患者リスト(一二一人)をもとに患者たちのその後を撮影。"生ける人形"の父松永善一(二任派)は撮影拒否 11月25日 桑原史成『写真記録 水俣病 一九六〇—一九七〇』一三四作品を朝日新聞社が出版、七一年日本写真協会年度賞。この写真集が知人を通じ米国の写真家ユージン・スミスへ
一九七一(昭46)	6月上旬 熊大二次水俣病研究班発足 熊本県委託で水俣、御所浦、有明町の検診、調査など一〇年後の水俣病に関する研究開始 9月7日 ユージン・スミスと妻アイリーンが水俣へ 桑原史成の写真集に触発され月浦の死亡患者溝口トヨ子方に借家し撮影開始(七四年十一月まで滞在) 9月29日 新潟訴訟で原告勝訴確定 公害被害者が加害企業に日本初の賠償請求権獲得(原告は賠償金上積みを法廷外で直接交渉、昭和電工は七三年6月原告の要求を丸飲みで補償協定) 12月5日 桑原史成が八回目の水俣取材 ユージン・スミスらと懇談、患者や工場を撮影 12月8日 チッソ東京本社座り込み自主交渉 川本輝夫ら新たに認定された患者と家族の行動に支援者多数
一九七二(昭47)	6月5日 水俣病患者が初の海外行動 宇井純の参加よびかけ運動にこたえて、坂本しのぶ、浜元二徳らが国連人間環境会議(ストックホルム)の人民広場へ
一九七三(昭48)	3月20日 熊本訴訟で原告勝訴 死者最高一八〇〇万円の慰謝料、見舞金契約は公序良俗に反し無効。チッソは判決前も控訴権放棄、判決後原告らがチッソ東京本社交渉を開始 5月22日 「第三の水俣病」熊本大二次研究班報告書の総括文に「第三の水俣病」の言葉がありその報道で不知火海、有明海の魚が市場取引を停止されるなど全国的な水銀パニックへ 7月9日 水俣病患者補償協定 医療費、年金、生活保障基金など熊本判決額に上積み、以後の認定患者にも適用
一九七四(昭49)	1月10日 水俣湾封鎖仕切り網設置作業 熊本県が水俣湾内の水銀汚染魚を封じ込めるとする工事を開始。湾の仕切り面積は三三〇万m²、初期設置費用一九〇〇万円(熊本県が支出) 1月17日 水俣湾で汚染魚の捕獲始まる 以後一九七七年十月まで汚染魚はチッソが買い上げドラム缶コンクリート詰め処理で水俣湾埋立地へ 4月7日 水俣病センター相思社 全国からの寄金で水俣市袋に落成、以後患者運動支援 8月25日 「生ける人形」命つきる 小児性患者松永久美子が死亡。失外套症候群(apallial syndrome)無動無言(akinetic mutism)で一八年間の二三歳、死者一〇〇人目
一九七五(昭50)	8月7日 「補償金目当てのニセ患者」 熊本県議二人が環境庁陳情の席で発言、問題となる
一九七六(昭51)	3月29日 水銀ヘドロ処理補償協定 熊本県と水俣市漁協(漁協員一四三人)が調印、補償金一六・九億円(工期が大幅に遅れ、八四年三月に二次補償一六・二五億円追加補償で合意)
一九七七(昭52)	1月15日 桑原史成が成人した胎児性患者を撮る 坂本しのぶや加賀田清子が成人式で晴れ着の女性らに平服で水俣病問題を考えるビラを配る風景など撮影(雑誌「世界」4月号グラビアに一枚掲載) 6月14日 公訴権乱用 チッソ元社員への傷害事件で起訴され東京地裁で有罪判決の川本輝夫被告に東京高裁(寺尾正二裁判長)が「国家もまた加害者」「訴追は偏頗、不公平」と公訴棄却(八〇年十二月最高裁で無罪確定)
一九七八(昭53)	7月1日 水俣病認定の新判断条件 水俣病認定検討会(椿忠雄座長)の見解により環境庁が県に通知。以後「患者認定を狭める切り捨て策」と患者支援運動側から批判が続く 12月5日 「宝子(たからこ)」を失う 在宅胎児性患者上村智子が21歳で急逝 12月20日 チッソ経営資金の公的支援始まる 熊本県議会が県債発行を可決(八五年以降無配で熊本判決前後から終始経営危機、九九年六月政府が行政責任否認のまま国費で支援と決定)
一九七九(昭54)	3月22日 チッソの刑事責任 元社長と元水俣工場長に有罪の判決(八八年2月最高裁で確定)
一九八六(昭61)	3月28日 司法認定 水俣二次訴訟判決で被害者の会の原告に補償協定より低額の賠償を認容 4月30日 桑原史成写真集『水俣 終わりなき三〇年——原点から転生へ』径書房が出版。七〇年以降の作品を主体に初期の撮影も。水俣事件三〇年の径変容を収録
一九八七(昭62)	3月30日 国と県の賠償責任で原告全面勝訴 熊本三次訴訟一陣訴訟(相良甲子彦裁判長)判決で食品衛生法不適用の責任を含め原告主張を認める(これ以降、地裁判決での国家賠償責任では熊本三次一陣、同二陣、京都で原告が全面または部分的勝訴、東京、大阪、新潟二次で敗訴)
一九八九(昭64・平成元)	9月19日 桑原史成『半世紀』(ソウル市朝鮮日報美術館)の中で、胎児性や小児性患者、船場岩蔵など二〇点。タイムスペース社主催
一九九〇(平2)	3月 水俣湾の水銀ヘドロ処理が終了 一五一万m³を浚渫、埋め立て五八ヘクタール、総工費四八五億円

年	事項
一九九〇(平2)	11月1日 「水俣の痛み」展 桑原史成がソウルの現代ギャラリア百貨店で、ソウルアイデア社主催。約八〇点。初めて水俣作品だけを韓国で展示
一九九三(平5)	1月4日 水俣市立水俣病資料館開館 桑原史成の水俣作品の一部を常時展示
一九九五(平7)	9月28日 連立三党の政治決着で政府の最終解決策 未認定者と訴訟原告計一万数千人を対象に、検討会で認めた人へ解決一時金二六〇万円と患者団体加算金をチッソに払わせ、行政は法的責任を認めずに総合対策医療事業の継続などで紛争停止（九六年五月までに関西訴訟を除く訴訟で加害企業と和解、行政責任を問われた被告の国と県については原告が訴訟取り下げ）
一九九六(平8)	4月10日 パリで水俣病写真展 桑原史成、芥川仁がパネル約一〇〇点を合同で展示、五月10日まで。水俣病公式発見の満四〇年で日本文化振興を事業とする Espace Japon 主催
一九九七(平9)	10月 仕切網撤去完了 七四年以来水俣湾の魚を封鎖？ 一〇年にわたる水銀汚染レベルの監視と安全宣言を経て二三年ぶりに湾内漁獲が可能に
一九九九(平11)	4月25日 『日本の公害二・桑原史成／水俣』 清里フォトアートミュージアム（山梨県）が初期から現在までの作品約一〇〇点を三カ月の長期展示、大半を自館に永久保存
二〇〇一(平13)	10月9日 桑原史成の個展「水俣」 草の根出版会編集で日本図書センターが出版
二〇〇四(平16)	4月27日 控訴審で国家賠償を認める チッソ水俣病関西訴訟大阪控訴審（岡部崇明裁判長）で、六〇年1月以降水質二法と県漁業調整規則で排水を規制しなかった国と県は違法の判決（九四年7月の大阪地裁一審判決では国と県の責任を認めず原告敗訴）
二〇〇五(平17)	10月15日 最高裁で国家賠償責任が確定 チッソ水俣病関西訴訟最高裁判決の第二小法廷（北川弘治裁判長）で四裁判官全員一致で国と県の上告を棄却、控訴審判決を一部修正して是認
二〇〇六(平18)	10月3日 新たな提訴 水俣病不知火患者会の五〇人が国、県、チッソに損害賠償を求める（最高裁判決後三〇〇人以上が認定申請、熊本、鹿児島両県認定審査会は委員を再任できず休止状態）
二〇〇六(平18)	5月1日 水俣病の公式発見五〇年 行政や諸団体が各種の記念企画、イベントなど
二〇〇七(平19)	4月30日 「水俣を見た七人の写真家たち」展 水俣市の水俣病資料館で。桑原史成、塩田武史、宮本成美、ユージン＆アイリーン・スミス、小柴一良、芥川仁、田中史子が参加
二〇〇七(平19)	10月11日 胎児性世代が提訴 水俣病未認定患者ら「水俣病被害者互助会」会員九人が、国と県、チッソを相手に二億二八〇〇万円の賠償を求め、熊本地裁に提訴
二〇〇九(平21)	7月8日 水俣病被害者の救済及び水俣病問題の解決に関する特別措置法（水俣病特措法） 参院本会議で可決成立（共産、社民は反対）、未認定患者の救済措置と原因企業チッソの分社化など一九九五年の政府解決策（約一万数千人が対象）以来二度目の政治決着を図る法律
二〇一一(平23)	1月12日 JNC設立 水俣病特措法に基づき、チッソを分社化してその事業を引き継ぐ新会社として発足（JNCは4月1日から営業開始、チッソは一〇〇％出資の持ち株会社となり、株式配当を原資に患者への補償金支払いや公的債務の返済をになう親会社へ）
二〇一二(平24)	7月31日 申請者数累計 六五一五一人。水俣病特別措置法に基づく未認定患者救済策への申請を締め切る
二〇一二(平24)	10月31日 一時金支給対象者累計 特措法救済申請が始まった一〇年五月から計二三三六五人
二〇一三(平25)	4月16日 二つの訴訟で、水俣病の認定棄却の行政処分を不当とする最高裁判決 第三小法廷（寺田逸郎裁判長）が五裁判官全員一致で、患者遺族側主張を認める。
溝口チエ（水俣市袋、七四年8月認定申請、七七年7月死亡、二〇〇一年12月熊本県を被告に提訴、熊本地裁で原告敗訴、福岡高裁で原告勝訴）について、熊本県の上告を棄却
Fさん（水俣市湯出出身、七八年9月認定申請、チッソ水俣病関西訴訟原告として二審と最高裁で国県の責任を認容、二〇〇七年5月大阪地裁に認定義務付けの行政訴訟提訴、二〇一〇年7月大阪地裁で原告勝訴、二〇一二年4月大阪高裁で逆転敗訴、二〇一三年3月死亡）について、二審判決を破棄、大阪高裁に差し戻す

（作成者・西村幹夫）

不知火海の地図　Minamata and the Shiranui Sea Area

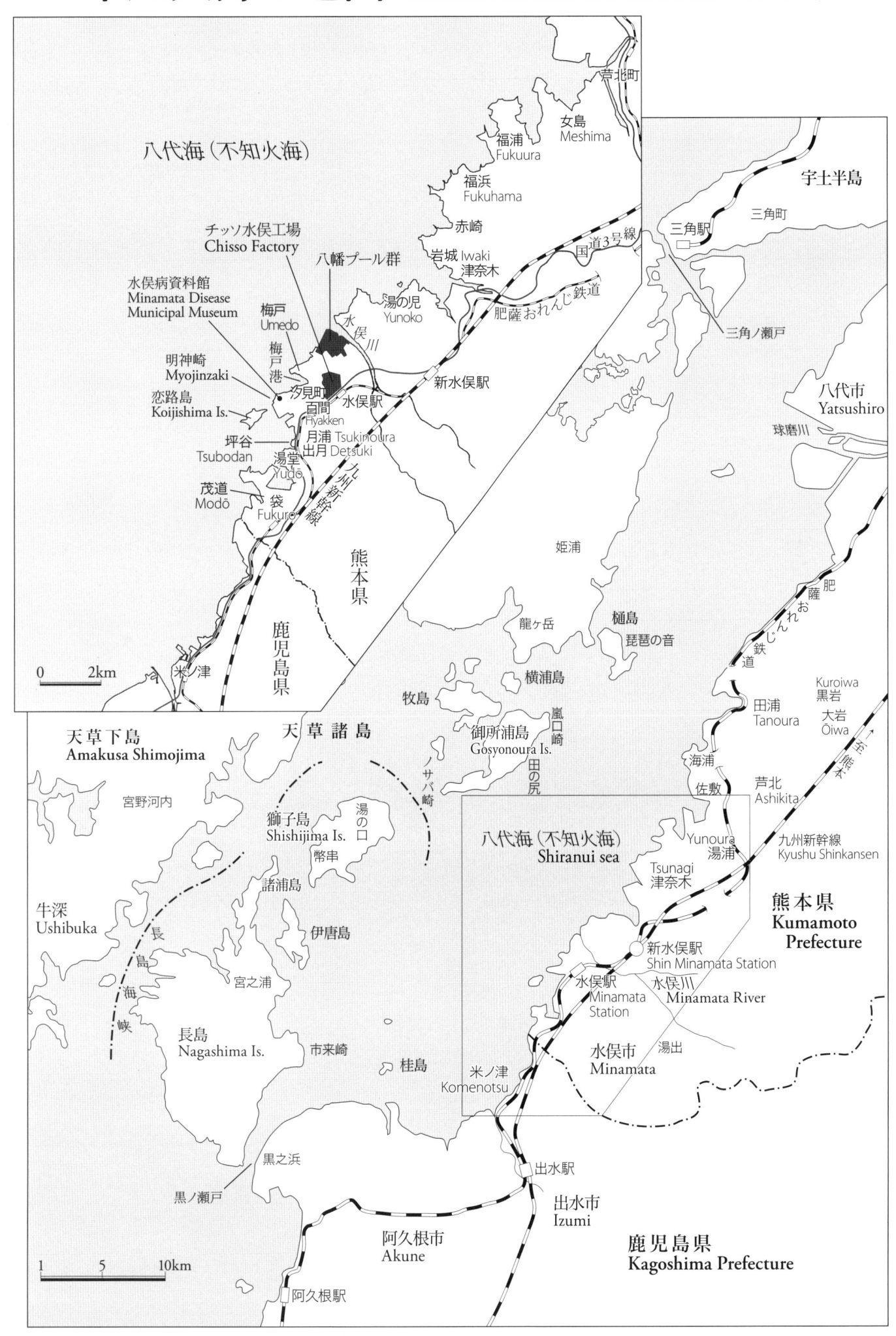

1972	5 Jun.	**Minamata disease patients mobilize overseas for the first time**
		Ui Jun as well as Sakamoto Shinobu, Hamamoto Tsuginori, etc. who answered Ui's request to participate in the movement go to the public assembly at the UN Conference on the Human Environment.
1973	20 Mar.	**Plaintiffs win in the Kumamoto Lawsuit**
		¥18 million ($67,712 USD) is the highest solatium payment made for a patient's death. Chisso renounced their right to appeal, and patients began negotiations at Chisso's Tokyo headquarters.
	22 May	**"The Third Minamata Disease"**
		There is a statement in a Kumamoto University Second Research Group report that there is a "third Minamata disease". Due to this information, there is a 'mercury panic', and all market transactions of fish from the Shiranui and Ariake seas are stopped.
	9 Jul.	**Minamata disease patient compensation agreement**
		The judicial decision from the Kumamoto Lawsuit is signed adding additional pensions, funds guaranteeing livelihoods, etc. This decision is also applied to previously and hereafter recognized patients.
1974	10 Jan.	**Installation of a blockade net to partition Minamata bay**
		Kumamoto Prefecture decides to begin the construction of a net to confine mercury-contaminated fish within the bay.
	17 Jan.	**Capturing polluted fish begins in Minamata bay**
		Chisso purchases the polluted fish and places them in concrete drums for disposal in the Minamata landfill from this time until Oct. 1997.
	7 Apr.	**The Minamata Disease Center Sōshisha**
		The Sōshisha is completed in Fukuro, Minamata using donations from all over the country for the patient support movement hereafter.
	25 Aug.	**The "Living Doll's" life comes to an end**
		Matsunaga Kumiko dies at age 23 after having apallial syndrome and akinetic mutism for 18 years. She is the 100th patient to pass away.
1975	7 Aug.	**"'Fake' patients seek compensation"**
		Two delegates from the Kumamoto Prefectural Assembly in say this at the Environmental Agency. It becomes a controversy.
1976	29 Mar.	**A compensation agreement for losing fishing grounds due to the disposal of mercuric sludge in Minamata bay**
		Kumamoto Prefecture and the Minamata Fishermen's Cooperative sign a compensation agreement totaling ¥1.69 trillion (approx. $5.64 million USD). Due to substantial delays in the dredging and landfill operations, there is a second, supplemental compensation agreement in Mar. 1984, totaling ¥1.625 trillion (approx. $5.42 million USD).
1977	14 Jun.	**Misappropriation of judicial authority**
		A patient, Kawamoto Teruo, is prosecuted and found guilty of inflicting bodily injury on the Chisso Company employees in a trial at the Tokyo District Court in 1975. The Tokyo High Court (Terao Shōji, presiding judge) dismisses the prosecution against the defendant saying "the government of Japan took little action on Minamata disease problems and then acted as a perpetrator on Mimamata victims...the prosecution engaged in illegal partiality." In Dec. 1980, the Supreme Court rules he is innocent.
	1 Jul.	**New diagnostic criteria for Minamata disease recognition**
		The Environmental Agency decides this based on medical opinions in favor of governmental policy. There is continuing criticism that it is a "policy of cutting down and restricting recognized patients."
1978	20 Dec.	**Public aid for Chisso's administrative funds begins**
		Kumamoto Prefecture and the national government lend capital aid to Chisso who is at risk of bankruptcy both before and after the Kuamoto legal decision.
1979	22 Mar.	**The responsible company's criminal liability**
		The former Chisso president and Minamata factory manager are found guilty in a trial at the Kumamoto District Court. The Supreme Court upholds the guilty verdict in Feb. 1988.
1987	30 Mar.	**The State and Prefecture's compensation liability is decided in a plaintiff's winning lawsuit at the Kumamoto District Court**
		Administrative error regarding the inability to prevent Minamata disease is investigated in additional district courts.
1990	Mar.	**Disposal of mercuric sludge in Minamata bay ends**
		1.51 million m³ are dredged, and a 58 hectare landfill is completed for a grand total of ¥48.5 trillion (approx. $316 million USD).
1995	28 Sept.	**Three parties agree to a solution**
		Tens of thousands of unrecognized patients and plaintiffs are the target of ¥2.6 million lump sum relief payment, and withdraw their legal disputes. The Kansai Lawsuit continues its demands for state compensation.
1996	10 Apr.	**The Minamata disease photographic exhibition in Paris**
		Kuwabara and Akutagawa Jin do a joint exhibition of 100 panels.
1997	October	**The partition net's removal is complete**
		Fish were blockaded in Minamata bay since 1974. Observations of the mercury pollution levels were continued for 10 years, and declared safe. It has been 23 years since fishing in Minamata bay was possible.
2001	27 Apr.	**State compensation is recognized in an appeal trial**
		In Kansai Lawsuit, the State and Prefecture are found liable for not regulating the effluent under the prefectural fishing regulations and the two water quality control laws. In the Supreme Court ruling on October 15, 2004, the State is found liable for compensation.
2007	11 Oct.	**The congenital generation sues**
		Nine people who are unrecognized congenital patients or from the same generation demand ¥228 million ($1.96 million USD) in compensation from the State, Prefecture, and Chisso in a lawsuit at the Kumamoto District Court.
2009	8 Jul.	**The Second Political Settlement**
		The Special Measures Law for the relief of patients is enacted by the government. The total number of new people seeking relief reaches 65,151 by Jul. 2012. On Oct. 31, 2012, the total number of people receiving lump sum payments under the new relief measure is 23,365.
2013	16 Apr.	**In two lawsuits, the Supreme Court rules that the administrative measures determining the rejection of recognition of Minamata disease are invalid.**

(© Nishimura Mikio, journalist)(Translated by Michelle D. J. Daigle)

1957	22 Mar.	**Cats bred for experiments become sick** At the request of Kumamoto University, fishing households in Minamata raise cats from Kumamoto City. All these cats develop the 'strange' disease.
	24 Jun.	**Advocacy for the term "Minamata disease"** In a Kumamoto University Study Group assembly, there is a description stating that pathologist Takeuchi Tadao temporarily renames Minamata's 'strange' disease to Minamata disease. Hereafter, the term "Minamata disease" spreads.
	11 Sept.	**"The Food Sanitation Law cannot be applied"** The Ministry of Health and Welfare (MHW) sends this as a written response to Kumamoto Prefecture's inquiry.
1958	4 Aug.	**Fear of the 'strange' disease reappears** A junior high school student who ate crabs from Fukuro bay becomes sick. Four new patients are medically identified this year.
	Sept.	**The effluent drainage outlet is secretly changed** The factory changes its drainage outlet for the mercuric effluent from the acetaldehyde production from the Hyakken Harbor to the mouth of the Minamata River. Fishermen around there and Tsunagi Village become sudden, onset patients from the spring of 1959.
1959	14 Jul.	**Attention to Mercury** Kumamoto University's Study Group reports on the contamination of marine products to the Ministry of Health and Welfare. Pathology professor Takeuchi Tadao asserts that the cause is organic mercury. The factory continually rebuts this claim several times.
	21 Jul.	**The Hosokawa Experiments** Hosokawa Hajime, the former director of the Shin Nitchitsu affiliated hospital, begins conducting experiments alone in which he directly feeds cats the mercury effluent. On October 6th, cat no. 400 develops Minamata disease.
	2 Nov.	**Shin Nitchitsu's Minamata Factory is broken into** Thirty-six fishermen's cooperatives surrounding the Shiranui Sea throw stones and damage the factory's office machinery, demanding compensation and a stop to the effluent discharge.
	30 Dec.	**The Solatium Agreement** The factory rejects a compensation agreement that would award each patient ¥3 million ($8,333 USD). An agreement mediated by Kumamoto Prefecture and Minamata City is signed. Patients receive ¥100,000 ($278 USD) annually from the onset of illness to death and ¥300,000 ($833 USD) for funerals. This contract stipulated that the victims will make no further demands for compensation should the factory's effluent be determined the cause of Minamata disease .
1960	30 Mar.	**An Independent Study** Ui Jun, a graduate student in the Department of Chemical Engineering at the University of Tokyo visits the Minamata factory. He decides to clarify the Minamata disease disaster.
	14 Jul.	**A young Kuwabara Shisei heads to Minamata aiming to be a photographer** Ōhashi Noboru, director of the Minamata Municipal Hospital, gives permission for Kuwabara to begin photographing in the hospital.
1962	27 Apr.	**Conflict at Shin Nitchitsu's Minamata factory** A 9-month battle starts. The labor union divides, forming a pro-company faction that renounced its right to strike. No.1 Labor Union sympathizers, who are destined to be discriminated against in the company, participate in the patient social movement from 1968.
	11 Aug.	**Kuwabara takes close-up photography of top-secret data** Ui and Kuwabara gather information from Dr. Kojima Terukazu at the Shin Nitchitsu affiliated hospital, and take close-up photographs of the section of a written report by the factory's internal research group on the causative agent of Minamata disease. Ui who deciphered the data grasps the real situation, and later summarized an enormous investigation record.
	15 Sept.	**The first photographic exhibition on the Minamata disease disaster** Kuwabara's *Minamata: Factory Effluent and Coastal Fishermen* (105 pieces) is exhibited at Fuji Photo Salon in Yūrakuchō, Tokyo.
	29 Nov.	**Doctors confirm congenital Minamata disease** The Minamata Disease Patients' Investigation Committee medically recognizes 16 congenital children after a heated discussion .
1964	12 Aug.	**Beginning a patient support movement** Nishikita Yumi and others members of the women student's Kumamoto Junior College Social Work Group activities to encourage children with Minamata disease. They exhibit Kuwabara's photos in Kumamoto City.
	Nov.	**Documentary film director Tsuchimoto Noriaki comes to Minamata** Nippon Television Network is triggered by Kuwabara Shisei's work to begin scouting for a location to film the television program *The Children of Minamata are Living*. Hereafter films on the Minamata disease disaster are repeatedly produced for 30 years.
1965	10 Mar.	**The first Minamata disease photo-documentary** Kuwabara publishes *Minamata* with San-ichi (31) Publishing Co., Ltd. In an introduction, Kuwabara criticizes the lack of mass media coverage and, in an afterward, Ui anonymously exposes the factory's top-secret experiments on Minamata disease.
	12 Jun.	**The second Minamata disease** Niigata University professor, Tsubaki Tadao et al. distribute a press release stating that there is an organic mercury poisoning that resembles Minamata disease in Niigata Prefecture.
1968	12 Jan.	**Founding of the Citizen's Council for Minamata Disease Countermeasures** Hiyoshi Fumiko and Matsumoto Tsutomu initiate the patient support movement for the Kumamoto Lawsuit prior to plaintiffs from the Niigata Minamata Disease Lawsuit visit Minamata.
	26 Sept.	**The government announces that organic mercury poisoning in Minamata and Niigata are pollution-caused illness** The president of Chisso apologizes at patients' homes. The patient support movement spreads all over the country.
1969	28 Jan.	**Ishimure Michiko's *Paradise in the Sea of Sorrow*** Published by Kōdansha. Twenty three of Kuwabara's photos are complied.
	5 Apr.	**The Minamata disease patient group splits** Patients are divided into two groups, one group decides to give unconditional authority over compensation to the Ministry of Health and Welfare, and the other group proceeds with civil action.
	20 Apr.	**Founding of the Citizen's Council to Indict for Minamata Disease** Trial support groups start in several places . Without Kuwabara's permission, the support movements carry Kuwabara's photos (relinquished by the Minamata City office) in street demonstrations.
	7 Sept.	**Founding of the Minamata Disease Research Group** The lawsuit group of Citizen's Council for Minamata Disease Countermeasures combines with scholars at Kumamoto.
	5 Oct.	**Ui Jun releases *Minamata: Documents for Minamata Disease Research* under the pen name Tonda Yarō** The Citizen's Council to Indict for Minamata Disease publishes a vast amount of records that is not for sale.
1970	25 May	**MHW's Compensation Committee's arbitration plan** Ui Jun, Tsuchimoto Noriaki and 11 others who object to the small compensation amount break in and are arrested. A settlement is decided on May 27th, and the patients' demands are drastically cut.
	18 Aug.	**Administrative appeal request** Kawamoto Teruo and other patients who were denied recognition petition to the MHW. The newly-established Environment Agency withdraws the certification rejection in August 1971.
	25 Nov.	**Kuwabara 's *Photo Record: Minamata Disease 1960-1970*** The Asahi Newspaper publishes 134 photographic works.
1971	Jun.	**Founding of the Second Kumamoto Minamata Disease Research Group in Kumamoto University's Dept. of Medicine** After 10 years of early research, under the Kumamoto Prefectural trust, **the research group** begins medical reexaminations and resurveys in Minamata, Goshonoura, and Ariake.
	7 Sept.	**Eugene Smith and his wife Aileen come to Minamata** Prompted by Kuwabara's photo-documentary, they rent a house in Tsukinoura and begin photographing. They stay until Nov. 1974.
	29 Sept.	**Court rules in favor of plaintiffs in Niigata Lawsuit** Pollution victims acquire the rights to compensation from the company responsible for the first time in Japan. Plaintiffs negotiate outside of the courtroom for additional indemnities . Showa Denko, Ltd. accepts without reservation the patients' demands in June 1973.
	8 Dec.	**Negotiations and sit-ins at Chisso's main office in Tokyo** Kawamoto Teruo's group mobilizes a great number of supporters.

page 148	Always alone. His own mother is not in the house for some reason. At home August 1960
149	Kazumitsu is 4 years old. He is the model for the young boy Mokutarō in Ishimure Michiko's *"Paradise in the Sea of Sorrow"*. He was born the year before the official discovery of the 'stange' disease, and was an unrecognized patient at the time of this photograph. His grandfather on his father's side, Taraki, stubbornly refused to apply for official recognition and died. At home in Hachinokubo July 1960
150-151	I ask the family, "How do you sleep?" All family members sleep in the living room. In the summer, Goza (woven rush mat) are their mattresses. At home July 1960
152	His father, Kazuki's (30 years old) fishing boat. Kazuki said, "I became sick at the end of the war". The Minamata Disease Patients' Investigation Committee, that strictly adheres to the "'strange' disease outbreak started from 1953" time-frame, officially recognized him 11 years later as having an unclear date of onset. Minamata Bay July 1960
153	When fishing was over they went to Hyakken Bay. They moored here, where there was a lot of factory effluent, so that oysters and barnacles would not attach to the hull of the boat. July 1960
154	Fish and seaweed were not lacking at this family's meals. At home July 1960
155	His father Kazuki (47 years old) and grandmother Sugiyo (81 years old) Their Japanese alcove (tokonoma) is handsome. After the Kumamoto lawsuit decision, the Patients' Tokyo Negotiation Group and Chisso finalized the patients' compensation agreement. Families like this one belonging to the former arbitration faction also received the appended compensation payment. At home January 1977
156	A small annex where Egoshita lived, a relative from his mother's side of the family, was a place where the 'strange' disease was discovered in Tubotani, Tsukinoura. His late grandfather, Miyoshi (73 years old, right), and uncle Kazumi (25 years old, left) Minamata Bay September 1970
157	His mother, Emiko (26 years old, left) returned to her natal family. His late uncle Mikazu (13 years old, center) and grandmother Masu (48 years old) Tubotani, Tsukinoura July 1960
158	His mother, Emiko (26 years old), waiting a train to meet her new husband. I learned years later that her new husband departed to work in Wakamatsu, Fukuoka Prefecture. Minamata Station Platform August 1960
159	His mother Emiko (77 years old) together with her husband, Miyamoto Takumi (former chairman of Minamata Disease Patient Council applying for official recognition) visited with Kazumitsu (55 years old). They became my photographic subjects on the day I photographed my commemorative album. Reclaimed land in Minamata Bay May 2011
160	Stele lined up erect at Otomezuka. Hiyoshi Fumiko, chairwoman of the Citizen's Council for Minamata Disease, erected them in March 2003 through donations and private funds. "Lamenting over the mercury pollution of the Shiranui Sea" and "Never forget the negative legacy of humanity" are Fuchigami Seien's calligraphy. Aileen Smith translated the prospectus carved into stone. Kaminokawa, Minamata May 2013

An Abridged Chronology of the Human-made Minamata Disease Disaster

1908	10 Nov.	**Founding of Japan Nitrogenous Fertilizers, Inc. (ref. to as Nitchitsu)**
		The company later responsible for the Minamata disease disaster begins Japan's electrochemical industry.
1910		**The Japanese annexation of Korea**
1927	May	**Establishment of Korea Nitrogenous Fertilizers, Inc.**
		Nitchitsu expands the electrochemical industry at Korea's Kōnan factory.
1930		**Medical literature on Organic Mercury Poisoning**
		A report from H. Zangger et. al. is published. Catalysts used in the acetaldehyde manufacturing process produce organic mercury. Organic mercury poisoning results in the diagnosis of chronic conditions such as heart disorders, polyneuritis, multiple sclerosis, and other malingering illnesses.
1932	7 May	**Mercury pollution begins**
		At the Minamata factory, they begin expelling untreated effluent into Minamata bay.
1941	13 Nov.	**The earliest congenital patient is born?**
		Suspicions that a girl born in Yudō, Minamata is a congenital Minamata disease patient are described in 1973.
1945	Aug.	**Japan's defeat in WWII**
		Nitchitsu's Korean operations are withdrawn to Nitchitsu's Minamata factory. In 1950, the company name is changed to Shin Nitchitsu. The name is later changed to Chisso in 1965. In 2011, the name is revised to JNC (Japan New Chisso).
1950		**The wildlife in and around the inland sea meet with a widespread, unusual phenomena**
		Fish floats, cats go mad, and crows and waterfowl fall from the sky in Minamata's hamlets of Modō and Yudō. In the following years, unusual phenomena are witnessed and reported in many types of literature.
1953	Dec.	**Successive occurrences of patients with sudden onset 'strange' disease**
		Fishermen and their families, disabled with mental disturbances, blindness, and motor ataxia, become gravely ill and die. They are misdiagnosed with alcoholism, mental illness, and neuritis, etc.
1955	Jan.	**Successive occurrences similar to the 'strange' disease of infants with cerebral palsy**
		Infants born with cerebral palsy-like symptoms are born one after another. There are no comprehensive survey to this day on the actual amount of stillbirths, miscarriages, abortions, and infant deaths.
1956	1 May	**The official discovery of Minamata 'strange' disease (later named Minamata disease)**
		A physician at the Minamata factory affiliated hospital notifies the Minamata public health center that "there is a strange disease that exhibits encephalopathy, and four people are hospitalized." After this, several newspapers report on the possibility of a contagious disease.
	28 May	**Minamata City establishes the Strange Disease Countermeasures Committee**
		The Minamata City Medical Association reexamines previous misdiagnoses. Patients are placed in isolation on July 27th. After this, their houses and wells are disinfected . Kumamoto University's Department of Medicine establishes the Minamata Strange Disease Study Group in August, and the Countermeasures Committee medically certifies 52 people by the end of the year.
1957	17 Jan.	**"Immediately discontinue discharging bad, polluted water"**
		The Minamata Fishermen's Cooperative voted to demand this in writing to the Minamata factory.
	4 Mar.	**Voluntary fishing prohibition**
		The Minamata Fishermen's Cooperative decides to voluntarily withdraw operations from the interior of Minamata bay.

118	Fishing boats on the shore are kept tied. Tubotani, Tsukinoura July 1960
119	Fishermen's cooperative members carry in their hands the day's food from fish caught outside of the bay in the early morning. Modō's shore September 1970
120	Here and there mothers say, "That child is strange. Even though she wasn't given fish." Morimoto Hisae (3 years old, below) was later found to be a congenital patient. Modō August 1960
121	Headed to the hospital with her highly feverish child. Iwasaka (later Ueno) Eiko is 33 years old. Her daughter was one year old, and she died at two years of age. She was recognized as a congenital patient after her death. July 1960
122	A patient comforts her daughter at the beach. Sakamoto Takae is 31 years old. Takae was an unmarried mother who was refused to enterance into her husband's family registry. Yudō September 1970
123	Hamada Ryōji (13 years old), a congenital patient playing alone by the drying sardines on the beach. His mother, Shizue, later on passes away at 64 years of age. The nurse who often came to the beach and loved fishing became his new mother. Egushi Fukuhama, Tsunagi September 1970
124	The entire family was affected. Kaneko Chikao (left), who developed Minamata disease as a child, is 19 years old. Kaneko Yūji (center), a congenital patient, is 15 years old. Their mother, Sumiko (right, 39 years old) was recognized as a patient 2 years later. Their father, Chikashi, died when he was 34 years old from sudden on-set of Minamata disease in 1955 before the official discovery of the 'strange' disease. At home in Myōjin September 1970
125	Husband and wife Tokiyoshi Masato (front) and Sachie. The problem regarding Izumi City's unrecognized patients is much more serious than in Minamata. His wife was recognized as a patient immediately following this photographic shoot, but he termed an alcoholic. He died a year and a half later an unrecognized patient. In their home in Shō, Izumi City January 1977
126 -127	The net partition is removed. The mercury-polluted fish were trapped inside the bay. Fish were caught and discarded, and it also took 23 years for the mercury in the bay to dilute within the fish. August 1997
128	The crow is his only friend. Yamshita Daizō (45 years old) is a recognized patient. So are his mother and older sister. Komenotsu, Izumi August 1997
129	Plaintiffs (congenital and those from the same generation) from the Second Generation Lawsuit. Patients from the winning lawsuit that obligates official recognition smile. In front of the Supreme Court 16 April 2013
130 -131	It's been 50 years for patients and their families. In this commemorative photo, I had each of the people I photographed line up holding old pictures. On the reclaimed land in Minamata Bay's harbor 1 May 2011

Section 16 Fish hawkers were able to sell in the mountainous region

I thought that the Minamata disaster is a story about the sea. Fifty two years after I first visited Minamata, I photographed for the first time the mountains where the mercuric pollution followed along the fish hawkers' trade route. The fishermen living in Yunoura, Ashikita, Tanoura, and Amakusa etc. are the ancestors of the Minamata fishermen. The fishermen in Minamata did not refuse to take Minamata Bay fish from fishermen living in Yunoura, etc., and the latter fishermen transported methyl mercury polluted fish to the mountainous region.

In the mountains where there was no news of the 'strange' disease, people ate the fish soup stock and sardines instead of throwing them away.

page 133	The body is strange. Numbness, stiffness, cramping in the feet all come and go. "I have many other symotoms. But I thought it's because of my age, and everyone says so. Ahh- I did not think it's because of Minamata disease!" Ōiwa, Ashikita May 2012
134	The pollution's root deep within the mountains. It is 500 meters above sea level. Forestry was once prosperous. A great number of applicants came forward for the Special Measures Relief Law. Kuroiwa, Ashikita May 2012
135	Ahh-, Hayashida, Kadomiya, Fujii---. "Ikki Don," was a nickname of a fish hawker who came from the sea. After drinking a cup of shōchū (Japanese liquor) "Ikki Don", vigorously shouldered a yoke, and climbed up the mountain road. The old folks of villages remembered well the names of hawker. "That sashimi was really delicious!" Kurozaki, Ashikita May 2012

Section 17 The Islands of Hidden Patients

Shishijima is 14 km directly in front of Minamata. The people on the island in the neighboring prefecture have a lifestyle and relatives close to that of Chisso's capital Minamata. Minamata disease was taboo on the island for many years. When officially recognized patients on the island came out in 1973, stones were thrown at them. Other fishermen who were officially recognized patients were immediately expelled from the fishermen's cooperative. Now approximately all the people on the island have become applicants for the Relief Law.

page 136	Sakaguchi Sumio (58 years old), an unrecognized patient. At an ironworks plant in Osaka, his left hand and arm were crushed 4 times in a pressing machine. He returned to the island after people said, "Your body is strange, is it not?" Goshonoura, Shishijima May 2012
137	The island's specialty is sea lettuce. Sensation in the fingertips was a problem when separating foreign materials from their products. Katasoba, Shishijima May 2012

Section 18 The Supporters

Eight years after Ui Jun and I went to Minamata from Tokyo, supporters of the Minamata disease victims spread throughout the country. The central government recognized Minamata disease as a pollution-caused illness, and name of the company responsible was announced to the entire world. In the 12 previous years, martyrs managed to live while concealing themselves from the world.

page 138 -139	Ui Jun (72 years old) protests at the Ministry of the Environment. Ui dies two years later. Matsumoto Tsutomu (73 years old) photographs Ui. Matsumoto dies five years later. At the patients' winning the Supreme Court lawsuit. Kumamoto Prefecture and the State loose their final appeal in the Chisso Minamata Disease Kansai Lawsuit. 15 October 2004
140 -141	Harada Masazumi (died 13 years later), Matsumoto Tsutomu (died 11 years later), Miyazawa Nobuo (died 13 years later), Shiraki Hirotsugu (died 5 years later), Togasi Sadao and Akagi Hirokatsu and others at a relaxed talk at the conference for the Minamata Disease People's inn Suitensō, Minamata January 1999
142 -143	Hiyoshi Fumiko (left of center) and Ishimure Michiko welcomed by supporters on the Tokyo station platform. They proceeded to the capital for the inauguration of Tokyo Citizen's Council to Indict for Minamata Disease. June 1970

Section 19 The International Conference on Mercury

"The International Conference on Mercury as a Global Pollutant" was held in Minamata in October 2001. Researchers from many countries reported on and displayed their basic research. The Ministry of the Environment handled its management. However, at an unaffiliated session planned by civilians, a diverse satellite conference was also opened, and foreign delegates participated.

page 145	Foreign female researchers came dressed in Japanese kimono on a day when the conference held a friendship party. The Minamata City gymnasium October 2001
146 -147	One conference scene. International delegates voiced their disappointment that, in Japan where the Minamata disaster occurred, there is almost no research data on mercuric trace pollution based on long-term, continuous surveying. Plenary session, Minamata October 2001

Section 20 One Congenital Patient's Family

When one sorts through Han'naga Kazumitsu's photographs, you can see bits and pieces of 50 years of walking with agony. In Yauchi's family (a relative), there are more than ten officially recognized patients. There are also many people who have already passed away. Kazumitsu has been living alone for long time in a institution for patients called Meisuien. He occasionally visits his mother who for some reason married another man.

85	A seriously ill patient (67 years old) who lies on the floor without climbing into a bed. One year 9 months later, he dies of general prostration. July 1960
86	Hospital Director Ōhashi Noboru makes his rounds to Morimoto Hisae, a congenital patient. Hisae is nine years old. Next to her is Nishikita Yumi (21 years old) who, in 1964, supported activities that encouraged children with Minamata disease. The Yunoko Municipal Rehabilitation Center opened in 1965 as the first specialized hospital of its kind in Japan. All of the patients in Minamata Municipal Hospital Ward transferred here. May 1966
87	Walking practice. Maeda Emiko (12 years old) who became sick after birth Rehabilitation Center May 1966
88	Nagai Isamu (19 years old), a congenital patient At Meisuien, a municipal institution exclusively for Minamata disease patients January 1977
89	Onoue Mitsuo (53 years old) At his home in Hyakken Town September 1970
91	Kagata Kiyoko (front) was an unrecognized congenital patient at the time. At home in Detsuki, Tsukinoura August 1960
92-93	Citizens crowd for the first Kumamoto University Department of Internal Medicine on-site medical exam by interview. Modō Community Hall July 1960
94	Sisters who were unrecognized congenital patients at the time. Iwasaka Mari is four years old (front, died at six years of age) and Sueko is two years old. At home in Yudō August 1960
95	Siblings who became sick after birth. Watanabe Matsuyo (10 years old, center) and Eiichi (7 years old, front). Inside is their mother Matsu (32 years old). At home in Yudō August 1960
96	Matsuda Tomiji (11 years old), he became sick after birth. He is the model for the boy Yamanaka Kyūhei in Ishimure Michiko's *"Paradise in the Sea of Sorrow."* He could not see and he enjoyed baseball and sumō by listening to the radio as an "expert sports commentator." At home in Yudō August 1960
97	Tanaka Toshimasa (4 years old), he was an unrecognized congenital patient at the time. He died when he was 13 years old. Inside is his grandfather, Kanosuke, and his father, Hajime. His grandfather avoided applying for recognition as a patient and died. His grandmother and parents were recognized as Minamata disease patients more than 10 years later. At home in Yudō July 1960
98-99	Fuchigami Masae (44 years old) carries her daughter, Hifue (3 years old), an unrecognized congenital patient at the time, on her back. The two girls in left are Hifue's sisters. At their home settled on the ruins of Modō's former naval gunpowder magazine August 1960

Section 12 The Niigata Minamata Disease Disaster

The calamity occurred a second time with the same cause. This time it happened to people who ate river fish in Niigata Prefecture. Ui Jun, a researcher who investigated the Minamata disaster, stated:"Mr. Kuwabara and I must lay a part of the responsibility on ourselves. Knowing the results of Chisso's secrete experiments on the causative agent of Minamata disease, we could have prevented the second Minamata disease outbreak in the Agano River." (Ui Jun, *Minamata disease*)

page 101	Showa Denko's Kanose factory holds responsibility. There was acetaldehyde production that discharged the same kind of organic mercury effluent as in the first Minamata disaster. The calamity became an issue in 1965 when there was a move to stop manufacturing process. Kanose, Niigata Prefecture June 1967
102	Medical examination of residents' body in the Agano River basin. It is a different scene from the examination by interview in Minamata City that happened in 1960. At Ōkawa and three places, Niigata City June 1967
103	Niigata University professor Tsubaki Tadao examines Furuyama Chieko, an unrecognized congenital patient at the time. She was officially recognized as a Minamata disease patient three years later. At Ōkawa and three places, Niigata City June 1967
104	Agano River fishermen The bank of the Agano River July 1967
105	The volume of water in the lower reaches of the Agano River is the highest in Japan. The river fish are huge. The woman holding the fish is the daughter of Kuwano Tadago, a seriously ill patient. The bank of the Agano River July 1967

Section 13 The factory labor strike and the transformed town of Minamata City

In 1962, two years after the Mitsui Miike coal mine strike, a confrontation between laborers and factory management engulfed the town. The joint labor unions made a general comment on a pressed arrangement that stated "absolutely no more strikes during which time we promise a stable wage increase" in Chisso's (a member of the Japan Federation of Economic Organizations) proposal is a revocation of basic labor rights. Local laborers and business owners were also divided by the long and drawn-out lockout and strike.

page 107	Wives of first labor union members formed the vanguard of the demonstration in front of the second labor union's (new union) office. Laborers who supported the Minamata disease patients' court battle were born after the company's 10 years of antagonistic discrimination towards the first labor union. The center of Minamata City August 1962
108	At the front gate of the factory, the first labor union set the striking picket line and formed a demonstration parade. I photographed the dispute, but Ui Jun, who accompanied me, investigated Minamata disease without acknowledging the strike. August 1962
109	Ishimoto Torashige (41 years old) a fisherman who was employed by the company during the 1960 negotiations for Minamata disease compensation. He was a member of the first labor union, and watched from his boat for members of the second union who attempted to break the strike and go to the factory by landing on the shore from the sea. He hid that he was a Minamata disease patient, but was recognized in June 1973. Minamata Bay August 1962

Section 14 The first Kumamoto Minamata disease lawsuit

The beginning of support activities for patients started after Ui Jun and others appealed for a visit to Minamata from patients in Niigata in January 1968. The Citizen's Council for Minamata Disease Countermeasures was founded, and, in September of the same year, the central government passed formal recognition of Minamata disease as a pollution-caused illness. Patients from the litigation group sued for compensation the following year, and the social movement went national.

page 110 -111	Demonstrators parade holding portraits of victims against their chests. The first labor union that did not acknowledge the Minamata disease problem send out a "declaration of embarrassment" in August 1968, and union members also participated in the demonstration. The center of Kumamoto City July 1970
112	The leaders of the patient and supporter demonstration carried my photographs without permission. The Tokyo Citizen's Council to Indict for Minamata Disease was established. Metropolitan Tokyo June 1970
113	Patients proceed to the capital and stage the first sit-in. The litigation group protests the small amount of money offered as compensation to the arbitration group from the Ministry of Health and Welfare. In front of Chisso's Tokyo headquarters close to Tokyo Station May 1970

Section 15 Hell in the Sea of Sorrow

"To us, it was Hell. Nobody helped us." The money eagerly received from the solatium contract with the company (end of 1959) was subtracted from the cost of protecting one's livelihood. The fish catch averaged 460 tons yearly between 1950 and 1953. In 1958, it decreased to 41 tons. In 1959, customers buying fish disappeared.

page 114	Protecting against "poaching." The Minamata Fishermen's Cooperative operated to voluntarily prohibit fishing in the bay, and they guarded their patrol boats at night. August 1962
115	Members of small fishermen's cooperatives working under the cover of darkness in the outside of the bay, where there were no voluntary fishing prohibitions. August 1960
116	Fish taken from outside the bay are peddled to fishing villages in Minamata by bicycle. The father of the "living doll", Matsunaga Zen'iti (44 years old), is buying them. July 1960
117	Out of place fishermen. Everyday was a painful holiday. At the home of a Yudō fisherman July 1960

46-47	"May I photograph your hand?" I asked, and he stuck his hand in front of the camera lens for me. Iwazō died in general prostration one year three months later. Rehabilitation Center September 1970
48	Their three grandchildren and mother Emika visit Iwazō and his wife Tsuyo's hospital room. To a fishing family who cannot sell fish, the hospital's meal of rice was a feast. Minamata Municipal Hospital Ward August 1960
49	At the end of Tōkichi's first ceremony commemorating his death (obon) Iwaki, Tsunagi August 1960

Section 6 A shipwright family became the impetus for the 'strange' disease's discovery.

In April 1956, Tanaka Yoshimitsu and Asao carried their third daughter, Shizuko (5 years old) to the Chisso affiliated hospital when she could no longer use chopsticks with her hand. Their forth daughter, Jitsuko (2 years old) also continued to get sick. The head of the hospital, Hosokawa Hajime, and staff came to conduct a survey in Tubotani, Tsukinoura, and discovered similar patients among the young children. On May 1st, they sent this information to the Minamata public health center. Later, this date became the day that Minamata disease was officially discovered.

page 51	Since leaving the Minamata Municipal Hospital ward and up until now, she has received home care. Jitsuko is 13 years old. Her mother Asao (44 years old) gently loosens her hand. At home October 1966
52-53	Since the inland sea came right in front of the house, they had as many side dishes for rice as they liked. But, the children were scared, so could not fish from the edge. At home July 1960
54	Shizuko died when she was 8 years old the previous year, and her younger sister, Jitsuko (7 years old) survived. Nursing Jitsuko became her parents' reason to live. Minamata Municipal Hospital Ward July 1960
55	Women gathering Japanese horse mussels for meager wages in the front of the house. They were used as food in the Kumamoto University Department of Medicine's cat experiments. Tubotani Jetty, Tsukinoura July 1960
56	Jitsuko is 32 years old. She dressed in a Kimono for me to take a photograph. For some reason, both of Jitsuko's hands always make the same shape. At home February 1986
57	In the year that followed seeing Jitsuko in her kimono, her father Yoshimitsu (76 years old) and her mother Asao (69 years old) died. At home February 1986
58-59	Her older sister Ayako holds and supports her when Jitsuko walks. The jetty in front of her home February 1986

Section 7 Nakamura Arazō, fishnet owner

In Fukuro Modō, a community separated from the town of Minamata, there were four families of fishnet owners. Nakamura Arazō knew about striped mullet. I repeatedly received Nakamura's good will. Even when he could not fish due to the Minamata disease catastrophe, he would take me out on his boat so that I could photograph the fishing landscape. The entire community suffered.

page 60	Striped mullet fishing. Within the fish bait balls at the fishing grounds is each family's secret recipe. Modō Bay September 1970
61	Arazō (58 years old) is basket fishing for striped mullet. The glittering fish in the basket are striped mullet. Modō Bay September 1970
62	Fingertips are life when fishing in the dark. Their fingers often suffered from paralysis caused by Minamata disease. Modō Bay August 1962
63	Arazō (48 years old) and Ayako's (44 years old) third daughter, Chizuru (3 years old). This is two years before she is recognized as having congenital Minamata disease, but I thought she was a patient at the time. At a Kumamoto University medical exam by interview, Modō Community Hall July 1960
64	Chizuru is thirteen years old. Her mother Ayako is 54 years old. She is carried to her distant home from the rehabilitation center. Yunoko, Minamata City September

Section 8 Sugimoto Eiko: Modō's female fishnet owner who acted better than an actress

I thought, "I want to listen to that flowing speech together with her chanting the Heike Monogatari to a biwa accompaniment." Storytellers who use the local Minamata dialect to draw out sobs, admiration, and anger tell their story in strong voices to people from the Capital who do not know about the Minamata disease disaster. Locals from Minamata also really enjoyed local theatrical performances with handmade costumes and dancing. She passed away in February 2008 at 69 years of age.

page 65	In the midst of the Strange disease disaster, they begin their newly-married life. Eiko (21 years old) and Takeshi (20 years old) Modō Beach July 1960
66	Rowing mellowly. Eiko is 27 years old. Modō Bay May 1966
67	Her mother Toshi brought Eiko to fishnet owner Sugimoto Susumu when they married. Susumu raised the young Eiko to be a female fishnet owner. At home August 1960
68	Striking the sea water, they herd fish into the nets. Modō Bay August 1960
69	Eiko is 38 years old. She becomes an accredited master of the Hanayaji school of Japanese dancing. At home in Modō 1977

Section 9 The Chisso Minamata Factory

With the manufacturing process converted in the 1970s, the factory continued to be downsized, and it is now the JNC Minamata Manufactory Works. Its chief enterprise is producing liquid crystals, etc. as raw materials. The old equipment was removed, and the landscape completely changed. The mercuric effluent that caused Minamata disease flowed from 1932 until 1968.

page 70-71	The old central part of the factory looking from the hill behind Minamata station September 1970
72-73	Looking in the direction of the Chisso Minamata Factory from Modō's mandarin orange hills September 1970

Section 10 Congenital patients become adults and the years that follow

Children born during the years Minamata disease was discovered become adults. Congenital patients, who hand out fliers to the same generation dressed in their best clothes, are also at the ceremony that the municipal city office held. "We received compensation money, but we, young patients, are not relieved. Would it be possible for us to receive your strength, and for you to once again think about this problem?"

page 75	Takishita Masafumi (right) and Onizuka Yūji (left) In front of the Minamata City Public Hall 15 January 1977
76-77	Handing their own handmade fliers to the new adults. Sakamoto Shinobu (center) and Kagata Kiyoko (left) In front of the Minamata City Public Hall 15 January 1977
78	Shinobu is 41 years old. Fujie is 72 years old (right). Going to the beach on the day the net partitioning Minamata bay to imprison the mercury polluted fish is removed. Yudō August 1997
79	Shinobu is 56 years old (center). Supporters from the winning lawsuit are delighted. In front of the Supreme Court 16 April 2013

Section 11 Patients at the hospital ward exclusively for Minamata disease and in their home

I entered to do an on-site photo-shoot in July 1960, and I remember that 18 people were hospitalized in the exclusive hospital ward. By the end of the same year, 34 people out of the 87 officially recognized patients died from sudden-onset Minamata disease. There were also people who died shortly after I photographed them. Other home care patients close-by were secretly struggling alone unassisted, and congenital patients went unrecognized.

81	Izumi City's seriously ill fishnet owner (57 years old). He died three months after I took this photograph. Minamata Municipal Hospital Ward July 1960
82	She collapsed in the hospital ward's hallway. Kawakami (her surname changed to Murano after her divorce) Tamano is 46 years old. She died at 62 years of age in an institution on Amakusa island. Minamata Municipal Hospital Ward August 1960
83	She had a seizure even in sleep. Minamata Municipal Hospital Ward August 1960
84	Ikoma Hideo is 17 years old. He places food in his seriously ill father's mouth. There is no family to look after his father who is an unrecognized patient. He had his father transferred to a bed in the same hospital room as his. August 1960

Photograph Explanation

Section 1 The Minamata Disease Disaster: exceeding half a century, towards the Supreme Court decision

16 April 2013: The Supreme Court of Japan ruled that Kumamoto Prefecture's procedural dismissal for formal recognition as a Minamata disease patient is invalid in two administrative lawsuits. Kumamoto Prefecture lost its final appeal against the late Mizoguchi Chie (Minamata City) after she won at the Fukuoka High Court. The Supreme Court repealed and sent back the appeal court ruling against the late Mrs. F (born in Minamata City) decided in the Osaka High Court.

page	
4	Sixty years have already passed since the dreaded 'strange' disease spread along the sides of the seashore. Sign for the old Satsuma road.
5	The late Mizoguchi Chie holding her grandchild when she came to undergo an on-site medical exam by interview in Kumamoto. I realized that Chie was in my first roll of film 50 years after photographing her. Minamata City, Fukuro July 1960
6-7	Among the many frames of film, this photograph is the only one in which a physician has a stethoscope. It appears that Chie is imploring, "Examine my grandchild's body." Kumamoto University Department of Internal Medicine's first medical exam July 1960
8	Bereaved family and supporters after the winning verdict supporting the demand to formally recognize Chie In front of the Supreme Court 16 April 2013
9	A branch of the family holding the photograph that I took of Chie while she was alive. At the bereaved family's home in Fukuro, Minamata May 2013
10-11	The bereaved family of the late Mrs. F, who finally had the decision sent back, is crowded by journalists and mass media. In front of the Supreme Court 16 April 2013

Section 2 Two Memorials

Every year on May 1st two memorials begin simultaneously in Minamata. One memorial service held by the Minamata Disease Mutual Aid Society at the Barrow of the Maiden (Otomezuka) is in its 33rd year. This is a place where all the sacrificed lives are enshrined together. At the Victims' Memorial Ceremony that began dozens of years later by Minamata City and other sponsoring committees, senior officials from the central government and prefecture as well as Diet members attend lined up on the Minamata Bay landfill.

page	
13	This is the first time a prime minister participated in the governmentally supported Memorial Ceremony. Hatoyama Yukio 2010
14-15	The center-front row at the memorial ceremony is always reserved for senior government officials and Diet members. Koike Yuriko, Minister of the Environment, and others 2006
16-17	A patient approaches Hosono Gōshi, Minister of the Environment. The security police move suddenly. 2012
18-19	The Administration changes, but nothing else does. Ishihara Nobuteru, Minister of the Environment (right), and Hosono Gōshi, former Minister of the Environment (left) 2013
20-21	Patient supporters at the memorial service in plain clothes, silent 2013
22-23	The memorial service at Otomezuka 2013
24-25	Lawyers from the Mizoguchi Lawsuit in front of the governmentally supported memorial ceremony say, "We want a word with Minister Ishihara." Local city officials block them. 2013
26-27	Patients, bereaved and extended family members, and representatives of uncertified patients in attendance at the memorial ceremony 2013

Section 3 Takarago (Precious Child)

A mother, whose first-born child has congenital Minamata disease, told me: "This child is my precious child. Thanks to her absorbing the mercury in my body, her six younger siblings are healthy and my symptoms also became light." Kamimura Tomoko, the precious child, was cared for by her patients at home from beginning to end. At 21 years, 6 months, she moved on to the next world.

page	
28	The road to Otomezuka where Tomoko is enshrined. It is on the boarder with Kagoshima Prefecture. 2012
29	Her father Yoshio holds Tomoko at her Coming of Age party. Tsukinoura, Tsubodan 15 January 1977
30-31	The Kamimura's living room when I first met them. At rental property in Tsukinoura, Detsuki July 1960
32	"All right, Tomoko, keep trying!" Tomoko (4 years old), her mother Yoshiko (26 years old) July 1960
33	"Older sister does nothing but lie down." July 1960
34-35	Family and relatives who gathered for the Coming of Age party. Tomoko died 324 days later. She is the 234th governmentally recognized patient to die. At home 15 January 1977

Section 4 The Living Doll

I was unable to take my eyes off of one beautiful little girl in the Minamata Municipal Hospital ward exclusively for Minamata disease. Matsunaga Kumiko was 9 years, 8 months old at the time. I thought surely she was a heavenly nymph. She was born healthy, but suddenly became bedridden at 5 years, seven months of age. She had apallial syndrome and akinetic mutism for 18 years. Kumiko died when she was 23 years, 9 months old, and was the 100th governmentally recognized patient to pass away.

page	
37	The third daughter of a fisherman came to be called the "living doll" by someone. At 11 years of age. Minamata Municipal Hospital Ward August 1962
38	For a short time, her father Zen'ichi (44 years old) and her mother Masa (44 years old) nestle their daughter. Minamata Municipal Hospital Ward August 1960
39	"Eat slowly so that you don't choke." Meals lasted for hours. Minamata Municipal Hospital Ward August 1960
40	"We took shrimp flowers blooming from the net." Shrimp were Kumiko's favorite food. Her father and mother worked as net fishermen in Minamata Bay. Yudō Bay August 1960
41	I wanted to beautifully capture Kumiko. During my fifth stay in Minamata, I was able to photograph her eyes. Is she looking or not looking at something? Minamata Municipal Hospital Ward October 1966
42-43	"Kumi, you look pretty today!" Minamata Municipal Hospital Ward August 1960

Section 5 The 'strange' disease that struck down the second generation of fishnet owners in a village to the near north of Minamata

The Shin Nitchitsu (later renamed Chisso, and JNC) Minamata Factory secretly changed the mercuric effluent's drainage outlet from Minamata bay to the mouth of the Minamata river in September 1958. The following year patients with severe, rapid onset Minamata disease successively appeared from around the mouth of the river to Tsunagi, a neighboring village to the north. In reality, this was a poisoning experiment on living people. When Funaba Tōkichi, a Tsunagi fishnet owner, was hospitalized, villagers came out to rise and see him off. "This means a send-off for a soldier leaving to the front," his wife Emika said. Soon after Tōkichi's father, Iwazō, was also hospitalized. In December 1959, Tōkichi died at 34 years of age. Iwazō died in December 1971 at 79 years of age after 12 years of being bedridden. During that time, they never returned home again. In October 1960, I received a letter from Emika that said this: "I strongly do hope many journalists will come from Tokyo, the political center, and they will see the reality of this crisis. And yet, the people lying in sickbeds as living corpses hope to make complete recoveries without further delay…If it is possible, for the sake of this Minamata disease, I humbly ask for you to widely spread this information so that Kuwabara's precious photo-journalism does not end meaninglessly…"

page	
44	In recent years, Iwazō's 'hand' has become a symbol at exhibitions of all sorts. Meiji University Campus September 2010
45	Fingernail scratches that Tōkichi etched into the hospital room wall while in agony Minamata disease Municipal Hospital Ward August 1962

180

Kuwabara met with Ōhashi Noboru, director of the Minamata Municipal Hospital and requested to "be allowed to take photographs of patients." "How can photographs help?," retorted the director. He simply replied, "I want to become a photographer and take photographs of patients." Perhaps it was Kuwabara's *nōtenki* utterance that touched the heart of the director.

The first time he photographed patients was at Kumamoto University Department of Medicine's mass medical examination by interview. When I look at the entire file, it is not a scene in which the bodies of fishermen are being examined. And yet, mothers who ask for their children to be examined are sitting with absentminded faces. The children who did not eat fish wear summer clothes that are seemingly new bought with the factory's solatium money (p.5, 63). Doctors who could not distinguish these children from ordinary cerebral palsy stubbornly would not recognized them as having Minamata disease, and said that it is impossible for poisons to pass through the placenta.

In a different film series, there are also scenes showing fish caught from outside Minamata brought by bicycle to be sold in fishing villages (p. 116). The fish in the sea directly in front of the villages were frightening, and no one would eat them. However, there are photographs in which you can almost hear the voices of the fishermen saying, "I can't live a life without eating fish." In fact, photographs such as this are practically still unpublished. With his idea to reconsider these points in a "record of photographs with this special quality," Kuwabara proceeded to select photographs. The result is this photo-documentary.

These images of patients in the hospital, etc. are not photographs that were printed in the pages of mass media. The reason their tragic images were not published is the same reason war journalism could not publish images of dead bodies. Thus, Kuwabara's work, which did not have a market, has become a singular, record of the present. He was destitute.

It was August 1962 when Kuwabara and Ui seized the definitive evidence that laid the blame on the responsible company. Dr. Kojima Terukazu left top-secret company documents out right in front of them when he was called out of his office by telephone during a visit to the Minamata factory affiliated hospital. Kojima was perhaps hinting that it was okay for them to read the documents. Ui flipped through the secret records, and Kuwabara took close-up photographs of each one. In a recording, Ui deciphered the documents saying, "This is the data that conclusively confirmed the experiments that the cause of Minamata disease is the organic mercury in the company's effluent." Ui did not allow the major journalist publishers to print this information until he began writing *Minamata*, a publication that later became a record of the motive for the social movement. As for Kuwabara, close-up photography of letters did not make photographs. He, in his *nōtenki* way, handed over all his film negatives to Ui.

I shall write about the genuine greatness of *nōtenki*.

Kuwabara's exhibition "Minamata: factory effluent and coastal fishermen" (Tokyo, Sept.1962) was a triumph. He quickly became a rising-star in photography. He sent as a 'donation' all his photographic panels to the Minamata city office. Kuwabara also worked in Korea and Vietnam for over 10 years, and, during that time, he was convinced that his works on Minamata were accepted in the city office. However, Kuwabara's photographic panels were left abandoned in community hall's underground storage, covered in dust. In reality, this produced an amazing effect.

The second organic mercury-poisoning disaster occurred in Niigata. The government officially recognized Minamata disease as a pollution-caused illness in 1968. Patient and supporter led social movements broke-out suing for the right to damages. Support groups for patients found Kuwabara's dust covered photographs and carried them in the vanguard of street demonstrations without Kuwabara's permission (p. 112).

One member of a patient family, who compromised with the responsible company instead of suing got angry about this unauthorized usage even though this person once invited Kuwabara to stay overnight in his home. The family informed Kuwabara that they would break off their friendly relationship with him.

The director of the Municipal Hospital bought 100 copies of Kuwabara's debut photo-documentary *Minamata* (1965), and distributed them at his discretion. The director also gave dozens of copies to someplace in the city office, but the city administration, which wanted to contain Minamata disease, probably hid the books. Kuwabara did not care how those books were handled. The sharp-sighted person who found these photo-documentaries was Hiyoshi Fumiko, the person in-charge of support groups. In 1969, many schoolteachers came to Minamata to learn about Minamata disease. "I know where you have hid Kuwabara's photo-documentaries! Turn them over!" Hiyoshi cried in a thundering voice to the city office staff, and they gave the books to the teachers. The photo-documentary was circulated to schools all over the country, which manifested powerfully in the support campaign for patients.

Kuwabara's photographs were the trigger for well-known American photographer, Eugene Smith to also photograph Minamata and spread it to the world. However, how are all the patients who he photographed 50 years prior doing now? Kuwabara is the only one who can remember each and every single person and family from that time. Within the present photo-documentary, photographs have been carefully arranged so that the passage of such an era can be understood.

Kuwabara is a photographer, not a scholar of the Minamata disaster. He writes his words with *nōtenki*, and, in them are outrageous factual mistakes and slips of the pen that can be said to verge on serious trouble. Compositions that he wrote were not well respected in Japan. Perhaps it is from now that the value of Kuwabara's work, with the inclusion of previously unpublished prints, will truly grow. (Nishimura Mikio, July 2013)

---

[1] Translator's note: All names that appear in this volume follow the Japanese convention of surname first followed by given name. All other names follow the Western tradition.

The Minamata Disaster
Abridged translation of the expository essay on photographer Kuwabara Shisei[1]

Nishimura Mikio, journalist
(Michelle D. J. Daigle, translator)

A half-century has passed since news photographer Kuwabara Shisei began photographing the Minamata disaster. This man-made disaster came to a head as Japan sought to rebuild herself out of the social chaos caused by her loss in the Second World War. In southern Japan, the result was Chisso's chemical factory, the company responsible for Minamata disease in Minamata, Kumamoto Prefecture on Kyushu, discharging organic mercury into Minamata bay. Even though the Japanese government knew, it took 12 years for them to conclude this fact. This is a disaster that humanity experienced beginning in the 20th Century, and its effect is also extending into the 21st Century.

In 1960, two young men came from Tokyo to Minamata, and were thrust from separate directions, unaided into this bizarre catastrophe in which all fish, people, and other living things were poisoned. These two young men were Ui Jun, a graduate student in Tokyo University's Department of Engineering, and Kuwabara Shisei, a photojournalist in the making. Together they warned the world about the Minamata disaster.

It was declared long ago that it is now safe to eat the fish. However, this does not mean that all the damage caused by harmful rumors and misinformation has disappeared. This past June, I heard the voices of fishermen saying, "We must continue shouldering the burden of 'Minamata' for our lifetime." From now on, many people will also be forced to carry the burden of 'Fukushima,' Tokyo Electric Power Company's nuclear meltdown and catastrophic explosion at their Fukushima plants.

This photo-documentary is a compilation of photographs selected anew from Kuwabara's vast collection of film. I try to express Kuwabara's special quality of unknowingness.

I say this while deeply respecting him. One special characteristic of Kuwabara's activities can be called '*nōtenki*.' *Nōtenki* is a several hundred year-old Japanese colloquialism meaning "a thing or person that is happy-go-lucky and frivolous". Kuwabara is now 76 years old, and it is rude of my 73 year-old self to call him *nōtenki*. However, if *nōtenki* also becomes extraordinary as in Kuwabara's case, then, should enough time and circumstances permit, this prodigious quality surely becomes an immense virtue. I think the fact that the Minamata disaster came to be a weighty concern to the world is thanks to Kuwabara's *nōtenki*.

Kuwabara was born in a poor village in Shimane Prefecture in 1936. During his childhood, Kuwabara lost his right eye in a high-temperature gas explosion after peering into an inadequately maintained car he found in the village. His father who worked at the town office bought his one-eyed son a camera as a gift that was expensive and of high quality at the time.

In his youth, a member of the communist party suddenly came to power in the conservative village. Consequently, Kuwabara knew Left wing terminology such as 'organizational cells' since he was a child. However, he was not an adult-like child that would appeal to the Left wing, but was rather thickheaded when it came to politics. When the village headman was banished and the General Headquarters' American military police boarded a car to the village, Kuwabara approached wondering if they had chocolates. Maybe it is because he had such experiences as a youth that, in his later career, his photography would pursue images of people amongst war and upheaval. According to his father, he entered the Tokyo University of Agriculture, but he also enthusiastically studied at the Tokyo College of Photography.

In May 1960, Kuwabara searched for his photographic theme without full-time employment. He was astonished by an article in the *Weekly Asahi* titled "Look at Minamata Disease!" He thought, "This disaster, where scores of causalities are appearing, is my theme," but he did not think it would be difficult to publish the photographs of the harsh reality of the patients in newspapers and magazines. He wrote this after: "Even 15 young children who did not eat Minamata's fish have fallen, stricken with Minamata disease's congenital form. They rapidly succumbed to states in which they are unable to move their bodies under their own will" (Kuwabara Shisei 1989).

There are in fact mistakes in this description. The urge to go to Minamata is true, but the circumstances surrounding the "suffering of Minamata disease's congenital patients" are wrong. At this time, medical scientists had not yet recognized that there were victims of a congenital Minamata disease. This here is one of Kuwabara's *nōtenki* compositions. He pointed his lens full speed at these tragic children during a time when medical science was not considering their profundity. Thus, Kuwabara became the foremost person to have photographed the "world's first nightmare which invaded the environment of the womb."

Just a short time before the coastal fishermen burst into the Minamata factory, the source of the pollution, compensation for the inshore fishery, and the patients' solatium contract was passed. Fishermen who joined in the trespassing incident were arrested in droves, and the incident ended. The investigation into Minamata disease came to a close.

During the period when the incident was smothered socially,

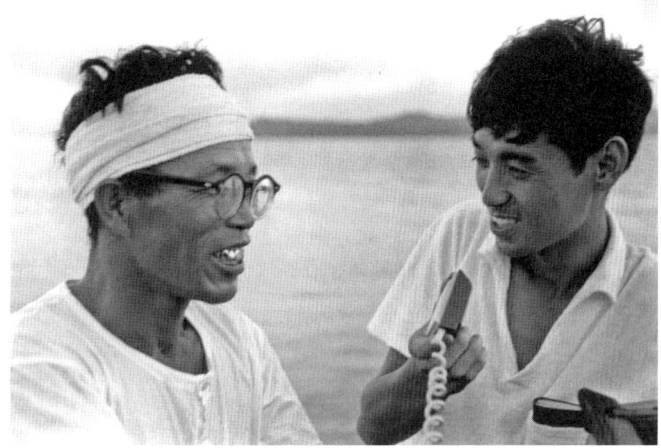

Photo by Shinzō Hanabusa

1962年、2度目の水俣取材時に「生ける人形」の父、松永善一さん（左）を漁場でインタビュー。友人の英伸三君が撮影。

An interview at the fishing wharf with Matsunaga Zen'iti (left), the father of the 'living doll', in 1962 during Kuwabara's second stay in Minamata. His friend, Hanabusa Shinzō, took the photograph.

著者紹介

桑原史成（くわばら・しせい）
フォトジャーナリスト。
1936年島根県生まれ。1960年、東京農業大学・東京綜合写真専門学校卒業。
主な著書に『報道写真家』（岩波書店）、『桑原史成写真全集』（水俣、韓国、ベトナム、筑豊・沖縄の全4巻、草の根出版会）。
郷里の津和野に「桑原史成写真美術館」が1997年開館。
kuwabara-shisei.com

Profile

Kuwabara Shisei
Photojournalist
Born in Shimane Prefecture in 1936. Graduated from the Tokyo University of Agriculture and the Tokyo College of Photography in 1960.
Principle Works: *News Photographers* (Iwanami Shoten Publishers), *The Complete Photographic Works of Kuwabara Shisei* (Four volumes: Minamata, Korea, Vietnam, Chikuhō/Okinawa; Kusa-no-ne Publishers)
The Kuwabara Shisei Photographic Museum opened in his hometown of Tsuwano in 1997. kuwabarashisei.com

The MINAMATA Disaster
Kuwabara Shisei
©Fujiwara-shoten Publishing Company, 2013

水俣事件　The MINAMATA Disaster

2013年9月30日　初版第1刷発行©

著　者　桑　原　史　成
発行者　藤　原　良　雄
発行所　株式会社　藤　原　書　店

〒162-0041　東京都新宿区早稲田鶴巻町523
電　話　03（5272）0301
ＦＡＸ　03（5272）0450
振　替　00160-4-17013
info@fujiwara-shoten.co.jp

印刷・製本　図書印刷

落丁本・乱丁本はお取替えいたします　　Printed in Japan
定価はカバーに表示してあります　　ISBN978-4-89434-924-7

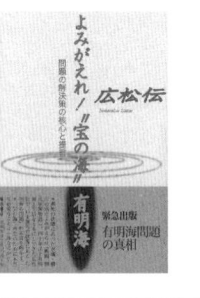

新しい学としての「水俣学」

水俣学研究序説
原田正純・花田昌宣編

医学、公害問題を超えた、総合的地域研究として原田正純の提唱する「水俣学」とは何か。現地で地域の患者・被害者や関係者との協働として活動を展開する医学、倫理学、人類学、社会学、福祉学、経済学、会計学、法学の専門家が、今も生き続ける水俣病問題に多面的に迫る画期作。

A5上製　三七六頁　四八〇〇円
（二〇〇四年三月刊）
◇978-4-89434-378-8

メディアのなかの「水俣」を徹底検証

「水俣」の言説と表象
小林直毅編
伊藤守／大石裕／烏谷昌幸／小林義寛／藤田真文／別府三奈子／山口仁／山腰修三

活字及び映像メディアの中で描かれ／見られた「水俣」を検証し、「水俣語」。四十年以上有明海と生活を共にしてきた近代日本の支配的言説の問題性を問う。従来のメディア研究の"盲点"に迫る！

A5上製　三八四頁　四六〇〇円
（二〇〇七年六月刊）
◇978-4-89434-577-5

有明海問題の真相

よみがえれ！"宝の海"有明海
〈問題の解決策の核心と提言〉
広松 伝

瀕死の状態にあった水郷・柳川の水をよみがえらせ（映画『柳川堀割物語』）、四十年以上有明海と生活を共にしてきた広松伝が、「いま瀕死の状態にある有明海再生のために本当に必要なことは何か」について緊急提言。

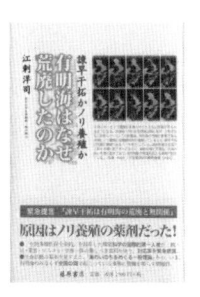

A5並製　一六〇頁　一五〇〇円
（二〇〇一年七月刊）
◇978-4-89434-245-3

諫早干拓は荒廃と無関係

有明海はなぜ荒廃したのか
〈諫早干拓かノリ養殖か〉
江刺洋司

荒廃の真因は、ノリ養殖の薬剤だった！「生物多様性の国際的保全条約」を起草した環境科学の国際的第一人者が、政官・業界・マスコミ・学会一体の驚くべき真相を抉り、対応策を緊急提言。いま全国の海で起きている事態に警鐘を鳴らす。

四六並製　二七二頁　二五〇〇円
（二〇〇三年一一月刊）
◇978-4-89434-364-1